REPRESENTATIONS OF HEALTH, ILLNESS AND HANDICAP

REPRESENTATIONS OF HEALTH, ILLNESS AND HANDICAP

Edited by

Ivana MARKOVÁ

Department of Psychology, University of Stirling, Stirling, FK9 4LA

and

Robert M. FARR

Department of Social Psychology, The London School of Economics and Political Science, Houghton Street, London, WC2A 2AE

harwood academic publishers

Australia • Austria • Belgium • China • France • Germany • India • Japan • Malaysia • Netherlands • Russia • Singapore • Switzerland• Thailand • United Kingdom • United States

Harwood Academic Publishers
Poststrasse 22
7000 Chur
Switzerland

British Library Cataloguing In Publication Data.

Representations of Health, Illness and Handicap
I. Marková, Ivana II. Farr, Robert M.
362.1

ISBN 3-7186-5657-4 (hard cover)
ISBN 3-7186-5658-2 (soft cover)

Includes bibliographical references and index.

CONTENTS

Contributors   vii

Preface   ix

Acknowledgements   xi

Part I — Representation of Health, Illness and Handicap   1

ONE   **Representation of Health, Illness and Handicap in the Mass Media of Communication: A Theoretical Overview**   3
Robert M. Farr

TWO   **The Self and Media Messages: Match or Mismatch?**   31
Janet E. Stockdale

THREE   **The Face of AIDS**   49
Jenny Kitzinger

FOUR   **Representations of Learning Disability in the Literature of Charity Campaigns**   67
Caroline B. Eayres, Nick Ellis, Robert S. P. Jones and Beth Miller

Part II — Professional and Lay Representations of Health, Illness and Handicap   91

FIVE   **Professional and Lay Representations of Health, Illness and Handicap: A Theoretical Overview**   93
Robert M. Farr and Ivana Marková

SIX   **The Self and the Other: Perception of the Risk of HIV/AIDS in Scottish Prisons**   111
Ivana Marková, Kevin J. McKee, Kevin G. Power and Eleanor Moodie

SEVEN   **Clinical Diagnosis and the Joint Construction of a Medical Voice**   131
Karin Aronsson, Ullabeth Sätterland Larsson and Roger Säljö

EIGHT   **The Mentally Ill Person and the Others: Social
             Representations and Interactive Strategies**   **145**
             Bruna Zani

NINE   **Lay Explanations of the Causes of Diabetes in India
             and the UK**   **163**
             Mary Sissons Joshi

             *Part III — Representations of Human Agency and of the
             Quality of Life*   **189**

TEN   **Human Agency and the Quality of Life: A Theoretical
             Overview**   **191**
             Ivana Marková

ELEVEN   **Quality of Life: Hope for the Future or an Echo from
             the Distant Past?**   **205**
             Andrew Jahoda

TWELVE   **Quality of Life and Mental Health: Evaluating the
             Impact of Long-Term Care**   **225**
             Margaret M. Barry and Charles Crosby

THIRTEEN   **Coping and Human Agency**   **249**
             Ladislav Valach

             Subject index   **267**

CONTRIBUTORS

Karin Aronsson
Department of Child Studies, Linköping University, S–581 Linköping, Sweden

Margaret M. Barry
Department of Psychology, Trinity College, Dublin, Eire

Charles Crosby
Department of Psychology, University College of North Wales, Bangor, Gwynedd, LL57 2DG, UK

Caroline B. Eayrs
Department of Psychology, University College of North Wales, Bangor, Gwynedd, LL57 2DG, UK

Nick Ellis
Department of Psychology, University College of North Wales, Bangor, Gwynedd, LL57 2DG, UK

Robert M. Farr
Department of Social Psychology, The London School of Economics and Political Science, Houghton Street, London, WC2A 2AE, UK

Andrew Jahoda
Strathmartine Hospital, Dundee, DD3 0PG, UK

Robert S. P. Jones
Department of Psychology, University College of North Wales, Bangor, Gwynedd, LL57 2DG, UK

Jenny Kitzinger
Glasgow University Media Group, 61 Southpark Avenue, Glasgow, G12 8LF, UK

Kevin J. McKee
Department of Psychology, University of Stirling, Stirling, FK9 4LA, UK

Ivana Marková
Department of Psychology, University of Stirling, Stirling, FK9 4LA, UK

Beth Miller
Department of Psychology, University College of North Wales, Bangor, Gwynedd, LL57 2DG, UK

Eleanor Moodie
Department of Psychology, University of Stirling, Stirling, FK9 4LA, UK

Kevin G. Power
Department of Psychology, University of Stirling, Stirling, FK9 4LA, UK

Roger Säljö
Department of Communication Studies, Linköping University, S–581 83 Linköping, Sweden

Ullabeth Sätterland Larsson
Department of Communication Studies, Linköping University, S–581 83 Linköping, Sweden

Mary Sissons Joshi
Psychology Unit, Oxford Brookes University, Gipsy Lane, Headington, Oxford, OX3 0BP, UK

Janet E. Stockdale
Department of Social Psychology, The London School of Economics and Political Science, Houghton Street, London, WC2A 2AE, UK

Ladislav Valach
Psychiatrische, Universitätspoliklinik Bern, Murtenstrasse 21, 3010 Bern, Switzerland

Bruna Zani
Dipartimento di Scienze del l'Educazione, Universita degli Studi di Bologna, Via Zamboni 34, 40126 Bologna, Italy

PREFACE

The promotion of health and the prevention of disease and disability are among the main concerns of the modern world. With the advances in medical science and in medical technology it is now possible to detect future hazards to the health of the unborn baby at very early stages of pregnancy. The prospective parents can decide whether to continue with the pregnancy or have an abortion. At the other end of the life cycle it is now possible, in some instances, to prolong on a life support system a severely diseased body beyond what was previously imaginable. Health and youthfulness into old age have become expectations of more and more people. Fitness classes, health foods, physical exercise, yoga and meditation have all become part of their daily routine.

Scientific facts and medical knowledge concerning health, disease and disability do not exist *in vacuo*. They are embedded in social reality. In the minds of professionals and lay people they interact with cultural values, social traditions, morals, conscious and unconscious beliefs, images, social constructions, conventions and with customary ways of thinking. In other words, in social reality they become representations of health, illness and handicap. Although the semantic difference between 'disease' and 'illness' is sometimes subtle and one should not be dogmatic about the use of these terms, disease has more to do with medical facts and organic disorder whereas illness, according to the Oxford English Dictionary, appears to be associated with 'wickedness, depravity, immorality'.

Similarly, there is a semantic difference between the terms 'disability' and 'handicap'. While disability refers to a restricted ability to perform a particular ability, in comparison with a normal range of ability, handicap is usually considered to be in people's attitudes — or representations. As a poster produced by The Spastics Society implies, it is not the disability as such, but other people's representation of cerebral palsy that makes people with such a disability handicapped: our biggest handicaps are other people's attitudes. As we are primarily concerned with the way in which society makes life difficult for those who are disabled, we frequently use the word 'handicap'.

The term 'representations' in the context of this volume does not refer to a particular theory. While some authors use the term 'representations', others refer instead to socio-culturally established images, constructions, explanations and to socially held widespread beliefs and attitudes. Some authors discuss representations in terms of social representations (Moscovici), others in terms of attribution theory, still others in terms of socio-anthropological, sociological and constructivist approaches. The range of uses of the term 'representations' reflects the interdisciplinary nature of the volume with its international cast of contributors. The majority of the authors are social scientists.

The three parts in this volume are primarily concerned with lay representations of health, illness and handicap and how these relate, in the delivery of health care, to the representations held by health care professionals working either in institutional or community settings. Authors of individual chapters also show how lay and professional images of illness and handicap often reinforce and perpetuate existing representations. Part I is concerned with representations in the mass media of communication and also in people's minds. Part II discusses lay representations and their relationship to those of medical and other health care professionals, both in institutions and in the community. Part III focuses on the representations of illness and of handicap in terms of the quality of life and of human agency. It is closely related to the issue of de-institutionalisation and the switch to stressing care in the community.

The present volume will be of interest to several kinds of reader. It could serve as a complementary text in courses of social psychology, the psychology of health and of disability, both at an advanced undergraduate and a postgraduate level. It could also be of interest to health educators and charities campaigning for a change in public attitudes toward disability, and to the providers and managers of health and social services.

Ivana MARKOVÁ
Robert M. FARR

Editors

ACKNOWLEDGEMENTS

We are grateful to the public relations officers of the following Agencies for granting their permission to reproduce publicity material from previous Charity Appeals or Health Educational Programmes: MENCAP (for material appearing in Chapters 1, 2 and 4); SCOPE (formerly The Spastics Society) (for material appearing in Chapters 1 and 2); The Royal National Institute for the Blind (RNIB - Chapters 1 and 2); The Down's Syndrome Association (Chapters 1, 2, and 3); The Terence Higgins Trust (Chapter 2); The Health Education Authority (Chapters 1, 2 and 3); AIDS Education and Research Trust (AVERT - Chapter 2); The George House Trust (formerly Manchester AIDSline - Chapter 2).

Professor Ivana Marková would like to acknowledge the generous support over the years by The Carnegie Trust in Scotland for her projects in the field of the social psychology of chronic illness and disability. Professor Rob Farr would like to acknowledge the generous support of his researches in the field of social representations over many years by the Laboratoire de Psychologie Sociale (LEPS) at the Maison des Sciences de l'Homme in Paris and the Economic and Social Research Council of the United Kingdom.

Part I — Representation of Health, Illness and Handicap

ONE   **Representation of Health, Illness and Handicap in the Mass Media of Communication: A Theoretical Overview**   **3**
Robert M. Farr

TWO   **The Self and Media Messages: Match or Mismatch?**   **31**
Janet E. Stockdale

THREE   **The Face of AIDS**   **49**
Jenny Kitzinger

FOUR   **Representations of Learning Disability in the Literature of Charity Campaigns**   **67**
Caroline B. Eayrs, Nick Ellis, Robert S. P. Jones and Beth Miller

CHAPTER ONE

Representations of Health, Illness and Handicap in the Mass Media of Communication: A Theoretical Overview

Robert M. FARR

Department of Social Psychology, The London School of Economics and Political Science, Houghton Street, London, WC2A 2AE

THE COLLECTIVE NATURE OF REPRESENTATIONS

In the course of this overview I wish to bring a particular theoretical perspective to bear on an aspect of social reality which without it, would remain mundane and rather prosaic; namely, the images of health, illness and handicap that appear in the mass media of communication. Durkheim (1898) first introduced the notion of collective representations almost a century ago. They differed sharply, in his view, from representations in the minds of individuals such as those that a psychologist might study. His distinction between collective and individual representations was an early attempt on his part to differentiate sociology from psychology. Collective representations are best understood in terms of culture. They belong to the public rather than to the private realm.

Durkheim was principally interested in the division of labour within society and in religion. He was concerned to understand what happens when the representations that hold a society together cease to be collective. They remain, for a while, as individual representations, collectively distributed, before dying out altogether. In his classic study of suicide, for example, Durkheim demonstrated how the break-up of common values (i.e. collective representations such as religion) resulted in pathological states of society such as anomie and egoism. Wundt was also interested in the study of collective representations. Language, religion, customs, myth, magic and related phenomena were the objects of study in his ten volume *Völkerpsychologie* (Wundt, 1900–20). For Wundt these were cultural rather than social phenomena. For an account of the links between Wundt and Durkheim see Farr (1983).

The specific representations studied by Durkheim and by Wundt are not particularly relevant in the context of modern society. Nor are they directly relevant to the topic of the present volume. This is scarcely surprising since both Durkheim and Wundt wrote almost a century ago. They based their respective theories on contemporary accounts by anthropologists and linguists concerning cultures and societies that were even less modern than their own. In modern societies science, especially medicine, has largely displaced religion and magic as the culturally approved means for controlling the forces of nature and for alleviating suffering. Wundt's vision of psychology as a truly comparative discipline has not stood the test of time (Danziger, 1983). Durkheim's notion of collective representations has fared somewhat better. In the period following World War II, Moscovici, in his theory of social representations, took up and modernised Durkheim's notion of collective representations. When representations are no longer collective in the full Durkheimian sense of the term then it is more appropriate, Moscovici argues, to describe them as social. In the eyes of some this semantic change would make Moscovici a postmodernist rather than a modernist. A postmodernist is likely to believe there are no longer any collective representations. Postmodernists are very much concerned with the fragmentation of knowledge.

Issues of Health and Illness

Many of the classic studies in the French tradition of research on social representations were concerned with issues of health and illness and hence are of direct relevance to the current volume. Moscovici (1961/76) launched this tradition of social psychology with his study of psychoanalysis. He wished to discover what happens when a new theory about human behaviour becomes public knowledge. He was not so much interested in the theory itself as in how it was reflected in the mass media of communication and in everyday discourse. He analysed the representations of psychoanalysis that appeared in some 241 different journals, papers and magazines that were published in France over a fourteen month period from 1st January 1952 to the 1st March 1953. His research was as much a contribution to media studies it was to social psychology.

Moscovici also sampled the opinions of various sectors of the French population concerning their knowledge of psychoanalysis. A new theory can be mildly threatening, as can the arrival of a new figure on the social scene, e.g. the psychoanalyst. Some of his informants thought of the analyst as a priest. In their minds being in analysis was rather like a secular version of the confessional. Others thought the analyst was some sort of doctor but one who listened to his patients talking rather than one who prescribed drugs. This latter representation, i.e. of psychoanalysis as a 'talking cure', is similar to the way in which it was talked about in the konditorei of its native city, Vienna at the turn of the century. The strange becomes less strange when it is linked to something with which people are more familiar. The process of anchoring is a key element in Moscovici's theory of social representations.

Another classic study was conducted by Herzlich (1969, English translation 1973). In *Health and Illness: A social psychological analysis* she employed open-ended interviews with a sample of 80 informants, the majority of whom lived in Paris. For them, health was a harmonious relationship between self and nature. Since this was a given, it did not need to be explained. Illness, however, was an event. It did have a cause. It called for an explanation. Her informants lived in a state of perpetual twilight somewhere between health and illness. They were neither ill nor healthy at the time of the interviews. Most suffered from some form of nervous exhaustion. Their dissatisfaction with life in the metropolis shaped their representations of health and illness – the artificial food, the unnatural rhythms of life, the noise of the city and the pollution of its atmosphere. 'Natural', for them, meant nature and nature meant the countryside. Herzlich demonstrated how these representations logically imply the notion of toxicity. It is clear from the structure of the representations she elicited from her informants that health is not the same as the absence of illness. Though the majority of her informants were not visibly ill at the time of the interview they did not claim to be healthy either. They reported that their bodily systems were poisoned. They often felt tired and rarely woke up refreshed. They were in a state of fatigue.

Herzlich went to great lengths to avoid imposing her own representations of health and illness on her informants. This was why she adopted the format of an open-ended interview. The uniformity of the accounts she collected led her, in the course of her study, to take two counter-measures (Farr, 1977). The first was to include a dozen villagers from Normandy. This, however, did not significantly alter the representations she elicited. Instead of speaking of the unnatural nature of life in the city the villagers spoke of the city invading the countryside. The other countermeasure she took was to ask, at one point in the interview, a direct, rather than an indirect, question. Surely medical science had done much to prolong life? This evoked the response that while people may now live longer the quality of their lives is less good than it was when most people lived in the countryside. The quality of life is a theme to which we shall return in Part III of the present work.

When I first read Herzlich's monograph I expressed the view that, if I were a capitalist and wished to make a profit, I could confidently, on the basis of her data, invest money in the marketing of Chambourcy and Loseley yoghurts to the middle-class denizens of Paris and London (Farr, 1977). Others have since followed this advice and, now, no doubt, are millionaires. The sale of health foods is a boom industry. One is delivering organically grown products into the very heart of the polluted metropolis. This marketing of health foods is directly in line with the representations of health and illness as set out in Herzlich's monograph. Whilst this is a familiar theme in the 1990s Herzlich first detected it in the 1960s. Managers in commercial organisations such as supermarkets know, through their marketing departments, how to exploit people's representations of health and illness in order to sell their products. The rural/urban contrast is often used in the marketing of health foods to correspond to the contrast between health and illness. One can purchase health by buying the advertised product. These same representations and images are also invoked in the marketing of products injurious to health. This is discussed more fully below. Within the metropolis a similar contrast exists between the leafy suburbs and the run-down inner cities. Here we are concerned with the marketing of real estate rather than of health foods. By buying a home with a garden in the suburbs of London, for example, one purchases a small piece of rural England for the sake of the health of one's family.

A weakness of Herzlich's original study was that she failed to include an analysis of the contents of the mass media on the issue of health and illness. This failure laid her open to the charge that she had not demonstrated the collective nature of the representations of health and illness which she described so vividly. The social representations may merely reflect the social psychology of her research interview and the positive self-concepts of her informants (Farr, 1977). She could have avoided this particular criticism by inviting groups of people to discuss health and illness rather than interviewing individuals. Group discussion is a useful way of sampling the stock of arguments available within a particular culture where the researcher is interested in the arguments produced rather than in the individuals producing the arguments. The dynamics of group talk are akin to those which, in a wider context, lead to the formation of public opinion. It is very different to the inter-personal dynamics of a one-to-one interview upon which Herzlich so depended in her study of social represeantations. A discussion group is 'the thinking society' (Moscovici, 1984) in miniature. It is a singular virtue of this French tradition of research in social psychology that it is centrally concerned with the study of people's thinking in regard to social issues and with sampling and analysing the information that circulates in society, mainly through the mass media, concerning the object of study.

Herzlich, in collaboration with Pierret, went on to examine illness within a wider societal and historical perspective (Herzlich & Pierret, 1984, 1987). Here, in the historical sections of their book, the authors do analyse written material, especially the diaries of famous invalids. This time they also interviewed those who were ill at the time of the interview. It is clear from this further study the extent to which modern medicine has transformed the experience of being ill. The experience of illness today is dramatically different to what it was in those simpler societies that interested Durkheim. It is more appropriate, in the light of the study by Herzlich and Pierret, to talk of social rather than of collective representations of illness. The experience of illness is infinitely more diverse today than it was in former times. In the eyes of some, for example Stainton Rogers (1991), this makes Herzlich and Pierret postmodernists rather than modernists. The French edition of their book was published (1984) just as AIDS was appearing on the human scene. They were unable to include this topic in their discussion. In their book they noted how a medical conception of illness had replaced a religious one. They would be interested to note how, with the arrival of HIV/AIDS, images of the plague and of divine retribution reappear, mainly in the mass media of communication.

The Role of the Media in the Generation and Spread of Representations

The notions of society and of culture in the writings of Durkheim and of Wundt respectively need to be revised to account for more than just the importance of science in the modern world. The media of communication today are dramatically different to what they were at the turn of the century. Wundt had a prescient appreciation of the importance of language and he sought to establish its origins in gesture (Wundt, 1973). Anthropologists appreciate the importance of distinguishing societies with a written as well as an oral tradition from those with only an oral tradition. Print and literacy were crucial forces for change in European culture at the time of the Reformation (McLuhan, 1962). In modern, as distinct from traditional, societies the mass media of communication play a key role in both the generation and the spread of representations. There is a greater range and variety of representations in modern society than ever before. We live in an age of representations (Moscovici, 1984). We react to the representations rather than to the reality they represent. It is no exaggeration to claim that, education apart, the media, collectively, comprise the representation industry *par excellence*.

This development is so recent that its full force has yet to be appreciated. McLuhan, like the voice of one crying from the wilderness, foretold it (McLuhan, 1951, 1962, 1964, 1967). He was a harbinger of the revolutionary changes in both culture and society brought about by the introduction of the modern media. In many respects the world today is like a global village. The Gulf War, for example, was fought out in our sitting rooms rather than, like the crusades in the Middle Ages, in some far distant land. The same is true of the war against HIV/AIDS. In part this is fought out in research laboratories; in part also, on television in our sitting rooms (Farr, 1993). In many respects HIV/AIDS is quite unlike the Black Death in the Middle Ages, despite evocations of the plague by those who work professionally in the media.

Modern Governments embark upon different campaigns to those waged in the Middle Ages. Its own citizens are often the targets of these campaigns, especially in the field of health. Governments in the modern world have a veritable arsenal of weapons at their disposal when it comes to waging a propaganda war. In this section of the volume we are mainly concerned with health education campaigns in the field of HIV/AIDS (Chapters 2 and 3) and with the advertising campaigns of various voluntary bodies concerned with providing services for those with disabilities (Chapters 1, 2 and 4). The main media involved are television images, posters, leaflets and the various print media.

The French anthropologist Sperber (1985, 1990) has proposed a new framework for collaboration between anthropologists and psychologists. He calls for an epidemiology of representations. This proposal is quite separate from, though compatible with, the work of French social psychologists involved in the study of social representations. Sperber's suggestion is an intriguing one. It is taken up and discussed more fully below in the context of HIV/AIDS. The essential point to note here is that it is concerned with the distribution of a representation within a given society and with changes over time in both the representation and its distribution. Clearly the media play an important role in determining both the form of a representation and its distribution. We are concerned here with the social psychological study of widespread beliefs (Fraser and Gaskell, 1990). In my treatment of social representation as a form widespread belief I have tried to make the role of the media explicit in both the creation and the diffusion of representations (Farr, 1990a).

It is singular virtue, in my opinion, of modern French research on social representations, that the social psychologists involved are interested in analysing both the information and the images that circulate in the mass media of communication concerning the object of their study. Many studies routinely include a content analysis of the mass media. The theory of social representations explicitly recognises that representations are in the media as well as in people's minds; they form part of culture as well as cognition – and they need to be sampled and analysed in both contexts. In many respects Moscovici's theory of social representations is a retro-revolution, i.e. it is a return to an earlier time in the history of social psychology in America when there was a healthy symbiosis between social psychology and media studies (e.g. Katz and Lazarsfeld, 1955).

There are now other forms of social psychology, besides the study of social representations, where social psychologists are producing work that is of interest to those who work in media studies. Billig's rhetorical approach to social psychology is a case in point (Billig, 1987). He is very critical of the attempt by experimental social psychologists in America to turn rhetoric into a science. Billig's work is particularly relevant in relation to debate and argument. It is slightly less relevant when dealing with the effects of the printed word or of images *per se*. This is because he is primarily concerned with the nature of the relationship between arguing and thinking. The work of Potter and Wetherell (1987) on discourse analysis is another good example of a form of social psychology relevant to media studies. We do not take this up further here since, in the present context, we are more directly concerned with the analysis of images than we are with the analysis of discourse *per se*. Livingstone (1990), in her recent book *Making Sense of Television*, focuses mainly on how audiences interpret televised drama, especially the soap opera. Here viewers establish a set of proto-relationships with a whole cast of characters often over a period of years. This model of viewers as active interpreters is highly compatible with the theory of social representations and includes visual as well as linguistic aspects of social communication.

As editors we very much hope the present book will stimulate an interest in the media on the part of health professionals, especially those involved in the field of health education. Whilst French studies in the field of social representations routinely include content analyses of the mass media of communication, there is little or no reflection in that same literature on the nature of the media themselves and of how the theory of social representations relates to those media. I have made a start in regard to what Sperber calls the epidemiology of representations (Farr, 1990a). In the present contribution I focus mainly on interpreting images of handicap in posters. I here link this form of cultural critique to an older tradition of scholarship in media studies i.e. McLuhan's work on *The Mechanical Bride* (McLuhan, (1951).

The representations of handicap that *actually* form in the minds of those who view these posters is a purely empirical matter. Much relevant evidence concerning this is contained in the contributions by Stockdale and by Eayrs, Ellis, Jones and Miller. In this theoretical overview I have sought to highlight how Moscovici, Herzlich, Herzlich & Pierret and Jodelet have modernised Durkheim's notion of collective representations by extending it to include science and the practice of modern medicine. Moscovici's main theoretical contribution has been to talk of social rather than of collective representations. He believes this is a necessary refinement in the modernisation of Durkheim's notion. There is, however, a powerful trend in the modern media that runs directly counter to Moscovici's objective. This is the tendency on the part of people who work in the media to convert social representations into collective representations. This is why they are referred to, collectively, as the *mass* media of communication. The aim is to convey representations to a mass audience. The fierce competition to make social representations collective contributes to the impression that we live in a postmodernist age.

In interpreting advertisements and posters it is important to inter-relate image and text. There is often a subtle relationship between the two. Any analysis of the images and representations of health and illness in advertising copy is likely to produce paradoxical results in terms of the social representations of health and illness as described by Herzlich (1969). Images of health, on the one hand, are often associated with the marketing of products injurious to health, e.g. tobacco and alcohol. Images of death and of illness, on the other hand, are frequently associated with health education campaigns, e.g. the 'Grim Reaper' series of adverts on Australian TV in connection with the HIV/AIDS campaign; similar images of tombstones and of icebergs in the British campaigns, etc. A great deal of psychological sophistication has been involved in the marketing of products injurious to health. The manufacturers of such products have had the benefit of advice from psychologists for well over a century now. Health educators are comparative newcomers when it comes to advertising. Statutory health warnings from the Government about the dangers of smoking, for example, can even be incorporated into advertisements by skilled copy-editors as though they were an official endorsement of the product. Now that Western Governments are placing increasingly stringent restrictions on the advertising of tobacco products tobacco companies are turning their attention elsewhere – to the countries of Central and Eastern Europe where there are few, if any, such restrictions on advertising and also to the Third World.

It is only in recent times that the creative talents of marketing agencies and of social psychologists have been harnessed for the promotion of health rather than for the marketing of products that undermine it. The talent often follows the money. Some Governments are now prepared to invest money in promoting health. In this respect the UK Government has a good track record. Prevention may turn out to be cheaper than cure and in some instances, e.g. HIV/AIDS, until an antidote to the virus is discovered, there may be no realistic alternative to containing the spread of the virus.

The theory of social representations is relevant to the devising of successful campaigns. The outcome of a campaign, however, may be the opposite of that intended. This is especially the case if those who devise a campaign fail to take into account the social representations of those who are its target. Kitzinger and Stockdale in their respective contributions to this volume cite examples of this from the field of health education campaigns concerning the risks of becoming infected with the HIV. It is not only in the promotion of health that campaigns can backfire. The voluntary organisations which provide services for the handicapped may unwittingly, in their advertising copy, perpetuate, rather than challenge, negative stereotypes concerning the nature of handicap. Examples of this are cited by Stockdale and by Eayrs and her colleagues in their respective contributions to this volume.

It does not matter, in our view, that several of the examples we cite of bad practice are no longer current. We believe a number of conceptual problems need to be worked through if health is to be marketed more effectively and if care in the community is to become a reality for those who are mentally ill or those with a disability. We all learn by our mistakes and this applies to agencies as well as to other actors in the social scene. Understanding the social representations of health, illness and handicap may be a good place to start.

CHANGES IN SOCIAL REPRESENTATIONS OF THE HUMAN BODY

Since social representations are cultural phenomena they change over time. Another early study in the French tradition of research on social representations was Jodelet's study of changes in the representation of the human body (Jodelet, 1984). She demonstrated, over an interval of some fifteen years, an increase in openness and in flexibility in people's discourse about their bodies. The discourse of men in particular became more centred on their own bodily experiences. Woman were more likely, at the later point in time, to rebel ideologically against both social definitions of their status and the equally constraining images of the female body portrayed in the mass media of communication. These changes corresponded to the growing influence of the feminist movement. The body is talked about more openly and more freely. People are much more knowledgeable about their bodies than they were previously. This is due, in part, to the diffusion of a knowledge of biology, mainly through the educational system.

As the relations between the sexes change so, too, does the relation of each sex to its own body. Jodelet found that men were less inhibited than previously in talking about their bodies. These changes in the public discourse about the body can be related to changes in society and to social movements such as the feminist movement or the green revolution. The body also features prominently in advertising. The sylph-like figures of women preferred by modelling agencies and in advertising copy create pressures on their own sex to be slim. This is part of the ideology against which they rebel, as reported in Jodelet's study. Although this is clearly part of culture (a collective representation in the full Durkheimian sense of the term) it may even feature as a significant element in the aetiology of such modern disorders as anorexia nervosa and bulimia.

In medical practice it is generally the body that is treated and there are even medical specialists for the various parts of the human body. Problems arise when it is the mind rather than the body that needs to be treated. This, in large measure, is because the mind is invisible. Science, including medical science, is dominated by vision as the principal modality of investigation. It is difficult to envisage the mind and its workings. When psychiatrists treat the mind they often do so by means of psychotropic drugs, i.e. they use agents that affect the mind through the body. Mental illness was rarely mentioned spontaneously by Herzlich's informants. This, almost certainly, is because illness, in the public mind, is more closely associated with the body than it is with the mind. It is also difficult, as we shall see, to portray mental illness effectively in a poster, which is a highly visual medium of communication. There are, then, conceptual (i.e. representational) problems in portraying certain forms of illness, especially those which do not assume a bodily form. In the overview to Part II we note how stigma (a form of social representation with negative valence) are related to stigmata (visible symptoms of illness and disability). This is also why it is conceptually difficult to convince readers and viewers that healthy looking people may be HIV antibody positive (Chapter 3).

Lay representations of the body are likely to affect the clinical picture, especially in the field of psychosomatic medicine. In his early studies of hysteria, for example, Freud noted that it was the patient's notion of a hand or arm that was paralysed, not the neurologist's conception of the same organ. Freud had been trained as a research physiologist. He was used to exploring nature visually. At one point he was even cutting open eels in order to search for their testes. For purely domestic reasons he had to relinquish his ambition to become a research physiologist. On his own admission, he became a reluctant clinician. His primary interests, however, were still in research. He spent the rest of his career listening to people talking about themselves and their bodies. This was discourse about the body rather than examining the body *per se*. He had dramatically switched the modality of his investigations from vision to speech. He was now a listener, rather than merely an observer. Psychoanalysis is the form of psychology he devised to enable him to interpret what his patients told him.

Vision is the preferred modality of investigation in science. By the criteria of the Vienna Circle psychoanalysis was not judged to be a science. Marie Jahoda claims that psychoanalysis is a psychological language for talking about the human body (Jahoda, 1977). When it diffuses within a culture, in the manner described by Moscovici (1961), then it will affect the discourse about the human body, in the manner described by Jodelet (1984). Thus we come full circle:

> *Not only does a person's representation of his own body influence his clinical symptoms, but the science which is then fashioned to 'interpret' these symptoms itself constitutes a psychological representation of the human body which, once it is published, diffuses within a culture and becomes the basis of still further changes in the social representation of the body (Farr, 1981, p. 310)*

It is also possible, with the benefits of hindsight, to detect in Herzlich's monograph on health and illness (1969) the first stirrings of the green revolution (Farr, 1993). Her data were collected in the mid-60s. The concern of her informants with the artificiality of life in the metropolis, with its pollution and unnatural rhythms of life, is clearly evident. So, too, is their nostalgia for life in the country. Their preoccupation with the state of their own health, however , is not, necessarily, a morbid preoccupation. It could represent a yearning to adopt a healthier style of life. A social movement gains momentum when familiar objects are seen in a new light. This may even include one's own body. Moscovici reminds us that there were trees before there were ecologists. Ecologists enable us to see those same trees in a different light. Health educators may enable us to view our our bodies in a different light. A social movement may originate in the change of a social representation. Changes in how the human body is represented are related to changes in one's conception of health and changes in the latter can also affect the former.

HIV/AIDS AS A NEW FORM OF THREAT TO HUMAN LIFE

This threat is so new that Herzlich and Pierret (1984) were unable to include it in their survey of illness down the ages. There may be little or no relation between HIV/AIDS and representations of HIV/AIDS within a particular culture at a particular point in time (Farr, 1993). It is important to distingusih between the two. The relationship between the virus and its representation might be as tenuous as that between psychoanalysis and the representations of psychoanalysis which Moscovici studied in France in the mid-50s.

In the case of HIV/AIDS it is important to study the social representations of the virus (if that is what it is) as well as to study the virus itself, especially if one wishes to conduct an effective health education campaign. These are two quite different forms of study (Farr, 1993). The concern is not so much with the public understanding of science as with using a knowledge of social representations to contain the spread of the virus. Until medical science comes up with an antidote to the virus the only effective way of containing its spread is to use our existing knowledge of social science to ensure safe practice in regard to those behaviours involved in transmitting the virus, i.e. to encourage the practice of safe sex and to issue warnings about the dangers of sharing syringes. This is the primary objective of most of the health educational material we review in the present volume. Each campaign is usually aimed at achieving a specific behavioural objective. It is an exercise in the application of social science. It is far removed from basic medical research into the nature of the virus itself, if virus it be.

At the outset in the early-80s, it was difficult to gauge either the nature or the extent of the threat to human life. This involved at least two very different forms of medical science. The first is concerned with identifying the nature of the threat. Is it a virus? Where did it come from? How is it transmitted? Is there an antidote?, etc. Here the primary medical specialisms are those of virology and immunology. The second is concerned with assessing the extent of the threat. Here epidemiology plays the lead role. The pattern and spread of the disease will vary from one society to another. As a consequence so, too, will the representation of the disease. The disease also unfolds over time and so it assumes a different form at different times within the same society. It is important, in my opinion, to appreciate the nature of the relationship between these two forms of medical science. Within medical circles they influence each other, and rightly so. The health educational programmes in the media, however, are driven almost exclusively by the epidemiological research. This has important consequences which I discuss further below. The history of the disease within a particular society is unique even if the virus that causes it (if, indeed, it is a virus) is universal.

The acronyms AIDS and HIV emerged in the context of basic medical science. An acronym *per se* is hardly life threatening. What it stands for, in this instance, is a virus that attacks and destroys the human immune system. How it is represented, however, may or may not be threatening. Representations, as well as viruses, can be threatening. They threaten the well-being and life styles of certain categories of individual. Indeed they will not be effective in changing those life styles unless they are threatening. Viruses, on the other hand, threaten the bodies of those they infect. Once formed, representations lead a life of their own. The mechanisms of their transmission and transformation, however, are dramatically different to those of the actual virus, if that is what it is. This is because the medium of transmission of a representation is different to that of a virus. Sperber (1985), in his Malinowski lecture, is at some pains to point out a key difference between the two forms of epidemiology that he discusses – a representation is transformed when it is transmitted whereas a virus remains the same.

Epidemiological research establishes the form and progress of a disease within a particular human population up to a particular point in time. It is a picture that unfolds over time and continually needs to be updated. The epidemiological evidence can identify the groups that are most at risk at any particular point in time. This is important when it comes to targeting health educational campaigns. The representations of a disease, however, are likely to reflect the history of the disease within that particular culture or society. When the phenomenon was first identified in the early-80s it was associated with the gay community. This was probably just an epidemiological fact. By labelling it as a gay disease, however, the heterosexual majority may have felt less threatened. When it is established that the virus is transmitted through sexual intercourse then popular representations of the disease take on the connotations of other sexually transmitted disease such as syphilis (Marková & Wilkie, 1987). The representation carries with it strong moral overtones.

Those who work in the media play a key role in the creation, transmission and transformation of representations. A threat remains vague until it assumes a tangible form. At an early stage HIV/AIDS was related, at least in Europe, to images of the plague. This evokes collective memories of the Black Death in the Middle Ages. Once these images are evoked and begin to circulate in the media it becomes easier to identify and to blame certain groups as being responsible for the introduction and transmission of the virus. This is where representations can so easily assume a life of their own that is quite unrelated to the nature of the epidemiological and medical evidence.

Even purely epidemiological evidence can lead to the scapegoating and stigmatising of certain human groups. This would be less likely to occur if the predominant attitude in medical circles were that of the scientist *vis-à-vis* an, as yet, unknown virus. If the epidemiological evidence is not interpreted by a scientist it is likely to re-enforce, rather than to challenge, pre-existing attitudes towards certain groups in the community. The "evidence" is not released into a neutral world. I am not suggesting that the evidence should be withheld. I think, rather, that those who work in the media have a professional responsibility to their various publics to ensure they themselves understand the nature of the evidence before they write about it or broadcast it.

The media campaigns concerning HIV/AIDS which are reported in Part I need to be understood within a particular historical and societal setting. The work of Kitzinger and of the AIDS Media Research Project in Glasgow is aimed at ascertaining what the public understanding is of being HIV antibody positive. The scientific problem is the gap in time (which could be years) between becoming infected by the virus and revealing the symptoms of AIDS. A person may be HIV positive without knowing this. His or her sexual partners may be unaware that he or she is HIV positive. This may lead both partners to believe they can practice safe sex without using a condom. This is possible because people believe they can recognise someone who is HIV positive. The whole purpose of the particular health education campaign Kitzinger and her colleagues are evaluating in the Glasgow Media Project is to persuade people that they can't tell the diffrence. The message, naturally, is itself threatening. It also may not be very credible, because those who are HIV positive will, with time, come to reveal the symptoms of AIDS and people will then forget the symptom-free period which preceded the onset of AIDS. The task of Kitzinger and her colleagues is to ascertain the credibility of the message amongst various at-risk groups and a few low-risk groups. This is an important area of applied research.

REPRESENTATIONS OF HANDICAP IN POSTERS

McLuhan (1951), in *The Mechanical Bride*, described advertisements as part of the folklore of an industrial culture. It is, quite literally, possible to read the signs of the times. In that book he presented an advertisement on one page and his own commentary upon it, usually on the page opposite. I propose to do the same with respect to a small sample of posters produced by various Voluntary Organisations working with the handicapped. McLuhan's work is a particularly fine example of the point made above, i.e. that representations are in the media as well as being in people's minds. It is also interesting that his 1951 book is classified in the Library of Congress Catalogue as social psychology. It is certainly compatible with the research reported above on social representations. It is, of course, a much earlier and quite independent tradition of research.

The posters cited below are selected to illustrate a range of different handicaps. Many of them are now quite dated. This does not matter from my own particular point of view. It is sufficient for my purposes that they once formed part of a public representation of that particular handicap. My illustrations are drawn from material that appeared in the public domain. If I were to confine my commentary to the posters that are currently in use I would lay myself open to charges of seeking to influence public donations to the different Charities. This I do not wish to do. I am more interested in the social psychology of handicap in general than I am in the social psychology of any particular form of handicap. It would of course be interesting to explore through the medium of posters changes over time in the representations of a particular handicap. These changes are often made because the Charity concerned is dissatisfied with its current "image". An "image" in this sense is a social representation. It is important to distinguish between the image of the Charity (e.g. its logo) and the image of the disability it exists to serve.

The posters I have reviewed were all commissioned by Voluntary Organisations responsible for looking after persons with a particular form of handicap. In the main, they are designed to elicit donations to the charities concerned. Occasionally, the posters are intended to educate the public about the nature of a particular handicap or to change our existing social representation, e.g. mongolism. Sometimes they seek to achieve more than one objective. How successful the various campaigns are is a purely empirical matter and I do not have access to any information on which to base a sound judgment. My concern here has been simply to explore the representations of handicap as portrayed through the medium of posters. I have attempted to educate the reader in how to read posters portraying handicap in much the same way as McLuhan coached his readers in how to interpret advertisements as the folkore of an industrial society.

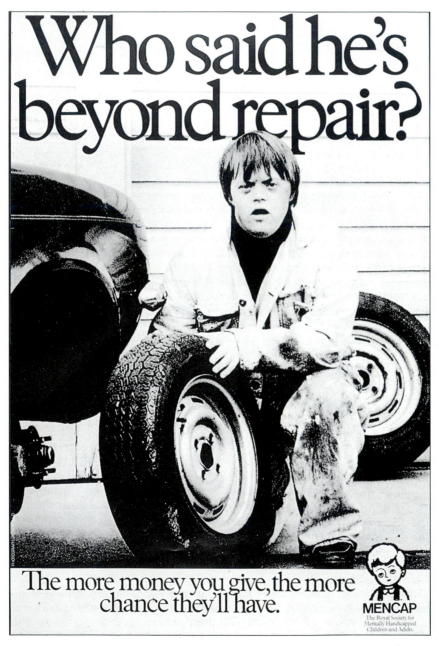

Figure 1.1   "Who said he's beyond repair?"

Figure 1.1
"Who said he's beyond repair?"

This is a deeply perplexing poster. It shows a mentally handicapped adult who is gainfully employed in a garage changing the wheels of a car. "Who said he's beyond repair?" To whom is this question addressed? Who says "Who said he's beyond repair?"? Surely this is not something said in the presence of the person to whom it refers? He would appear to be excluded from any conversation that might be held about him. This is deeply alienating. Provision is often made for those with a mental handicap without involving them in dialogue.

Perhaps the question expresses a thought rather than being the opening gambit in a conversation? If so, whose thought is it? Is it one ever likely to have occurred to the viewer of the poster? Is it the purpose of the poster to refute the question it raises? If so, how does it achieve this objective? The person who is the focus of the picture is referred to in the third person singular. The viewer or reader is not told his name. This contrasts with the young boy in the poster for The Down's Children's Association (see below) about whom we are told "His mates call him David".

The phrase "beyond repair" is an acoustic pun. It depends upon the pictorial context and on his job as a repair man at a garage. It is the twin poster of "Jane is wanted by the police" which is discussed by Stockdale and also by Eayrs et al. in their contributions to this volume. In what sense might a human being, as distinct from a motor car, be "beyond repair"? Does the text refer to the person's occupational status or to his mental status? Is he in danger of being thrown on the scrapheap as being unemployable? Is his mental condition hopeless? What thoughts *does* the phrase "beyond repair" evoke in the minds of the average reader or viewer? This is a purely empirical question.

"The more money you give, the more chance they'll have". Notice the switch in the text from the third person singular to the third person plural. The text no longer refers to the nameless person in the picture. He is merely one of many – the mentally handicapped. Why are members of the public being asked to donate money if he is gainfully employed? Is he being under-paid for the work he does? Why should we, as members of the public, further improve his employer's profit margins by donating our hard-earned money?

It is no longer fashionable to talk of mental handicap. However the Charity cannot avoid this as it forms part of its own title and logo. In 1992 the Society replaced its 'Little Stephen' logo and changed its image (Chapter 4). Elsewhere in this volume we refer to people with the same disability as experiencing difficulties in learning.

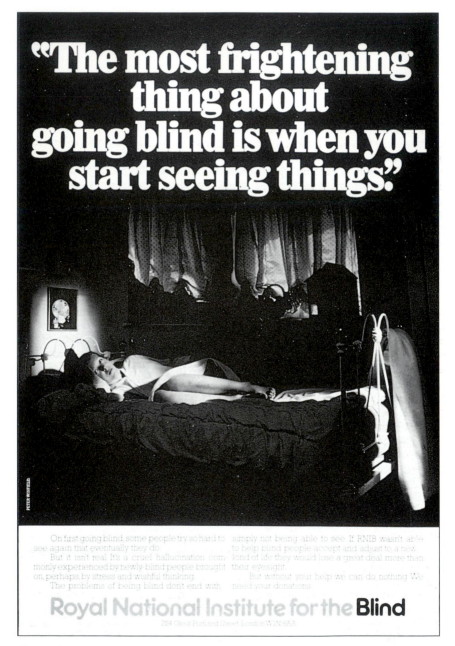

Figure 1.2   "The most frightening thing about going blind is when you start seeing things."

Figure 1.2
"The most frightening thing about going blind is when you start seeing things."

An arresting statement designed to capture the attention of passers-by in the hope that they will stop and read more of the text. It depends on a paradox – that seeing again when you are going blind is disturbing. This is described, in the text below, as "a cruel hallucination". It is a direct quote. A blind person tells us, from her own experience, what it is like to go blind. The "you" in the quote is ambiguous. It could refer to the reader as well as to the speaker. It could be the opening of a dialogue. The viewer, however, can only participate by reading. This further highlights the difference between the blind and the sighted. The blind appeal to the sighted through the medium of the printed word. Perhaps the reader can be thankful that he or she is not going blind. This momentary sense of gratitude might elicit the charitable response that the rest of the text invites.

The passer-by may pause to reflect on the nature of blindnes as an afflication and not just on his or her own good fortune. The rest of the text is informative in this regard. "On first going blind, some people try so hard to see again that eventually they do. But it isn't real. It's a cruel hallucination commonly experienced by newly-blind people brought on, perhaps by stress and wishful thinking". Perhaps the poster has an educational as well as a financial purpose? This is re-enforced by the image of a blind woman curled up on her own bed. The popular image is of a blind man or woman with a stick needing help from members of the public to cross the street. This is a situation that evokes a great deal of spontaneous help. The picture introduces us into a very different world – the private world of the blind. What it is like when the blind are alone with themselves and confront their hopes and fears for the future in the privacy of their own room. There is a great deal more to blindness than needing help in public places. The text elaborates on what the picture and the quote can only suggest:

"The problems of being blind don't end with simply not being able to see. If RNIB wasn't able to help blind people accept and adjust to a new kind of life they would lose a great deal more that their eyesight".

They might lose their minds as well as their sight and thus be multiply handicapped. There is, however, one organisation which knows what to do. Fortunately RNIB is able to help... "But without your help we can do nothing. We need your donations'. RNIB is as dependent on donations from the public as the blind are dependent on RNIB.

The text suggests that the blind need to learn to be blind. This is a theme that Scott (1969) discusses at some length in his book. *The Making of Blind Men.*

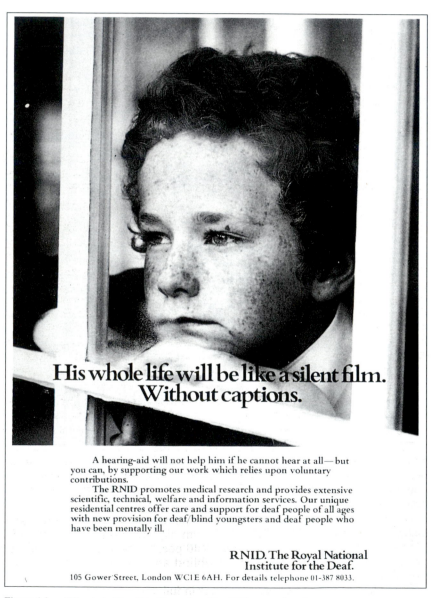

Figure 1.3   "His whole life will be like a silent film. Without captions."

Figure 1.3

"His whole life will be like a silent film. Without captions."

The statement is in two parts. It is written in the third person rather than in the first person. This contrasts with the RNIB poster. It is easier to switch from the first person singular to the second person singular than it is from the third person singular to the second person singular. As a consequence there is less of a dialogue between reader and poster in the RNID poster than in the RNIB one. The poster is thus more impersonal, though not as impersonal as the MENCAP poster. This may reflect the greater difficulty of establishing a dialogue with someone who is deaf than with someone who is blind.

Perhaps it is difficult to convey the nature of deafness visually, i.e. through the medium of a poster. RNID produce audio tapes which enable normal hearing persons to gain some idea of what it might be like to be deaf. The caption tries to build a bridge between the reader and the boy in the picture. "His whole life will be like a silent film". Note the use of the future tense. His life lies ahead of him. The simile (the use of the word "like") constitutes the bridge. The particular simile will be more meaningful to an older generation than to the young – since the days of the silent film are now long gone. If the first part of the statement is meaningful then the second part re-enforces that meaning. It is even worse that you imagined because there are no sub-titles to the silent film. Perhaps the deaf are even more handicapped than you imagined. This is a recurrent theme in some of the other posters sponsored by RNID. There is a pane of glass between the viewer and the boy. He lives in another world. A silent world. There are physical barriers to communicating with him. There are no easy answers even if the poster does arouse your sympathy:

"A hearing-aid will not help him if he cannot hear at all – but you can, by supporting our work which relies upon voluntary contributions".

We are then informed about the services that our money will support:

"The RNID promotes medical research and provides extensive scientific, technical welfare and information services. Our unique residential centres offer care and support for deaf people of all ages with new provision for deaf/blind youngsters and deaf people who have been mentally ill".

The stress is on high status institutions, e.g. medical, scientific and technical facilities. The emphasis on youth highlights the life-long nature of the commitment. Again, as in the RNIB poster, there is the suggestion of multiple handicaps, e.g. the deaf/blind and also the deaf who are mentally ill.

The logo of the Institute is spelled out in full followed by the address to which to send donations.

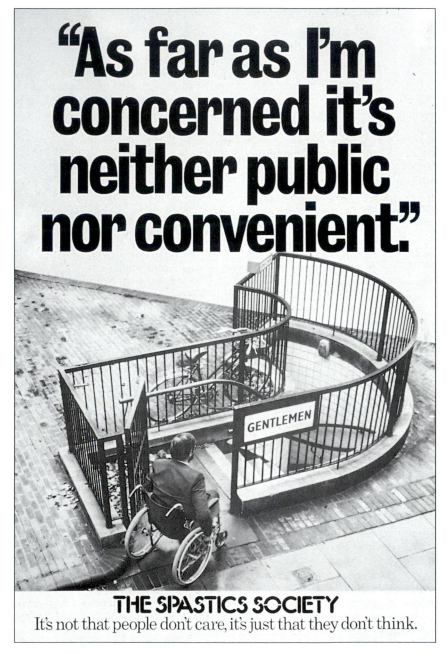

Figure 1.4   "As far as I'm concerned it's neither public nor convenient."

Figure 1.4
"As far as I'm concerned it's neither public nor convenient."

This poster is elegant in its simplicity. The verbatim quote and the visual image say it all. The quote is in the first person singular. A handicapped person expresses an opinion. It is a point of view that the reader may not have previously encountered. If so, then it is provocative, in the best sense of the word. It depends for its force on the shared cultural knowledge that a public toilet is also called "a public convenience". Hence the acoustic pun. There is a subtle relationship, here, between the image and the opinion expressed; between vision and speech. The reader needs to articulate the opinion from the printed text in order to appreciate the acoustic nature of the pun. It is no less forceful for being expressed by someone who has his back to us. The empathy which this poster engenders is mediated visually. We are able to assume the role of the other *because* he has his back to us. We are able to see for ourselves just how inconvenient this particular toilet is. The word "public" in the quote means people in general, i.e. the travelling public. It may not include you, however, if you travel in a wheelchair. Some people are excluded from this particular public convenience.

The punch line is clear "It's not that people don't care, it's just that they don't think". The poster is designed to re-educate the public – to get them to think about what it would be like to be confined to a wheelchair. It does not ask for donations. There is not even an address to which donations could be sent. The poster asks for understanding instead. Nor does it accuse the public of being callous; merely of being unthinking. It is not people in general who are unthinking but rather those who commission and those who design public facilities such as toilets. In a number of the other posters we consider there is too much text in relation to the image. This tends to be generally the case in posters for RNIB and RNID. Here, in this poster for The Spastics Society, text and image complement each other perfectly and the viewer/reader is left to think. There is a single statement of opinion and a single image.

The visual image is compelling. How could one possibly descend a spiral staircase in a wheelchair? The bicycle propped against the railings is also highly suggestive. Some people can conveniently leave their means of transport behind before descending the steps in order to relieve themselves. Others cannot. Especially spastics. People in general create handicaps for the handicapped because they don't think. The poster does not accuse them of not caring – but of not thinking. Indeed the poster assumes they do care. It makes you think, doesn't it?

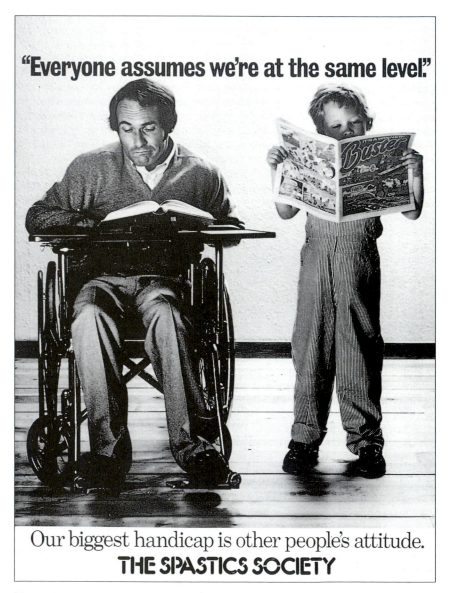

Figure 1.5   "Everyone assumes we're at the same level."

Figure 1.5

"Everyone assumes we're at the same level."

Again, the message is elegantly simple, though a bit more complicated than the poster about the public convenience. The verbatim quote here is in the first person plural. "Everyone assumes we're at the same level". The person in the wheelchair would appear to be the author of this thought. The thought is divisive since it differentiates between the two persons portrayed in the photograph. Clearly the person in the wheelchair is not speaking on behalf of both of those portrayed, even though he does use the pronoun "we". The poster is a device whereby the viewer can read the thought of the person in the wheelchair.

The physical location of the quote emphasises that the two persons portrayed are of similar height. The stated assumption is that they are both at the same level. The unstated assumption is that they are also at the same intellectual level. That they are not is suggested by the difference in their respective reading material. The boy is reading a comic *Buster* which combines pictures and text. Since comics are produced for a mass readership they assume only a restricted vocabulary on the part of their readers. The person in the wheelchair is reading a substantial tome. It implies a much higher level of education. The weighty tome rests on the table of the wheelchair and cannot be held aloft for reading like the altogether more lightweight comic. Both readers are about half way through their respective tasks.

The poster is designed to force members of the public to distinguish between spastics and those who are mentally handicapped. This is done in an indirect and subtle way that is not offensive to those who are mentally handicapped. Many spastics are well qualified in terms of their education. The poster is a warning against assuming that people in wheelchairs are mentally as well as physically handicapped.

The punch line is clear "Our biggest handicap is other people's attitudes". This is a theme that recurs in a number of the posters sponsored by The Spastics Society. Spastics face discrimination when they seek employment commensurate with their qualifications. The poster campaign is designed to alter that state of affairs. It is not asking for charity. Nor is any address provided to which donations could be sent. It calls, instead, for a change in attitude on the part of the public. It's the stereotypes of spastics in the minds of the public that need to be challenged and changed. This is the theme that Goffman (1963) treated in his book *Stigm: Notes on the management of spoiled identity*. Let's not further handicap those with a handicap by virtue of our attitudes towards them. Here the word handicap refers to the nature of the relationship between the spastic and members of the general public. It does not refer to the spastic alone. As with the other poster on behalf of The Spastics Society the aim is to encourage the public to think about the nature of the handicap.

Members of the Spastics Society recently voted to change the name of the Society. It's now called SCOPE. This suggests that, in the view of its members, the word spastic conveyed negative overtones they did not wish to perpetuate in the name of their Society.

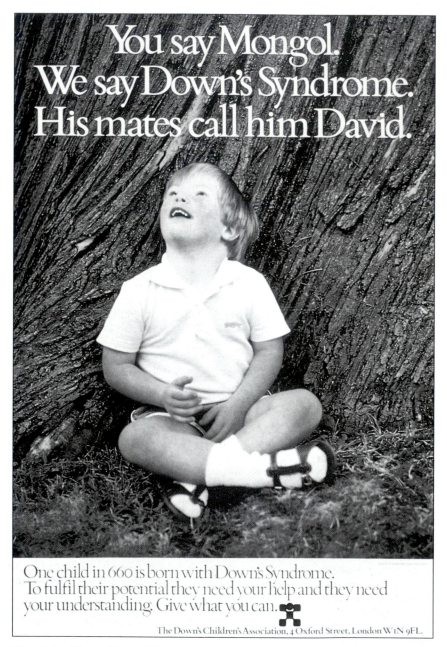

Figure 1.6   "You say Mongol. We say Down's Syndrome. His mates call him David."

Figure 1.6

"You say Mongol. We say Down's Syndrome. His mates call him David."

This triple caption arrests the attention of passers-by and invokes at least three distinct worlds, each marked by a different personal pronoun. The addressees "you" are members of the public who are inclined to call David a mongol. They are informed by the Charity whose poster it is that the correct term is "Down's syndrome". Mongol is no longer an acceptable representation. The aim is to educate the public at large in the correct use of the term. The term corresponds to the name of the Charity so the poster is also an exercise in establishing a brand image within the Charities' market. The Charity distances itself from the popular stereotype of mongolism. It offers instead a more medical and technical term for the handicap – Down's syndrome – as a replacement in the minds of the public for the ethnic term. The switch from the second person plural – "you" – to the first person plural – "we" – marks a distinction between two groups. "We" is a linguistic marker for the "in-group", i.e. the Charity; "you" is a linguistic marker for the "out-group", i.e. the public. The third world – marked by the use of the third person singular – is the world of David himself and of his friends. The Charity acts as a self-appointed mediator between David and members of the public. The poster introduces David to the public. Pronouns are a linguistic device for switching the attention of the reader or the listener (Farr, 1990b, 1991). The double switch in the use of pronouns within the triple caption enhances the inter-active effect of the poster.

The photographic image is highly pleasing visually. The original is in colour and is taken by the world-famous photographer, Lord Lichfield. The relation between image and text is both elegant and simple. In this respect it is like the "As far as I'm concerned it's neither public nor convenient" poster for The Spastics' Society which we considered earlier. Colourfully dressed and sitting cross-legged beneath what might be a giant oak tree David appears like any other normal, healthy boy of his age. His attention could be attracted by some movement in the branches over his head. The angle of his head helps to ensure it appears of normal size. It would be unfortunate, in this particular poster, if the photograph were to reinforce, rather than to challenge, popular stereotypes of mongolism. The contrast with the Mencap poster considered earlier is quite marked. The visual image here is a highly pleasing and colourful one and we know the name of the person in the photograph.

The didactic tone of the text is perpetuated in the sub-text. We are informed that "one child in 660 is born with Down's syndrome". Like acorns they, too have the potential to grow. Note the switch to the third person plural. To fulfil their potential they need two things from us – our help and our understanding. The former is probably a euphemism for our money. An address is conveniently provided to which we can send our donations. To this extent the poster is less altruistic than those for The Spastics Society which we considered above. Alternatively, if we have no disposable income, we can provide understanding. We have a choice. We can at least stop saying mongol as we are enjoined to do by Sarah in the related poster.

Whether or not the handicapped themselves approve of these campaigns on their behalf is an interesting question from a social psychological point of view. The answer is likely to vary all the way from The Spastics Society, where, I understand, spastics themselves were the main pressure group behind the campaign to educate the public about the nature of their handicap, to Mencap, where it is extremely unlikely that the mentally handicapped were directly involved in devising the particular campaign considered here. This is a state of affairs that at Mencap has almost certainly changed as a consequence of the launch of their new image in 1992.

It is possible, of course, to gauge the impressions that form in the minds of those who view and read these posters. This is done in Stockdale's contribution to the present volume and, in the case of mental handicap, in the contribution by Eayrs and her colleagues. The extent to which the posters evoke a sympathetic response from viewers and readers can also be assessed. A more important question concerns whether the images used reinforce or challenge existing stereotypes. This is an issue raised by two of the three contributors to this section of the book. Stockdale also looks at the issue of match and mismatch in relation to a range of media messages, including those concerned with HIV/AIDS.

Eayrs and her colleagues have analysed charity advertising on behalf of people with learning disabilities. They present the results of several experimental studies. Their research suggests that the images which elicit the greatest commitment to donate funds are those most closely associated with feelings of guilt, sympathy and pity. In their contribution to this volume they discuss how these negative images of mental handicap hinder the integration of the handicapped into the community. This is theme to which we shall return in Part III of the present volume where Jahoda raises the issue of the quality of life of those with a handicap who now live in the community but who previously lived in an institution. This is also a central theme in Zani's contribution to Part II.

Charities invest, over time, in the marketing of their logos (this includes the name of the Charity). It is not easy to change an exisiting logo or to patent a new one. The quality of life of those with a handicap is likely to depend upon the level of services provided by the State as well as by voluntary organisations and on how the particular handicap is represented socially. Charity advertising plays an important role in regard to the latter. A successful advertising campaign may improve the level of services but tarnish the image. Eayrs et al. point to some of the contradictions involved here. The ideal, of course, is to improve both the level of services and the image. Changing existing stereotypes that are negative and fostering news ones that are positive are laudable aims. There are probably limits to just how far one can improve the quality of life of those with a handicap by effecting changes in the image of the handicap. I suspect one can reduce levels of dissatisfaction with life by such changes without positively promoting satisfaction with life. This would be in line with Herzberg's theory of work motivation (Herzberg, Mausner, and Snyderman, 1959; see the theoretical overview to Part II). Improving the quality of life of those with a handicap should not depend upon purely semantic changes. This relates to the name both of the handicap and of the

Charity providing for those with a particular handicap. The notion of mental handicap, in particular, has come under increasing pressure in recent decades. A cascade of new euphemisms (Luckmann, personal communication) for the same form of handicap is unlikely significantly to improve the quality of life of those affected.

REFERENCES

Billig, M. (1987), *Arguing and Thinking: A rhetorical approach to social psychology.* Cambridge: Cambridge University Press.

Danziger, K. (1983), Origins and basic principles of Wundt's Völkerpsychologie. *British Journal of Social Psychology*, **22**, 303–313.

Durkheim, E. (1898), Représentations individuelles et représentations collectives. *Revue de Metaphysique et de Morale*, **VI**, 273–302.

Farr, R. M. (1977), Heider, Harré and Herzlich on health and illness: Some observations on the structure of 'représentations collectives'. *European Journal of Social Psychology*, **7** (4), 491–504.

Farr, R. M. (1981), On the nature of human nature and the science of behaviour. In P. Heelas & A. Lock (Eds.), *Indigenous Psychologies: The anthropology of the self.* (pp. 303–317). London: Academic Press.

Farr, R. M. (1983), Wilhelm Wundt (1832-1920) and the origins of psychology as an experimental and social science. *British Journal of Social Psychology*, **22** (4), 289–301.

Farr, R. M. (1990a), Social representations as widespread beliefs. In C. Fraser & G. Gaskell (Eds.), *Psychological Studies of Widespread Beliefs.* (pp. 47–64). Oxford: Clarendon Press.

Farr, R. M. (1990b), The social psychology of the prefix 'inter': A prologue to the study of dialogue. In I. Marková & K. Foppa (Eds.), *The Dynamics of Dialogue.* (pp. 25–44). London: Harvester/Wheatsheaf.

Farr, R. M. (1991), Bodies and voices in dialogue. In I. Marková & K. Foppa (Eds.), *Asymmetries in Dialogue.* (pp. 241–258). London: Harvester/ Wheatsheaf.

Farr, R. M. (1993), Common sense, science and social representations. *Public Understanding of Science*, **2**, 111–122.

Fraser, C. & Gaskell, G. (Ed.). (1990), *The Social Psychological Study of Widespread Beliefs.* Oxford: Clarendon Press.

Goffman, E. (1963), *Stigma: Notes on the management of spoiled identity.* Englewood Cliffs, New Jersey: Prentice-Hall.

Herzberg, F., Mausner, B. & Snyderman, B. B. (1959), *The Motivation to Work* (2nd ed.). New York: Wiley.

Herzlich, C. (1969), *Santé et Maladie: Analyse d'une représentation sociale.* Paris: Mouton.

Herzlich, C. (1973), *Health and Illness: A social psychological analysis.* London: Academic Press.

Herzlich, C. & Pierret, J. (1984), *Malades d'hier, Malades d'aujourd'hui: De la mort collective au devoir de guérison.* Paris: Payot.

Herzlich, C. & Pierret, J. (1987), *Illness and Self in Society.* Baltimore: The Johns Hopkins University Press.

Jahoda, M. (1977), *Freud and the Dilemmas of Psychology.* London: The Hogarth Press.

Jodelet, D. (1984), The representation of the body and its transformations. In R. M. Farr & S. Moscovici (Eds.), *Social Representations.* (pp. 211–238). Cambridge: Cambridge University Press.

Katz, E. & Lazarsfeld, P. F. (1955), *Personal Influence: The part played by people in the flow of mass communications.* New York: The Free Press.

Livingstone, S. M. (1990), *Making Sense of Television: The psychology of audience interpretation*. Oxford: Pergamon.

Marková, I. & Wilkie, P. (1987), Representations, concepts and social change: The phenomenon of AIDS. *Journal for the Theory of Social Behaviour*, **17** (4), 389–409.

McLuhan, H. M. (1951), *The Mechanical Bride: Folklore of industrial man*. New York: Vanguard Press.

McLuhan, H. M. (1962), *The Gutenberg Galaxy: The making of typographic man*. London: Routledge & Kegan Paul.

McLuhan, H. M. (1964), *Understanding Media: The extension of man*. London: Routledge & Kegan Paul.

McLuhan, H. M. (1967), *The Medium is the Message*. New York: Random House.

Moscovici, S. (1961), *La Psychanalyse: Son image et son public* (Deuxième édition: 1976). Paris: Presses Universitaires de France.

Moscovici, S. (1984), The phenomenon of social representations. In R. M. Farr & S. Moscovici (Eds.), *Social Representations*. (pp. 3–69). Cambridge: Cambridge University Press.

Potter, J. & Wetherall, M. (1987), *Discourse and Social Psychology: Beyond attitudes and behaviour*. London: Sage.

Scott, R. A. (1969), *The Making of Blind Men*. New York: Russell Sage.

Sperber, D. (1985), Anthropology and psychology: Towards an epidemiology of representations. *Man (New Series)*, **1**, 73–89.

Sperber, D. (1990), The epidemiology of beliefs. In C. Fraser & G. Gaskell (Eds.), *The Social Psychological Study of Widespread Beliefs*. (pp. 25–44). Oxford: The Clarendon Press.

Stainton Rogers, W. (1991), *Explaining Health and Illness: An exploration of diversity*. New York: Harvester/Wheatsheaf.

Wundt, W. (1900–1920), *Völkerpsychologie: Eine Untersuchung der Entwicklungsgesetze von Sprache, Mythus und Sitte*. Leipzig: Englemann.

Wundt, W. (1973), *The Language of Gestures*. The Hague: Mouton. (with an introduction by A. L. Blumenthal and additional essays by G. H. Mead and K. Bühler).

CHAPTER TWO

The Self and Media Messages: Match or Mismatch?

Janet E STOCKDALE

Department of Social Psychology, The London School of Economics and Political Science, Houghton Street, London, WC2A 2AE

CONTEXT AND ISSUES

This chapter addresses some of the issues raised by poster campaigns designed to affect people's attitudes and belief systems and to influence their behaviour. A basic question is whether we can develop effective methods of conveying information that will engage the attention of its audience, stimulate awareness, challenge stereotypes and influence both the way we construe our environment and how we behave within it. The idea of neutral information is illusory. Information carries with it the ideology, values and intentions of the communicator, and its interpretation reflects the recipients' understanding and biases, and the social and cultural environments to which they both belong. This is very evident in the media, which are in the business of representing ideas and images, and which themselves form part of the cultural framework for understanding social issues and defining their personal significance. The interaction between the individual and society, and among 'social facts', as portrayed by the media, and the individual's self image and group identity are of prime importance in the analysis of media campaigns designed to raise people's awareness of and reactions to societal issues.

The links between information, attitudes and behaviour are problematic. The assumption that information is sufficient to generate a change in either attitudes or behaviour is unfounded. A change in attitude is no longer seen as the trigger for behavioural change. Behaviour occurs in a social and cultural context and therefore we need to understand the environment in which beliefs and behaviour are legitimised. Yet media campaigners sometimes fail to appreciate that knowledge is insufficient to guarantee a change in status on the part of the reader or viewer from mere observer to actor. The recognition of information as relevant to you – rather than to everyone else – and the activation of decision-making steps necessary for behavioural change depend on how people view the problem with which they are confronted and who they are. This implies at least two things.

First, the media messages must force the individual to recognise that there is a problem. As Marková (1990) suggests, this occurs only when the individual's mind wakes up from its customary somnolent state and becomes engaged. Individuals have to be reflexive about their reactions to media messages and the relationships between public and private representations of the issues and their behaviour. Second, we must appreciate the active role played by individuals' self-perceptions – their personal and social identity – and their personal priorities, sources of vulnerability and responses to social pressures. This approach recognises the perils of neglecting the social environment and the importance of interpreting 'social' in its widest sense (cf. Doise, 1978; Himmelweit, 1990). It highlights both the inadequacy of a limited explanatory focus when dealing with social phenomena and the pivotal role of the social environment in generating and maintaining behaviour.

How successful are media messages in encouraging reflexivity, and a questioning of beliefs and behaviours, rather than in endorsing customary linguistic, conceptual and behavioural routines? How successful are they in changing their audience from passive observers into active participants? On a practical level, what affects reactions to charity advertising and how far are reactions to posters mirrored in donations to the charities the posters represent?

I shall consider some answers to these questions with illustrations from research into the role played by the visual images and captions in posters representing various charities and other agencies[1]. I shall begin with examples from poster campaigns relating to representations of handicap. I use the term 'handicap' advisedly, and I shall return to the issue of labelling later. I shall also refer to campaigns concerned with the promotion of safer sex, in relation to the risk of HIV infection. The campaigns share common goals of education, raised awareness and change of attitudes. Both types of campaign aim to affect behaviour, whether it be in public, in the way that people behave toward those labelled mentally or physically handicapped or through the donation of money, or in the way people behave in the privacy of a sexual relationship. Such campaigns face similar problems: stereotyping, which exists in the media as well as in people's heads, and which the media have done much to create and reinforce; stigma,which is as much in the eye of the beholder as it is in the mind or body of the person being stigmatised; and the fears and vulnerabilities we face when dealing with people who are seen as 'different', or when we are asked to question our beliefs and actions in our intimate relationships.

REPRESENTATIONS OF HANDICAP

In seeking to improve the quality of life for those whom society defines as handicapped, it is necessary to set about changing social representations, as well as working with those with disabilities. Social representations refer to the shared, consensual beliefs which make up our social reality (cf. Moscovici, 1981; 1984; 1988). They refer to the products of our social thinking and interaction, and are expressed in our language, in our communication and in the cultural artefacts of a society. They are conventional and prescriptive but, at the same time, are dynamic and changing. They are the means by which we understand and communicate about events and issues which confront us in our daily lives. They are, in effect, the collective and active memory of individuals living together in a social environment. The media can both reflect and help to change social representations which are common currency in our society and which shape our understanding of what life is like for those with disabilities.

The first phase of the research examined people's representations of handicap. The second phase focused on the images and messages conveyed by poster campaigns commissioned by five relevant charities. (The respondents numbered 55 in all, and consisted of 21 students who took part in the preliminary study (Stockdale & Farr, 1987) and 34 non-students who participated in the replication study). In the initial phase of the research respondents were first asked what they understood by the term 'handicap' and to generate examples. The majority representation of handicap emerged as: "a disability, disadvantage, insufficiency or lack; where the individual has difficulty doing things, is restricted and constrained and not able to live life to the full; as an affliction which means that the individual is separated and alienated from society". The recurrent theme was a comparison with 'normality' – whatever that may be. Physical handicaps were generated as examples twice as often as were mental handicaps, with blindness and lack of normal physical movement and function being the most frequently mentioned.

The study then focused on how people represent and react to five specific handicaps: blindness, deafness, being spastic, i.e having cerebral palsy, being mentally handicapped or having Down's syndrome. While all respondents had a relatively accurate perception of blindness, deafness and mental handicap, there was a notable lack of understanding of the terms 'spastic' and 'Down's syndrome'. There were other contrasts: people who are deaf or blind are seen as more integrated into society than people with other handicaps. People feel that they can cope with blindness and deafness, while mental handicap and physical abnormality, involving lack of motor control or function, are difficult to come to terms with and create feelings of apprehension and unease. These perceptions form the backdrop against which posters promoting relevant charities are perceived.

What Messages do the Posters Convey?

The second phase of the study involved the collection of both qualitative and quantitative data concerning the images and messages conveyed by ten posters, two examples of those issued by each of five charities: The Royal National Institute for the Blind (RNIB), The Royal National Institute for the Deaf (RNID), The Spastics Society, The Down's Children's Association (DCA) and MENCAP. Which of these posters are most successful and which of them are less well-received?

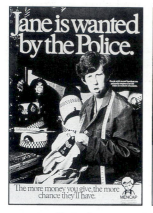

Poster 1

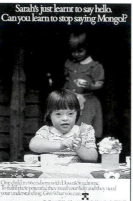

Poster 2

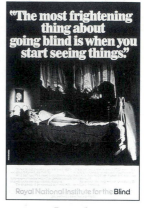

Poster 3

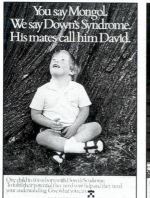

Poster 4

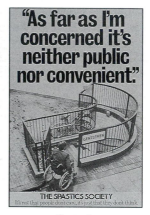

Poster 5

Poster 6

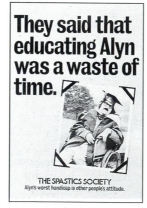

Poster 7

Figure 2.1   Seven posters depicting various forms of handicap.

Both our student and non-student respondents agreed about the posters they liked least: one from each of MENCAP, RNID and RNIB. The MENCAP poster "Jane is wanted by the Police" (Poster 1) conveyed a confusing and dubious message. Is Jane impersonating a Police Officer? If it means that mentally handicapped people can be employed, why do they need our money? While the poster has impact, is it for the right or wrong reasons? Some respondents thought it suggested exploitation of the mentally handicapped and questioned whether it was appropriate to use a play on words.

Two posters from the RNID and the RNIB produced similar negative reactions: the images are dark and depressing and the posters contain too much small print. The RNID poster "Where are deaf people usually sent? To Coventry" (Poster 2) is seen as sad and depressing and conveyed feelings of loneliness and isolation. The portrayal generated feelings of guilt but, perhaps, its message is too close for comfort. The RNIB poster "The most frightening thing about going blind is when you start seeing things" (Poster 3) was also seen as dark, disturbing and frightening. However, the image was powerful and personally meaningful: "I'd hate to be like that – I can imagine what it would be like". The simple, strong caption was effective in catching people's attention but ironically you have to have good eyesight to find out how giving money might help. There was a very positive response to the posters produced by the Spastics Society and the DCA. These four posters are liked most and are those which are most likely to make respondents think that society creates many of the problems people like this face (Posters 4 to 7).

Both the posters from the DCA were seen as simple, clear and effective, making people reconsider their attitudes and their behaviour. They are dramatically different from the previous examples. They respect the autonomy and selfhood of those with a mental handicap and they set out to educate the public. They are also more sophisticated from a psychological viewpoint. They are not just presented in the third person singular. The style is a much more interrogative one between self and other; between viewer and poster.

You say Mongol. We say Down's Syndrome.
His mates call him David. (Poster 4)

Sarah's just learnt to say hello.
Can you learn to stop saying Mongol. (Poster 5)

In addition to the emotive power of children, the stress on normality and naturalness, makes you see David and Sarah as real people whom you want to help. They are also visually pleasing and in colour, reinforcing the link with the real world. They seek to change public attitudes, to remove stigma and to generate new social representations.

The two posters from the Spastics Society were described as superb, excellent and effective. They each conveyed a clear, concise and simple message. The lack of access to the public convenience was easy to identify with and generated strong feelings of anger and frustration (Poster 6).

"Educating Alyn" (Poster 7) gave an equally direct message: people with cerebral palsy are intellectually able; they are not mentally handicapped but can live normal, fulfilled lives if given the chance by society. In short, they are both challenging and provocative posters. The main pressure group here is those who have cerebral palsy and who find themselves face to face with a social representation that is unhelpful to them: "Our biggest handicap is other people's attitudes". The campaign is designed to effect change in that social representation. It is not asking for sympathy. Neither does it ask for money. It is an educational campaign. The images are excellent and the copy is succinct. There is a subtle attempt to differentiate, in the minds of the public, between those with cerebral palsy and those with mental handicap. Yet this is not done in a way that would be offensive to those with a mental handicap.

Overall, these accounts show that the posters representing the DCA and the Spastics Society are perceived very positively, with those from MENCAP, the RNIB and RNID receiving a mixed response.

The final question was: How far are reactions to the posters mirrored by donations to the five charities they represent? When our respondents were asked to distribute £100 among the five charitable causes respresented, the RNIB and DCA attracted the highest funds overall, but the student and non-student groups in our sample responded somewhat differently (Table 2.1).

The RNIB was popular with both sets of respondents but, while the DCA touched our students, it was MENCAP that attracted our older, non-student respondents. On what are these decisions based? It is not just liking. It is not just whether there is a direct appeal for money. Donating money is complex. It depends on how we see the handicap, its personal significance, and the images and messages conveyed by the posters.

Although the RNIB posters are depressing and frightening, they have a clear and direct message: "We need your donations". Blindness is a condition with which people can identify and the posters which illustrate its impact are successful in invoking pity and the recognition that the blind do need help. The 'fear inducing' approach appears to be effective in raising funds when the handicap is one which people can imagine

Table 2.1 – **Allocation of money across charities**

| | Total | | Sample | | | |
| | | | Student (N=21) | | Non-student (N=34) | |
	£	Rank	£	Rank	£	Rank
RNIB	23.20	1	23.88	2	22.85	1
DCA	20.42	2	25.88	1	17.71	3.5
MENCAP	18.57	3	16.94	4	19.44	2
RNID	16.75	4.5	14.72	5	17.83	3.5
Spastics Society	16.36	4.5	18.88	3	15.03	5

happening to them. Children with Down's syndrome commonly encounter a less than positive response – people often feel awkward and ill-at-ease – but the DCA posters, with their positive images of happy and achieving children, are very successful in countering people's pre-conceptions. The images are reinforced by a clear and clever message which links the emotional response to donating funds: "...they need your help and understanding. Give what you can." The RNID posters are clearly asking for donations with the message: "Please help us to help the deaf...' and '...you can (help) by supporting our work which relies on voluntary contributions". However, these posters emphasise the depressing and lonely aspects of being deaf and, while social isolation is recognised as a problem for those who are deaf, it is not immediately clear how donations might help. The rationale for giving money – research, developing new technology, etc. – is either not explicit or relies on a close reading of the copy which is in very small print. Although the Spastics Society's posters were seen as effective in challenging the public's misconceptions and assumptions, they had less success in attracting money. In so far as the posters make no appeal for money, but rather emphasise the need for attitudes to change, they achieve their objective. The obvious, but at the moment unanswered, question is whether, had the posters made an explicit appeal for donations, they could have been successful in both changing attitudes and raising funds.

Those whom society deems mentally handicapped commonly evoke a negative reaction – fear, apprehension and avoidance – and the MENCAP posters do little to negate this view. The images were confusing and the captions too complex to be meaningful. Although people did recognise the call for donations with the appeal 'The more money you give, the more chance they'll have', it generated a mixed response. Research by Eayrs & Ellis (1990) focusing on people's reactions to ten MENCAP posters addressed the issue of whether it is possible for charity advertising campaigns simultaneously to stimulate donations and to represent people with disabilities as valued human beings. Their results suggest that images which elicit the greatest commitment to giving money are those most closely associated with feelings of guilt, sympathy and pity and are negatively associated with posters which illustrate people with a mental handicap as having the same rights, value and capability as non-handicapped persons. (The poster "Jane is wanted by the Police" was the only poster common to the two studies and it is worth noting that of the ten MENCAP posters used in the Eayrs & Ellis study this poster induced the least sympathy, guilt and pity and was rated as the least likely to elicit a donation of money. Similarly, in our study this poster was least likely to make respondents understand that people like this have the same feelings as anyone else or to make them want to do something to help.) However, the effectiveness of guilt inducing messages is not clear-cut. There is evidence that feelings of guilt are not successful in encouraging a stated commitment to increasing future donations or in effecting a change in attitude (cf. Bozinoff & Ghingold, 1983). Our results raise the question of whether it may be possible to represent people with disabilities in a positive way, while retaining the ability to promote donations. Charities are faced with a sophisticated market place. We are selfish – we will give money in response to a strong message about the effects of a handicap, such as blindness, which we dread but which we can imagine happening to us – especially as we get older. Donations may also serve to assuage some of the guilt we may feel about our inability to deal with certain forms of handicap. However, we will also put our hands in our pockets and donate to causes which challenge our prejudices and our ignorance with a positive message promising a fulfilled and happy life.

So, there is some consensus in the way people think about handicap and the images presented by posters relating to handicap. But, the representations in such posters do not necessarily mirror the dominant representations in society, and in fact can do much to counter negative perceptions and reactions.

To what extent is this true of posters produced by agencies concerned about the spread of HIV? How do people perceive images of HIV, AIDS and safer sex portrayed in campaign posters and how do these perceptions relate to people's self-perceptions?

REPRESENTATIONS OF HIV, AIDS AND SAFER SEX

Health education is designed to stimulate individuals to alter their behaviour. Much effort has been expended in Britain on the dissemination of information about the transmission of HIV but, as pointed out earlier, while knowledge is a necessary condition for behavioural change it is not a sufficient condition. A basic pre-requisite of campaigns relating to HIV is that members of target populations see the messages as relevant to themselves, accept the message and are motivated to change (cf. Rhodes & Shaughnessy, 1989; Stockdale, Dockrell & Wells, 1989). We must understand the ways in which people acquire a sense of identity, not only as unique individuals, but also by virtue of their group membership. We need to appreciate that people are embedded in their social environments, and that the self acquires meaning from membership of social groups and the emotional significance people attach to their social roles. Tajfel (1978) and Tajfel and Turner (1979) propose that social identity is constructed by a process of intergroup comparison, based on social categorisation, such that group membership becomes salient. The appropriate in-group identifications must be triggered by the media message for it to be considered relevant. Success depends on a match between the message and an individual's social or group identity.

A COMPARISON OF POSTERS AIMED AT HOMOSEXUALS AND HETEROSEXUALS

The first study focused on two major determinants of individuals' responses to posters and advertisements: reactions to specific campaign 'messages' about HIV/AIDS and the representations people use to organise

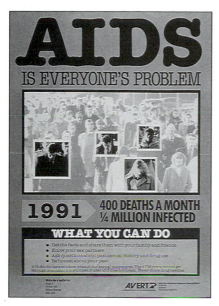

Poster 1

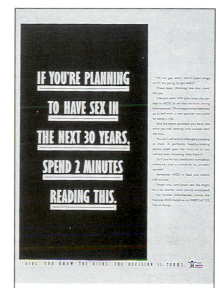

Poster 2

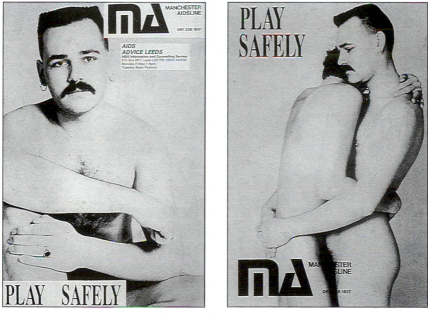

Poster 3

Poster 4

Figure 2.2　Four posters aimed at (a) a heterosexual (Posters 1 and 2) and (b) a homosexual population (Posters 3 and 4).

their response to media messages (Stockdale et al., 1989). One phase of
the study focused on the messages conveyed by specific posters aimed at
different target groups. In addition to answering a number of open-ended
questions about the posters, respondents rated the posters on a range of
attributes (e.g. personal relevance, relevance to the majority of the population, clarity, impact, fear inducement, information content and likelihood
of behavioural change). The other phase was designed to gain an understanding of people's perceptions of themselves and others within the population of those potentially at risk from HIV. The key questions this study
aimed to explore are: To what extent do individuals see posters as relevant
to themselves? What role does perception of self and perception of others
play in this process? (There were 24 respondents in total: 11 homosexuals,
2 bisexuals and 11 heterosexuals. They included males and females, some
in exclusive relationships and others without a stable sexual partner.)

Our results suggested that many of these early campaigns, although
successful in targeting their selected groups, achieved a limited impact
(Figure 2.2). Some of the posters, aimed at heterosexuals and on general
distribution, engendered fear. For example, the immediate response to the
poster: 'Aids is everyone's problem' (Poster 1), was despair: "Aids is
killing the human race". In response to the poster: 'If you're planning to
have sex.....' (Poster 2), one of our heterosexual respondents pointed out
that: "you cannot be sure of anyone", while another suggested that: "the
best – but possibly impractical – idea is to give up sex". In contrast, the
images found only in the gay press were described as sensual and erotic by
our homosexual respondents (e.g. Posters 3 & 4). This reflects the explicit
policy in many 'gay campaigns' of eroticising safer sex and making it a
behavioural norm rather than a negative directive, such that the costs to
pleasure outweigh the potential benefits to health. Pleas have been made
for similar campaigns aimed at the heterosexual population (cf. Wellings,
1987) and I shall look at the response to one such campaign later.

This research also indicated that, although heterosexual and homosexual
respondents agree about the groups that are more at risk than others, they
have a different 'cognitive map' of themselves in relation to others potentially at risk from HIV and hold a somewhat different view of the risks
they face. Homosexuals, including those in stable relationships, recognise
their potential susceptibility to HIV but feel that they have 'got the message'. However, heterosexuals still do not see themselves at risk. It is
someone else's problem. Those who are at risk are unlike them. Others are
likely to contract HIV, not them, and those others have only themselves to
blame. In the unlikely event that heterosexuals do contract HIV, it is not
their fault.

These differences in perspective have implications for the design of
media messages. It is pointless to aim a message at everyone. This does
not provide an adequate reference group for one's own behaviour.
'Everyone' is not perceived as at risk and therefore it is not surprising that
the messages are seen to have little personal relevance. Equally, messages
perceived as aimed at those with multiple partners are easily discounted as
irrelevant because people do not see themselves as promiscuous. Until we

can encourage a change in the way people perceive their own behaviours and lifestyle, heterosexuals will continue to see little match between their behaviours and those of people at risk, and to represent HIV from the viewpoint of an observer, rather than that of a participant with a positive role to play in preventing its spread within the sexually active population.

So how can we approach the problem? Is there any evidence that these insights have been applied to devise an effective poster campaign? The answer is a cautious "yes".

A POSITIVE APPROACH TO SAFER SEX

The tone and style of the safer sex campaigns, launched in recent years by the charity, the Terence Higgins Trust, are in marked contrast to those from the majority of other agencies including the Department of Health, whose efforts have ranged from the doom-laden and assumingly celibacy-inducing imagery of icebergs and graves to experts giving facts and figures about the spread of HIV infection. I shall take one such campaign to illustrate the approach. A series of six posters (Figure 2.3) portraying a variety of sexual activities and aimed at the young, presents the happy rather than the sombre face of sex. The posters are in line with the more explicit European advertising which assumes that most people enjoy sex. Moreover, a major aim of the campaign was not to marginalise the problems associated with HIV by perpetuating the idea that these problems are confined to minority groups.

How do people, especially young people, react to the new-style campaign? The overall response was positive. (Data were collected from 49 respondents: 17 students and 32 non-students: 16 aged 16 – 19 and 16 aged 32 – 45.) The message from the first poster 'Get set for safer sex' (Poster 1) was that safer sex is trendy and fun and is practised by attractive people. However, the poster lacks information on what practices constitute safer sex. The second poster "No risk in a kiss" (Poster 2) clearly conveyed the message: 'kissing is safe', but a majority of respondents were confused about whether those portrayed were male or female. "There is more to sex than penetration" was identified as the message in the next poster "As safe as playing on your own" (Poster 3). It was perceived as eye-catching and fun by the majority. However, some found it offensive and described it as rude or horrifying. The fourth poster 'Discover safer sex' (Poster 4) had impact but gained a mixed reception. Over half the respondents identified the message as: 'oral sex can be safe, enjoyable and is an alternative to intercourse'. Nearly half the respondents thought the poster might offend and a substantial minority considered it shocking and pornographic. (There has been some criticism of the posters. A number of schools, youth organisations and some health educators have deemed them offensive and have objected to their use.) The fifth poster "Wet your appetite for safer sex" (Poster 5) also produced some confusion and contradictory reactions. Some thought the image sensual, beautiful and loving, but others, mainly older respondents, thought the image degrading

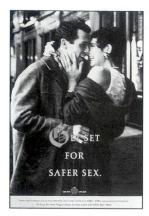

Poster 1

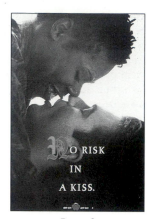

Poster 2

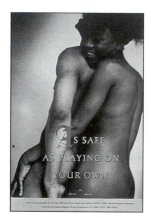

Poster 3

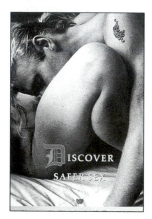

Poster 4

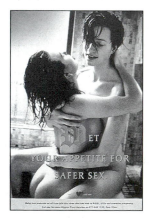

Poster 5

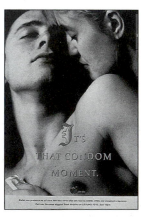

Poster 6

Figure 2.3   Six safer sex campaign posters.

and shocking. There was confusion about what the poster was trying to say, but the dominant view was that it was promoting lesbian activity as a variant of safer sex.

The final poster "It's that condom moment" (Poster 6) was described as amusing, erotic, striking and tasteful. It portrayed a situation with which respondents could identify and gave the clear message: "use a condom". "It's that condom moment" is the poster that emerges as the most informative, having the clearest message and the most preferred. Also, it was seen as the poster most likely to make people think about their sexual behaviour and to affect them whether or not they practise safer sex.

ISSUES AND FUTURE DIRECTIONS

These examples of poster campaigns and the images and messages they convey, or fail to convey, raise a number of issues of theoretical significance and practical importance. They provide pointers for future campaigns designed to increase public awareness and to affect our representations of societal issues and relevant behaviours.
The message to campaigners is clear. Posters *should:*

− Engage their audience
− Contain clear, succinct copy
− Convey a simple, unambiguous message
− Portray a positive and attractive image
− Challenge stereotypes and pre-conceptions
− Identify and match their target audience
− Encourage reflexivity and a 'new look' at the issues
− Broaden our horizons − both conceptually and behaviourally

Well-designed media campaigns have a significant role to play in stimulating awareness, providing knowledge, and influencing decision making. However, to do so they must engage our attention, make us question our beliefs and behaviours and supply new, positive directions for our social representations and behavioural repertoires.

Some of the first set of posters relating to disability − I use this term rather than handicap for reasons which will become clear in a moment − serve to highlight the powerful role of language in either perpetuating or challenging the stereotypical views which provide the basis for prejudice. The United Nations − after the World Health Organisation − defines disability as: 'Any restriction or lack (resulting form an impairment) of ability to perform an activity in the manner or within the range considered normal for a human being'. This is distinguished from handicap which is: 'A function of the *relationship* between disabled persons and their environment...Handicap is the loss or limitation of opportunities to take part in the life of the community on an equal level with others.' We create the handicap; it is not inherent in the person with a disability. However, in our everyday discourse our representations of disability and handicap merge and we rarely confront the ways in which our language, attitudes and behaviour transform a disability into a handicap.

Used inappropriately, language can foster a sense of a handicap. For example, 'spastic', as a noun, is not only misused as a term of abuse but also equates people with the condition that they are affected by and so dehumanises them. It cannot be overemphasised that anyone with a disability is first and foremost a *person* and not a disability. There has been some success in the field of mental handicap. The terms the 'feeble-minded' and 'mentally deficient' are rarely used and there is an expanding vocabulary reflecting increased knowledge of the issues.

The issue of labelling has become contentious with the accusation that some charities are insulting the people they represent with the terminology that they use. The term 'mentally handicapped' used by MENCAP in its advertising has been condemned as derogatory and 'politically incorrect' by a number of social workers and support groups. They insist people should be described only as having 'learning difficulties'. Although MENCAP posters sought to show that life can be enjoyed as much by people with a mental handicap as by the rest of the population, a number of people have argued that such campaigns are offensive and degrading, because they emphasise the handicap and limitations of people with learing difficulties, instead of highlighting what they can achieve. However, the Chairman of MENCAP has responded that the stigma will not disappear just because of a change in terminology. In his view, the term 'mental handicap' accurately describes the condition of many of the people the charity represents and to say otherwise would understate their condition and possibly deny them their welfare rights. The Department of Health has stopped the use of the term 'mental handicap', in response to external pressure, and now refers only to 'people with learning disabilities'. However, it has not gone as far as some organisations, expecially those in the United States, would like to see. There the preference is increasingly for the phrase 'intellectually challenged'.

Such changes and criticisms have not, however, received universal support. Many parents and others protest that to classify people who have a permanent condition of 'mental handicap' under euphemistic labels, such as 'learning difficulties or disabilities' denies their special needs. They argue that people who are capable of feeling insulted and distressed by the MENCAP campaign are not really mentally handicapped in their understanding of the term. In their view a relabelling of mental handicap creates a fool's paradise.

In recognition of the need to give the charity a more positive image, MENCAP has recently relaunched itself with a new identity. The charity has adopted a series of picture logos featuring people with disabilities and a new slogan: "Making the most of life". MENCAP has also initiated a 12-month consultation exercise with its members on the question of whether it should abandon the term 'mental handicap' in favour of a more positive expression. Such changes reflect both the fact that many of MENCAP's members have disabilities themselves and the need to project MENCAP as a modern business rather than as an old-fashioned charity. MENCAP's new image has not received a positive response from People First, a national organisation of people with learning difficulties which campaigns for self-advocacy. The organisation is critical of both the new 'positive' logos, which it argues deny the fact that people with learning difficulties encounter enormous problems, and the continued use of the term 'mental handicap', especially in the name of the charity. However, a change of name might jeopardise the charity's brand recognition and image and therefore its ability to raise money.

The Spastics Society has recognised that it also faces problems of labelling. Research carried out by the Society suggested that the name of the Society deters some people, particularly parents, from seeking the Society's help because they do not want their child labelled. The Society's consultative process with its members showed that although some people were apprehensive about a change of name because of the risks associated with an unknown and untested alternative, the majority recognised that the current name is out of date and offensive to people with cerebral palsy. This view was reflected in the overwhelming vote by the members of the Society in favour of choosing a new name for the charity[2].

These arguments touch on issues that charity advertising must at some stage confront: the enormous and growing disparity between the day-to-day work and the public sales pitch on behalf of the people charities represent. Although charities are moving away from just raising money and are recognising that they must respect the people they represent, much of their work depends on their ability to generate donations. Appeals are necessarily formulated to tap into emotions and donation is essentially a supportive act which does not always rest easily with the idea that 'victims' are also citizens with equal rights. Emotive advertising which makes people dip their hands into their pockets risks demeaning the very people it sets out to help. There is a need to educate the public and potential donors about 'societal issues' and the campaigns by the Spastics Society and by the DCA testify to the success of this approach. Equally, it must be recognised that such campaigns may reduce the attraction of powerful images of disability which evoke the reaction that 'I can do something' immediately and without involvement. This is the dilemma that many charities face today when deciding how to portray the people they represent, in an increasingly competitive arena.

The posters relating to handicap, or rather to disability, which seek to change our representations, are based on the premise that it is possible to change the way people perceive and react to those who are identified as 'different' on the basis of their disability. Posters, such as those produced by The Spastics Society and the DCA, articulate the problems faced by the people whom these organisations represent and for whom they seek justice rather than pity. In that sense they are more progressive than those posters, which although sometimes challenging, evoke guilt, fear, unease or apprehension and which, although often effective in money-raising terms, do little to suggest that people themselves have any power to change the status quo. People have to be involved and recognise that handicap is a societal and not just an individual issue. The equation that is commonly made between disability and handicap, is the cause of our failure to provide for people with a disability those life opportunities enjoyed by the majority. This disparity of opportunity is mirrored elsewhere in society and reflects the way in which people's representations of individuals with identifiable characteristics evoke inferences about abilities, needs and a whole range of uncorrelated attributes which then serve to justify discriminatory behaviour.

It is clear that with the sensitive, but not inappropriate or euphemistic, use of language and a considered choice of images, posters can be an effective medium for challenging current representations. They can encourage sensitivity rather than sensationalism; accuracy rather than apprehension; societal awareness rather than individual sentimentality; and they can emphasise empowerment without being patronising. Such challenges are necessary if we are to disturb the comfortable and convenient assumption that disability necessarily means handicap. As in the safer sex campaigns, viewers need to consider themselves as participants, not just observers, and to recognise that it is within their power to prevent themselves converting a disability into a handicap. The Spastics Society campaign is designed to foster such self-insight.

The conventional and prescriptive nature of our social reality and the consequent automaticity of much of our behaviour applies not only to the practised way in which we transform a disability into a handicap but also to health promotion – a growth industry. The advent of Aids, with its close link with sexual and drug-using behaviour, has put personal behaviour on public display and has reinforced the view that individuals play a major role in shaping their own destinies (cf. Kaplan, 1990). However, the determinants of health risks are too complex and forceful to succumb easily to efforts to inform the public and change its practices (Mechanic, 1990). Most behaviour, either conducive or detrimental to health, is influenced as much or more by the routine organization of everyday settings and activities as by the personal decisions of individuals. It is only necessary to consider smoking, drinking, and nutrition to appreciate the argument that almost all behaviours damaging to health flourish in contexts that routinely sustain them and usually require vigilance and conscious choice to resist. Similarly, sexual scripts define the appropriateness of a wide range of risk behaviours and affect compliance with safer sex guidelines (cf. Ford, 1987; Richardson,1989).

Sexual behaviour is inextricably linked with the norms characteristic of the social groups with which we identify. These norms shape the boundaries of permissible behaviour and define the limits of deviance. People, particularly the young, tend to see themselves as invulnerable (cf. Price, Desmond, Hallinan & Griffin, 1988; Eiser, Eiser & Lang, 1989). Also, being young is seen as a time to be free and to experiment. So, the perceived costs associated with safer sex may well outweigh any long-term benefits. Safer sex practices require negotiation, which is not always encouraged by traditional sexual roles. It is unrealistic to advise people – whether in heterosexual or homosexual relationships – to practise safer sex, without acknowledging the power imbalance that exists in many relationships. Moreover, some men may see protected or non-penetrative sex as a threat to their masculinity.

The expectations people have, both of themselves and of others, are embodied in the way they represent and practise sex. Campaigns such as those illustrated earlier provide an opportunity to reassess the meanings and pleasure of sex. Excitement and vulnerability are part of the appeal of sex – but they should also be made part of our representation of safer sex. The message must be positive and personalised. Health education efforts that ignore these principles are destined to failure. Clearly, the challenge lies in identifying points of leverage that heighten awareness of the link between lifestyle and health, and change the balance of influences so that everyday activities favour more positive patterns (cf. Mechanic, 1990). Effective health promotion requires a deeper scrutiny of communities, relationships and the routine activities of everyday life, combined with stronger interventions than those commonly used.

Mass media poster campaigns cannot be expected to achieve dramatic results. However, if carefully designed, they can generate an effective response from the public in terms of active involvement in the issues they raise and monetary support for the work of the charities concerned. More importantly such poster campaigns can foster change in how we represent and respond to those with disabilities and can influence health-related attitudes and practices.

NOTES

1. Some of the posters used in the research reported in this chapter, although current at the time, are now dated. Many of the organisations have modified their approach to take account of both new knowledge and feedback about the impact of poster campaigns.
2. From November 1994, the Spastics Society will be renamed 'SCOPE'.

ACKNOWLEDGEMENTS

I should like to express my thanks to Dr. L. M. Blud, Dr. J. E. Dockrell, Professor R. M. Farr, Ms. J. Rowley and Mr. A. J. Wells for their contributions to the research reported in this chapter.

REFERENCES

Bozinoff, L. & Ghingold, M. (1983), Evaluating guilt arousing marketing communication. *Journal of Business Research*, **11**, 243–255.

Doise, W. (1978), *Groups and Individuals: Explanations in social psychology.* Cambridge: Cambridge University Press.

Eayrs, C. B. & Ellis, N. (1990), Charity advertising: For or against people with a mental handicap? *British Journal of Social Psychology*, **29**, 349–360.

Eiser, C., Eiser, J. R., & Lang, J. (1989), Adolescent beliefs about AIDS prevention. *Psychology and Health*, **3**, 287–296.

Ford, N. (1987), Research into heterosexual behaviour with implications for the spread of AIDS. *British Journal of Family Planning,* **13**, 50–54.

Himmelweit, H. T. (1990), Societal psychology: Implications and scope. In H. T. Himmelweit & G. Gaskell (Eds), *Societal Psychology,* Newbury Park, CA: Sage.

Kaplan, M. S. (1990), AIDS: Individualizing a social problem. *Society,* **27** (2), 4–7.

Marková, I. (1990), Medical ethics: A branch of societal psychology. In H. T. Himmelweit & G. Gaskell (Eds), *Societal Psychology,* Newbury Park, CA: Sage.

Mechanic, D. (1990), Promoting health. *Society,* **27** (2), 16–22.

Moscovici, S. (1981), On social representations. In J. P. Forgas (Ed), *Social Cognitions: Perspectives on everyday understanding,* pp. 181–209, London: Academic Press.

Moscovici, S. (1984), The phenomenon of social representations. In R. M. Farr & S. Moscovici (Eds), *Social Representations,* pp. 3–69, Cambridge: Cambridge University Press.

Moscovici, S. (1988), Notes towards a description of social representations. *European Journal of Social Psychology,* **18**, 211–250.

Price, J. H., Desmond, S. M., Hallinan, C., & Griffin, T. B. (1988), College students' perceived risk and seriousness of AIDS. *Health Education, Aug/Sept,* 16–20.

Rhodes, T. & Shauhnessy, R. (1989), Selling safer sex: AIDS education and advertising. *Health Promotion,* **4** (1), 27–30.

Richardson, D. (1989), *Women and the AIDS crisis.* London: Pandora Press.

Stockdale, J. E. & Farr, R. M. *Social representations of handicap in poster campaigns.* Paper presented at the London Conference of the British Psychological Society, December 1987.

Stockdale, J. E., Dockrell, J. E., & Wells, A. J. (1989), The self in relation to mass media representations of HIV and Aids - match or mismatch? *Health Education Journal,* **48** (3), 121–130.

Tajfel, H. (1978), Social categorization, social identity and social comparison. In H. Tajfel (Ed), *Differentiation Between Social Groups,* London: Academic Press.

Tajfel, H. & Turner, J. C. (1979), An integrative theory of social conflict. In W. Austin & S. Worschel (Eds), *The Social Psychology of Intergroup Relations,* Monterey, CA: Brooks/Cole.

Wellings, K. (1987), Heterosexual spread of Aids – a challenge for health education. *Health Education Journal,* **46** (4), 143–147.

CHAPTER THREE

The Face of AIDS

Jenny KITZINGER

Glasgow University Media Group, 61 Southpark Av, Glasgow G12 8LF.

INTRODUCTION

It is December 1986 and Independent Television News (ITN) is presenting its annual end of year review. "How will *you* remember '86" asks the presenter "… what images will linger in the mind's eye – the image of '86"? A scene showing a white baby appears on the screen. "The Face of AIDS '86" says the presenter, "a British baby inheriting life and the promise of an early death from her infected parents." The camera shifts to show an emaciated black infant. "The Face of AIDS '86", repeats the presenter, "a baby in central Africa where it is now estimated a million people can expect to die from it within the next decade" and the camera zooms-in to show the face of a black man lying in bed, looking half-dead, staring into the distance (ITN Review of the Year, 30.12.86). This doom-laden message was, and is, the 'Face of AIDS' according to many parts of the media and it was these sorts of image that 'lingered in the mind's eye' of many of the people we spoke to in the course of our research. The Acquired Immune Deficiency Syndrome is personified by a haggard, painfully thin person dying of AIDS-related illnesses – a figure with jutting bones, sunken eyes and a listless expression of despair. In fact 'emaciation has become emblematic of AIDS' (Grundberg quoted in Crimp, 1992, p. 117). In this chapter I explore why such images are so popular and what impact they have on public understandings of AIDS and people's interpretations of health education messages.

IMAGES OF DEATH

The death's head image was evident in the British media coverage of AIDS from the very start. Photo-journalists deliberately sought out people with AIDS who looked particularly ill, rejecting healthier 'specimens' who volunteered to be photographed or filmed because they did not 'look the part'. The physical degeneration of the body was emphasised by before-and-after portraits of people with the syndrome. As early as 1983 newspapers such as *The News of the World* were printing photographs

showing once handsome faces of gay men juxtaposed against those
"ravaged by the progressive toll of the disease" (Wellings, 1988). The
pictures are reminiscent of the before-and-after images used in women's
magazines and slimming advertisements – except that here, instead of
plain-looking, plump women transformed into sylph-like, cover-girls,
young men at the peak of health are shown degenerating into skeletons.
The media reporting of Rock Hudson's illness and death in 1985 was
typical in this respect. The press luridly exploited the contrast between the
film star's original 'hunky' glamourous image and the 'frail skeleton' he
had become. Rock Hudson was portrayed as "a shadow of his former self"
(The Sun, 18.6.86). We were repeatedly presented with photographs
showing his previous "rugged good looks" as 'The Baron of Beefcake'
versus the image of him "As he is now ...a haggard, tired Rock
Hudson"(Daily Express, 25.7.85). This formula was endlessly repeated
with each new celebrity to succumb to the illness. One of the more recent
personalities to attract attention – Freddie Mercury – is shown healthy and
defiant on some pages ('flamboyant', 'outrageous' and 'flaunting' his
sexuality) only to have such photographs contrasted with references to him
looking "sad" and "haunted", "no longer able to enjoy the lifestyle he
craved" (The Sun, 25.11.91). The later photographs show him looking thin
and wan with captions such as "Ravaged...star Freddie on a rare outing in
April" (The Sun, 8.11.91) and "Last Battle: Doomed Freddie Mercury"
(The Star, 24.11.91)[1].

These images are often accompanied by language reminiscent of movies
such as "Frankenstein" or "Zombie Flesh-Eaters". One journalist,
describing a medical slide-show, writes of "images no Hollywood horror
film has matched (...) Here, in colour, are the ravages of AIDS (...) the
raw sores, bloated organs, shrivelled limbs and glassy stares of the walking
dead" (Washington Post, 19.6.90). Taken in by their own creations, some
reporters write as if the photographs are the reality, whereas the actual
people are merely reflections of these medical or media creations. When
one journalist met some people with AIDS he vividly described his shock
and sense of déjà vu. "There they are, *television images made flesh*", he
wrote, "men typically in their thirties, sunken-cheeked, some in
wheelchairs or with walking sticks, others with the purple blotches of
Kaposi's sarcoma – all united in facing an inevitable unpleasant death
soon." (Observer Magazine, 22.7.90)(my emphasis)[2].

People with AIDS are rendered speechless and anonymous – ruthlessly
exposed to the camera's scrutiny and stripped of their humanity. They are

---

[1] Such 'before-and-after' portraits appear to be particularly popular in the tabloid press.
However, the Guardian has used the same technique – although in a somewhat subtler and
perhaps more 'positive' way. When Ian Charleson, for example, died as a result of AIDS the
Guardian printed a tribute applauding his acting abilities and his fighting spirit. The article was
accompanied by two snapshots. One showed Charleson borne high on the shoulders of his team
mates in the victorious scene from the film "Chariots of Fire" – the other showed him rehearsing
for the final scene in "Hamlet" with the caption: "Sometimes he had scarcely enough strength for
the final duel" (Weekend Guardian, October 6-7 1990).

'the walking dead'. Indeed, within this style of reporting the objects of the camera's gaze do not even make eye-contact with the viewer. Their eyes are glazed, their tongues are not organs of speech but instead display boils and the thick coating of herpes; their bodies are no more than a collection of gruesome symptoms.

Why do the media dwell on such images? In part, I will argue, this style of representation is typical of a certain genre of photography but, in the context of AIDS, they also serve a very specific purpose: illustrating the consequences of 'deviant' and 'immoral' lifestyles.

PHOTOGRAPHIC GENRES IN THE MEDIA

Images of the 'Face of AIDS' in the media were not formed in a cultural vacuum. The focus on bodily decay and the before-and-after formula draw on an established history of medical photography (Watney & Gupta, 1990) and the attempt to personify a syndrome is also not unique to the media coverage of AIDS. Journalists routinely seek to give a 'face' to momentous events and concepts such as Starvation, Disaster, Revolution or War. During the fighting in the Gulf, for example, the Observer illustrated 'The Real Face of War' with a large photograph of the charred head of an Iraqi soldier who was burnt to death in his vehicle.

The obsessive lingering on physical decay and 'deformity' evident in the AIDS coverage echoes not only the tactics of horror movie directors but also fits into normal journalistic practice – at least on some newspapers. Chippendale and Horrie highlight the existence of 'Yuck journalism'; they point out that the production of 'eye-catching' images which both attract and repel the viewer is staple fare in tabloids such as *The News of the World* and *The Sun* which repeatedly publish photographs of 'physical freaks' and grotesquely injured survivors (Chippendale and Horrie, 1990, p. 167). For example, *The Sun's* controversial coverage of Simon Weston – who was severely burned in the Falklands war – included before-and-after pictures to illustrate his transformation from normality to abnormality and dwelt on his "hideous" scarring and other people's horror. Simon Weston himself had been trying to convey a message of hope, a story about the triumph of the human spirit in the face of adversity and a

---

[2] There is no room for hope of resistance in these representations. The message is one of endless despair, inevitable decay and certain death. The ITN review described at the beginning of this chapter included one single quote from Elizabeth Taylor: "These people are walking round with a noose around their neck", she said, "They are living time bombs." (ITN, 30.12.86) (Given Elizabeth Taylor's involvement in the politics of AIDS this is, of course, unlikely to represent her entire perspective on the subject – it was this one quotation, however, that was selected for broadcast in the review). Referring to a similar phenomenon within the North American context, Donald Crimp describes the way in which a CBS programme entitled "AIDS Hits Home" reinforced hopelessness: Whenever a person with AIDS is allowed to utter words of optimism, a voice-over adds a caveat such as: "Six weeks after she said this, she was dead." (Crimp, 1992, p. 120).

challenge to disablement. *The Sun* however totally warped his self-presentation, preferring to latch onto the 'yuck' potential of the story.

THE 'MORAL' DIMENSION

The media portrayal of AIDS 'victims' is, then, not a unique phenomenon. However, the AIDS story does have specific characteristics which add an extra dimension to such coverage and may make people with AIDS particularly vulnerable to such treatment by the media. Soldiers, such as Simon Weston, are firmly identified as 'normal' members of ordinary families by reference to the children, wives and sweethearts left behind. When 'our boys' are injured it is because they have been carrying out their duty, defending 'our values' and 'the great British way of life' (Glasgow University Media Group, 1985). People with AIDS, on the other hand, are routinely portrayed as 'outsiders' – abnormal, immoral and anti-social. There is a widespread assumption that they have become infected as a result of 'unnatural' practices such as homosexuality, injecting drugs or prostitution. HIV infection "is a disease avoidable by decent living" (Daily Express, 30.8.85).

This means that people with AIDS may be presented as deviant and 'guilty victims' who deserve to suffer and who endanger the lives of others. The focus on the degenerate body of the person with AIDS is particularly significant within this moral framework. The suffering represented in these photographs serves as a health warning. The message is clear: 'This is a horrible way to die – be careful or you might end up like this'. Such images are 'anti-AIDS' but they can also be anti-gay (or anti-prostitute, anti-drug user, etc). The danger is that the diseased body of the 'AIDS victim' becomes a gibbet-display warning others not only of HIV but also of the supposed consequences of 'deviance'.

The debilitated body of the adult 'AIDS victim' carries a heavy moral burden and the fetishistic promotion of such images draws on and reinforces the link between degenerate activity and the degenerate body – a link emphasised in Victorian phrenology, in early scientific dissections of 'the homosexual body' and in anti-syphillis campaigns (Boffin & Gupta, 1990; Brandt, 1987).[3] The focus on the visible stigma of AIDS-related illnesses is sometimes accompanied by textual references to gay or bisexual men who have become 'unmasked' by their fate – they can no longer pretend to be 'one of us' (see, for example, press coverage of Rock Hudson). They stand exposed as the pariahs they really are. There can even be a certain self-righteous satisfaction in the way that the media juxtapose references to the previous 'self-indulgent' lifestyle of 'AIDS victims' and the suffering that now awaits them – a suffering which is subtly signalled as their 'just deserts' from which neither fame nor money can protect them. The Star, for example, talked of Freddie Mercury as "the

---

[3] Portraits of children with AIDS can serve a quite different function: they are the innocents suffering for the sins of their fathers or mothers. In this way they serve as an indirect, but equally powerful, indictment of deviance or, in the case of the Romanian orphans, of a political regime.

bed-hopping millionaire" and referred to his "£4 million Kensington mansion where he retreated to end his flamboyant days as a gaunt recluse. Freddie shamed his family through the gay expoits which finally struck him down with AIDS" (The Star, 24.11.91). Some television coverage, too, echoes this formula – contrasting images from a 'homosexual' disco with those from an 'AIDS ward' for example. The former images focus on writhing bodies, hedonistic excesses and gay men's supposed narcissistic worship of the perfect male physique; the latter show the wretched plight of the man facing up to the 'consequences of a gay lifestyle' – enduring an agonising and ugly death.[4] The portrayal of physical affliction is intertwined with notions of sin, punishment, damnation and repentance. The ravages of illness are themselves sometimes used to symbolise corruption. One set of before-and-after pictures of Rock Hudson were captioned: "The two faces of Hollywood – vibrant, virile ...dissipated, corrupt, decadent – captured on the two faces of Rock Hudson..." (Daily Mail quoted in Watney, 1987, p. 89).

ALTERNATIVE REPRESENTATIONS

This is, of course, not the only sort of image of people with HIV and AIDS. People affected by the virus have united to demand a very different voice showing people with HIV as individuals with their own personal views and experiences and as part of a community which is defiant and angry (Miller & Beharrell, 1993). Organisations such as ACT-UP have created a distinct kind of spectacle for the television camera and there have been dramas and documentaries which offer alternative representations (most notably the TV programme *Remember Terry*). There are also striking examples of people with HIV being portrayed (at least in some segments of the media) as healthy and conventionally attractive. *Cosmopolitan*, for example, had an unusual article entitled: "My name is Denise...I'm HIV positive," this was accompanied by a traditional glamour photograph of Denise Hathaway – 'Hair and make-up by Sarah Adler at Models One.' (Hathaway & Kurtz, 1991). More recently the press reporting of a Birmingham haemophiliac who, knowing that he had the virus, had gone on to infect several women, was often accompanied with a photograph of the young man looking completely healthy and rather dashing (see press coverage June/July 1991).[5]

However, despite the existence of such alternative images, it was the

---

[4] The same sort of glee was shown by some of the media in printing a close-up shot of Michael Jackson – "his face ravaged by plastic surgery" and "hideously disfigured" (Mirror, 28.7.92). Here was a pop idol, a black man, who seemed to aspire to resemble a young Caucasian woman – and had ended up with "sunken cheeks and a pinched nose", a 'phantom with a face covered by scar tissue'. Using the language of investigative reporting The Mirror implied that they had "unmasked" the 'real' face of Michael Jackson. The paper published its 'exposé' picture along side another photograph of the way they alleged Jackson preferred to see himself – "in soft focus" – and they urged him to "Face Up to it, Michael" (The Mirror, 28.7.92)

[5] These latter images were used to illustrate a quite different morality tale – the tale of vengeful virus-carriers deliberately seeking to infect others. For further discussion, see Kitzinger, 1993.

traditional ravaged 'Face of AIDS' that seemed to dominate the imagination of large sections of the public – at least during the period of our field research. How did this happen? Why does one type of image rather than another come to represent an epidemic in the popular imagination? How did people come to adopt such images and what effect do they have on their understandings of HIV/AIDS? It is to these questions of audience understandings that I now turn.

SOCIAL REPRESENTATIONS OF AIDS IN GROUP DISCUSSIONS

The research into audience understandings involved in-depth discussions and a series of group exercises with 52 different groups of people from a range of backgrounds (Table 3.1). The data clearly show that it was the 'yuck' photographs which were remembered and, indeed, had come to 'represent' AIDS in many people's minds, rather than any images of 'normal' or 'attractive' people with 'the AIDS virus'.

When I asked questions such as "What image comes to mind when you hear the word AIDS?" research participants responded with descriptions such as: "...someone white and skeletal"; "disease-ridden, emaciated body sat in bed"; 'the image of a victim, forlorn and dying'; 'someone fading away and dying – because that's what you see – they're more like a vegetable than a (human being)'. (School students, group 1; Prisoners, group 5; Market Researchers).

Most people explicitly identified the media as the source of these images. As one man commented: "I've never seen an AIDS victim by the way. I've never seen one personally. I've read about it all the same. I've seen them looking all ghastly and I've seen how much weight they've lost. I've seen maybe photographs laid out." (Janitor).

In addition to structured discussion the research technique included a group exercise called 'the news game'. This involved giving people a set of photographs taken from the TV coverage of AIDS and asking them to write their own news bulletins. When first presented with the set of photographs research participants frequently looked through them to find the 'Face of AIDS' and made comments about signs of gauntness in several of the faces portrayed: "he's *definitely* got it"/"it looks like it, he's got it"/"*This* is the one, look"/"He's got it, he's not looking too well, he's got a bit more than flu I suspect" (Roundtable group). Although the news game photographs included one picture showing a man sitting up in a hospital-type bed this image was not the stereotypically lurid image of the 'Face of AIDS' which many research participants expected to see. Participants in one group, for example, complained about the absence of any graphic image of someone with AIDS among the set of photographs provided to them and said that I should have included a picture of "someone on their last legs" (School students, group 2). Even so the 'news bulletins' produced by the groups included references to people rapidly "wasting away", leading lives of "bitter despair", ending up "in hospital

Table 3.1
The range of groups participating in the study.

Group	No of groups of this type
I People with some occupational interest or responsibility	
Doctors	1
Nurses/health visitors	1
Social workers	1
Drug workers	1
SACRO* workers	1
Police staff	2
Prison staff	5
Teachers	1
African journalists (Nigeria, Zaire, Zimbabwe, Uganda)	1
Community council workers	1
II People targetted as 'high risk' or who have some special knowledge of the issue	
Male prostitutes	2
Gay men	2
Lesbians	2
Family of a gay man	1
Prisoners	5
Clients of NACRO and SACRO*	4
Clients in drug rehabilitation centre	1
Young people in intermediate treatment	1
III People who, as a group, have no obvious special interest or involvement in the issue	
Retired people	3
Women living on the same Glasgow estate	1
School students	3
Women with children attending playgroup	2
Engineers	2
Round table group	1
American students	1
Janitors	1
Market researchers	1
Cleaners	1
British college students (England, Scotland and Wales)	3
Total number of all groups	52

Note: *These acronyms stand respectively for the National and the Scottish Association for the Care and Resettlement of Offenders

with no hope" and suffering "agonising deaths". One group even chose two photographs (of different men) and used them to reproduce a before-and-after scenario. "This was when he first came into prison", they said holding up a photograph of a sturdy, healthy-looking prisoner, "and he subsequently became very ill" they continued – holding up the photograph of the thin man sitting in bed (Prison staff, group 5).

Such images of people with AIDS formed a central part of many people's earliest memories of the epidemic. When I asked a group of gay men how they had first heard about AIDS one man replied: "It was in 1984 in *The News of the World*. It had like this bloated face of some San Francisco person dying of it – was like *before* and *after* the AIDS effect" (Gay men, group 1) (my emphasis). Members of other groups had first become aware of AIDS during the Rock Hudson case. They too talked of before-and-after images:

> *These pictures of Rock Hudson at the end...they were really horrific (...) he looked really, really terrible (...) and when you remembered how he was in the films and that and saw ....it was horrific (Women with children attending same playgroup).*

Even when recalling more three-dimensional profiles of people with AIDS some of the research participants picked out the before-and-after scenarios as particularly memorable. Describing a recent television documentary about a woman with AIDS two school students emphasised their horror at how she looked:

> *...they followed her every couple of months, how she was dying and all that (...) it showed you in the last one what she'd looked like before - she had totally wasted away (School students, group 2). She was just like a wee stick and she couldn't work or anything, she was all white and Yuuurk (Exaggeratedly shudders) (School students, group 1).*

Such images may be recalled out of all proportion to their actual occurrence in the media. They are 'memorable' in a way that 'softer' images are not because, in the words of one research participant, 'they just looked so disgusting, they looked really horrible'. They capture the imagination of the audience for some of the same reasons that they attract media attention in the first place and are further imprinted in people's memories by the way such images are invoked in day-to-day interactions. Some research participants referred to playing a sort of 'spot the AIDS victim' game: speculating about people they saw in the street or at work who looked sick or bullying class-mates with 'disfigured' faces – accusing them of having AIDS. Indeed, the relish with which some participants in our research sought to reproduce the 'Face of AIDS' through acting it out – contorting their faces, squinting and drooling – suggests that such images can exercise a voyeuristic fascination. The 'Face of AIDS' has become absorbed into, and reiterated through, particular sub-cultures thereby receiving an exposure over and above that actually given to it in the press or on television.

THE COUNTER-PRODUCTIVE NATURE OF THE 'FACE OF AIDS'

But what is the effect of this 'Face of AIDS', as it is presented in the media and created, recalled and reproduced in public consciousness? Many of the research participants themselves thought that displaying such photographs was a good idea because it might terrify people into changing their behaviour. In fact some research participants called for a greater media focus on 'hard-hitting images' of people "decomposing" (School students, group 2). Recommending 'shock tactics' one prisoner said that if he were designing advertisements "I would get a guy with AIDS, right, that's dying and he's looking bad and go 'bang, this could be you'". (Prisoners, group 3). Indeed, the 'Face of AIDS' was evoked in some of the audience groups' news bulletins in ways which clearly articulated the 'health warning' import. A statement produced by one group, for example, read: "The effects of AIDS can waste away your body so much, so watch out you don't end up like him" (School students, group 2) while another group cautioned people to avoid risky activities or else "You could end up like this" (School students, group 3). Several research participants suggested that there was a direct correlation between the extent to which the media dwelt upon physical degradation caused by AIDS and the extent to which people – at least *other* people – would pay attention to health warnings and adopt safer practices. However, their *own* reactions to the 'Face of AIDS' belie such theories.

Firstly, it was precisely because such images were so frightening that some people were tempted to (or actually did) turn away from them – deliberately avoiding reading the article or watching the television item about AIDS. Fear is not necessarily a good strategy for health education. For example, two research participants who considered themselves to be at risk (a male prostitute and a woman who had been raped by several men) told me that they avoided reading or watching anything about HIV/AIDS because they found it too dreadful to think about. Both of them found the 'Face of AIDS' images depressing and disempowering. Such images, combined with a lack of media concern about the treatment available to people with HIV to delay the onset of symptoms, certainly does not encourage people to seek early diagnosis or help. HIV infection is simply equated with a death sentence.

Secondly, such images also appeared to alienate those who did not consider themselves to be at risk. This 'Face of AIDS' is not a 'human' face, it distances the viewer from that individual and renders the person with AIDS almost sub-human in their eyes. The 'faces' which journalists usually try to create for major tragedies are images with which the reader can identify and through which they can understand the individual joys and sorrows which make up part of the momentous event. Such 'faces' present 'the human dimension'. The 'Face of AIDS', however, offers a very different visage and the snap-shot of an objectified individual with a disfigured face can operate in precisely the opposite way. The focus on bits of the body and distorted features frames these people as monsters or aliens, not part of the human race. Because the 'Face of AIDS' resembles the mask created by the special-effects department on the set of some horror movie, it taps into a whole cultural repertoire which represents people who look different as threatening and villainous. The audience's own descriptions of people with AIDS as "vegetables", "a body sat in bed" or "living skeletons" demonstrate how they objectify and dehumanise the victim.

Thirdly, the 'Face of AIDS' is problematic because the monopoly such images have over many people's associations with the word 'AIDS' may obscure other ways of viewing the issue. AIDS is equated with the death of isolated individuals rather than, for example, with the scandal of government inaction or the triumph of gay solidarity in response to the tragedy. The word AIDS conjures up images of death rather than alternative images such as the drama of ACT-UP demonstrations or the memory of candle-lit vigils as whole communities celebrate the lives, and mourn the deaths, of their friends and family. The extreme close-up focus on the 'Face of AIDS' literally and figuratively effaces the social and political context of the epidemic.

Fourthly, and finally, the 'Face of AIDS' may be counter-productive because the emphasis placed on the distinctive 'AIDS-look' can undermine the crucial health education message that people with HIV ('the AIDS virus') do not look any different from anyone else. The contrasting before-and-after images suggest rapid deterioration and beg the question 'before' and 'after' what? Some of the pictures of people glowing with health may, in fact, be pictures taken while they were infected with HIV – but this is rarely pointed out. Instead we are repeatedly presented with images of 'AIDS carriers' who are visibly stigmatised and obviously look 'different'. The power of this image can undermine the message that 'you can't tell by looking who's got HIV'. This last point was most clearly illustrated in some people's 'readings' of one of the health education advertisements – and it is these which are discussed below.

THE HEALTH EDUCATION CAMPAIGN

The 1988/89 advertising campaign conducted by the English-based Health Education Authority focused on informing the public that people with HIV can look and feel perfectly well. This message was identified as crucial in the struggle against the spread of HIV because, without this knowledge, people might think that it was safe to have sex or share needles with anyone who looked healthy. To this end the Health Education Authority produced advertisements such as one showing a healthy young man with labels pointing out his clear skin and normal weight. The slogan read: "Before you sleep with someone, look out for the signs of HIV (the virus that leads to AIDS)". The small print made it clear: "A person can have HIV, the Human Immunodeficiency Virus, for years before any signs appear…". Another advertisement showed a stereotypically attractive woman with the slogan: "If this woman had the virus which leads to AIDS, in a few years she could look like the person over the page." (Figure 3.1a). The next page reproduced an identical portrait with the caption: "Worrying, isn't it?" (Figure 3.1b). Such adverts both drew on and attempted to challenge the mainstream images discussed above. The 'attractive woman' advert, in particular, relies for its effect on the before-and-after images in press and documentaries because, as McGrath (1990, p. 147) points out, those pre-existing images lead us to 'expect to turn the

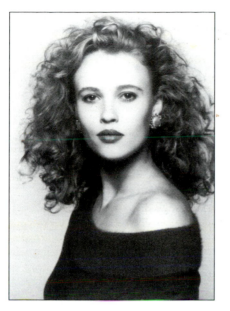

Figure 3.1a   If this woman had the virus which leads to AIDS, in a few years she could look like the person over the page.

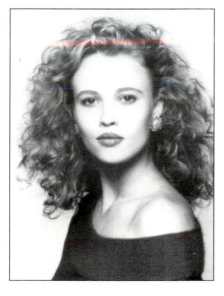

Figure 3.1b   "Worrying, isn't it?"
The virus that leads to AIDS is known as the Human Immuno-deficiency Virus. Or HIV. A person can be infected with HIV for several years before it shows any signs or symptoms. During this time, however, it can be passed on, through sexual intercourse, to more and more people. There are already many thousands of people in this country who are unaware that they have the virus. Obviously the more people you sleep with the more chance you have of becoming infected. But having fewer partners is only part of the answer. Safer sex also means using a condom, or even having sex that avoids penetration. HIV infection may be impossible to recognise, but it is possible to avoid.

page, see a grisly image of a woman who is a shadow of her former self'. The advert relies for its impact on the shock that we are supposed to feel when we see she is just as healthy-looking and attractive as before.

Ironically, but perhaps predictably, this campaign was attacked for promoting the wrong sort of image. *The Daily Mail*, for example, reproduced the 'beautiful woman' advert with the headline: "The Phoney Face of the War on AIDS" (Mail, 7.11.88). The tabloid press which had exploited the 'yuck' potential of the 'Face of AIDS' rejected this image of HIV anti-body positive people and called for "less appealing" and more "realistic" images (The Sun, 13.2.89). Underlying the furore was the assertion that the 'real' face of AIDS was the face of the dissipated, degenerate homosexual, not a normal, healthy, attractive heterosexual (Beharrell, 1993).

In order more fully to explore people's readings of health education advertisements one of the advertisements from this campaign was selected as a basis for discussion with research participants. Rather than select the 'attractive woman' advertisement which had received so much controversial coverage in the press we selected one of the apparently 'blander' images from the campaign. This advertisement simply bore the words 'Two eyes, nose, mouth' against a plain black background, and the main caption underneath read: "How to recognise someone with HIV". The message was that anyone might be infected, you can't tell by looking (Figure 3.2). This advertisement was more abstract than its stablemates. It was not narrowly targeted at either men or women, straight people or gays, and the main message was relevant both to needle-sharing and to sexual activity. It was felt therefore that this was a particularly appropriate advertisement to present to the wide range of groups with whom we were working (e.g including 'general public' groups, gay men, lesbians, ex-drug-users and prostitutes).

The advertisement was presented to the research participants in a step-by-step process. First, the groups were shown the top part of the advertisement, the eyes-nose-mouth motif, and asked to imagine what the caption underneath might be. Then they were shown the main slogan and asked to discuss what they thought of it. Due to lack of time this advertisement was shown only to 27 out of the 52 different groups involved in the research. Even so the results were quite striking.

Only 11 out of the 142 participants presented with the eye-nose-mouth advertisement could recall having seen it. However, most of the groups were able, on the basis of the motif alone, to invent a slogan along the lines of "you can't tell who's got AIDS – anyone could be infected". Most of them knew that the Health Education Authority was trying to convince them not to 'judge by appearances'. However, this did not mean that they abandoned the idea that there were visual cues which would alert them to the likelihood of any partner being infected. In spite of intellectually accepting the message of the eyes-nose-mouth advertisement many research participants still had mental images of the likely appearance of an 'AIDS carrier'. They drew on pre-existing class stereotypes and assumptions about the appearance of people who were gay or injected drugs in order to describe 'safe-looking' versus 'unsafe-looking' patients, punters, clients, or lovers. A male prostitute said he selected between punters, trying to assess which ones were safer than others and compared "the punter with the dirty penis" to "the big business men... You know they've no got AIDS if they are in big jobs like that". A social worker

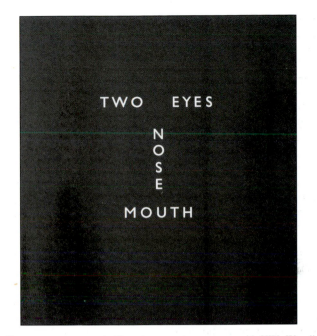

Figure 3.2 Two eyes, nose, mouth. How to recognise someone with HIV. We all know how devastating the effects of AIDS can be. But what are the signs of the Human Immunodeficiency Virus, the virus that leads to AIDS? The fact is, a person can have HIV for years without any signs developing. During this time they may look and feel perfectly healthy. But, through sexual intercourse, they can pass on the virus to more and more people. Already there are many thousands of people in this country who are unaware that they have the virus. Obviously the more people you sleep with the more chance you have of becoming infected. But having fewer partners is only part of the answer. Safer sex also means using a condom, or alternatively, having sex that avoids penetration. HIV is now a fact of life. And while infection may be impossible to recognise, fortunately it is possible to avoid.

compared "someone who is sort of down and out and looks like a drug abuser" with the 'safe' client – "the lady in the twin set and pearls with the poodle"; and a gay man commented that although he 'knew' that anyone might have the virus he had a residual image of the typical person with HIV: "You'd expect them to look scruffy with rips in their jeans, not fashionable rips made deliberately, but rips in old and unwashed clothing" (for further discussion of these data see Kitzinger, 1991).

More interestingly, however we found that a small number of research participants totally misunderstood the advertisement. Instead of taking it to mean that 'you can't tell by looking' some participants in five different groups interpreted this eyes-nose-mouth advertisement to mean that there were definite symptoms of HIV infection. For example, when I showed one group the eyes-nose-mouth motif part of the advertisement (without the slogan) they suggested that the slogan might be telling you to 'use your eyes to watch out for signs of the disease in others'. Once I revealed the real slogan – 'How to recognise someone with HIV' – they thought that the advert meant that people with HIV look very odd: 'Aye, their eyes are all black underneath'/ 'or red'/ 'His face is all skinny' (Male prostitutes, group 1).

The same sort of interpretation was reiterated in the other four groups. Two of the young men in the second group of male prostitutes said that the advertisement showed that "Their eyes are all dazzly" and they "froth at the mouth" (Male prostitutes, group 2). Some members of a club for retired people thought that the advert was intended to convey the fact that people with HIV "are inclined to sniff and have constant colds"/ "they often have sores all round about, and mouth sores"/ "nose running, eyes watering"/"...their hair drops out" (Retired people, group 2). Another group drew on similar sorts of images in their interpretations of the advert:

> Look at their eyes, look at their nose and look at their mouth and if they look queer you don't bother going near them/ If they are foaming at the mouth and blinking.../ and if their nose is all running all the time (...) and they've got scabs round their nose (Young people in Intermediate treatment).

Clearly there was an element of confusion about the difference between HIV and AIDS – a confusion that, for some people, could be compounded rather than challenged by this advertisement. People had such strong pre-existing mental pictures of the 'Face of AIDS' that this 'face' could become superimposed on the abstract and relatively unusual 'face of HIV' as represented in the eyes-nose-mouth advertisement. The vivid image of AIDS – the killer disease – swamps the supposedly neutral and less dramatic representation of 'the Face of HIV'. Instead of representing a normal and healthy face this advertisement comes to display the two eyes, nose and mouth of illness and disease.[6]

DISCUSSION

The 'Face of AIDS', by which I mean the visual representation of acute debilitation, is extremely powerful. The impression it makes on many people is so overwhelming that it may obliterate all other images – subverting and even inverting health education messages.

---

[6] In addition the ironical tone of the advertisement could backfire. In fact, some people who knew that there were no visible symptoms of HIV infection criticised this advertisement for giving out wrong information. Some participants, for example, claimed that the advertisement indicated that you should look out for signs such as "runny nose and constant colds". However, they did not accept this message because of other advertisements they had seen: "I don't know how you would recognise them...'cos there's an advert on the telly. Which one's got AIDS? I mean you can't tell" (Women with children attending same play group, group 2). Other participants attempted to reconcile the perceived message of the eyes-nose-mouth advert with messages they had received from other sources: people with HIV may look ill, they said, but "when they are covered with clothing you don't recognise it" or "it might be slimmer's disease" or "ordinary cancer" (Prisoners, group 5; Retired people, group 2)

The media-defined 'Face-of-AIDS' is sometimes identified as the only 'real' face of AIDS to the extent that a journalist can describe living people with the syndrome as 'television images made flesh' or challenge any alternative, attractive or healthy representation of 'AIDS carriers' as "phoney" (Daily Mail, 7.11.88). The same process occurs in some members of the audience – the 'real' face of AIDS is gaunt and hollow-eyed, any other image is reinterpreted to fit with their preconceptions.

This is true not only of some audience 'readings' of health education advertisments but it is also true of their 'readings' of real life. Indeed, television and newspaper representations are, for many people, the lens through which they view the reality of AIDS. Media images of the visible ravages of disease form the template for their perceptions of the world and of the people in it. They may have friends or acquaintances who are seropositive but they may be unaware that this is so. They do not think that they know anyone with the virus precisely because the person 'looks O.K' and does not disclose his or her anti-body status. On the other hand they may meet people who look very ill and then assume that they have AIDS. In fact when one of the male prostitutes (the only one out of six to do so) protested that he had seen some information saying that people with the virus might *not* look ill another young man countered with the statement: "A guy came up last night, his eyes were all black under there, his face all stinging, his face was all red there, wee scabs, his lips were all scabby ...they *do* look different!" The man's face resembled a photomontage of all those images of AIDS in the press and on television, the prostitute therefore assumed that this punter must have the virus (an assumption which, in turn, reinforced his belief in the media image). The media portrait of the 'Face of AIDS' is self-reinforcing; it can define 'personal experience, and 'real-life encounters' which, in turn, carry more credibility than might be accredited to media images on their own.[7]

The absence of representations of healthy, openly HIV-antibody positive people in the media (and in real life) undermines any attempt to inform people that those with HIV do not look any different from anyone else.[8] Discrimination and other people's ignorance often keeps HIV-antibody positive people in the closet.

---

[7] Personal experience of becoming infected with other sexually transmitted diseases can be an important counter-balance to this. One woman, for example, told me how she had caught herpes from a man who had looked entirely healthy even under close-examination during oral sex (He had a reputation for sleeping around so she had been "on the look out" for any signs of disease). She commented: "I mean that's how I can really understand the advert saying 'You can't tell by looking at someone.' Well, you can't (…) there was nothing there and yet that happened and it makes me more aware that you can't just judge (..) He looked so healthy!"

[8] The problem lies not simply in the power of the 'Face of AIDS' but in the weakness of the 'Face of HIV'. How does one represent the invisible? The health education campaign of 1988/89 in many ways was very successful in doing precisely this. The 'attractive woman advert' in particular was widely remembered – in fact it was the single advertisement most likely to be recalled by our research participants. Perhaps its 'success' on this level was partly due to the surrounding controversy and partly due to the fact that it, like the 'Face of AIDS', tapped into a whole set of pre-existing archetypes (the vamp, the witch, the femme fatale). There is some suggestion in our data that the use of radio to convey the message that "you can't tell by looking" may have been particularly successful because radio is an image-free medium.

Indeed, many of the famous personalities who have become infected have not dared to 'come out' until they can hide the fact no longer – until they, too, conform to the 'Face of AIDS' image.

This situation has changed recently with the new face that has become associated with AIDS – the face of Magic Johnson, a North American sportsman, who has come out as HIV antibody positive with massive accompanying media publicity. This happened after field work had been completed on the media project; however, I was subsequently involved in a study at the Medical Research Council, Medical Sociology Unit at Glasgow researching young women's sexual experiences. During the course of these interviews the women frequently talked about the impact that the Magic Johnson case had had on their perceptions of HIV/AIDS. Here was a sportsman who was respectable, apparently heterosexual and *healthy,* who openly admitted to having the virus. The signs are that he has dramatically changed the face of the epidemic:

> R8: *I always imagine them to be really drawn looking, white in the face, skinny. He's really tall and muscular and all that. You wouldn't expect him to be the person to have AIDS. Freddie Mercury you kind of guessed it because he was gay but for Magic Johnson (…) he's really healthy, full of muscle, you don't imagine him to have AIDS.*

> R3: *Think about Magic Johnson - it's more difficult to imagine someone who's clean and tidy, good-looking, charming to have AIDS than somebody who isn't clean and tidy and charming.*

> JK: *Do you have an image in your head of the look of someone with HIV?*

> R3: *Yes, a bit like the thing Freddie Mercury looked like. Honestly. Skinny, unshaven - gaunt and awful looking and horrid. That is AIDS really. That looks like AIDS (…) awful and ill and uurgh, uurgh (acting dopey).*[9]

CONCLUSION

The power of the 'Face of AIDS' lies, in part, in media news values and production processes and, in part, in the imagination of the audience. But its power for the audience lies not just in the potency of certain media representations; it is also rooted in the social structuring of personal experience and specifically in the discrimination against people with HIV infection and AIDS (and those in 'high-risk groups'). This means that attempts to transform public understandings need to include measures to

---

[9] In fact, Freddie Mercury was seen as 'the type' to 'get AIDS' even before he was known to be infected with HIV. Prior to any public disclosures about Freddie Mercury's antibody status, one research participant was trying to describe the type of person he would expect to have the virus. He said: "I've just got a preconceived idea to be honest, I have got a sort of Freddie Mercury preconceived ideas (…) you know, Queen type gay with a moustache" (Family group).

protect the rights of people with the virus (and those in traditional 'high-risk' groups) in order to enable them to 'come out'. Instead of, or as well as, continually refining ways of denoting particular messages, intervention must challenge the connotations surrounding AIDS – there is no such thing as denotation without connotation. Each health education message needs to be examined in its wider cultural context as it is affected by competing media images, previous health education campaigns, people's personal experiences and the surrounding political or social structures. There is also a need for broader 'health education' approaches that do not rely on advertising alone but adopt creative media and social intervention strategies which work on multiple levels to transform the symbolic face of AIDS, and ultimately to transform the actual profile of the epidemic.

ACKNOWLEDGEMENTS

I would like to acknowledge the financial support of the ESRC (grant ref no. A44250006). Thanks also to my colleagues on the project - Peter Beharrell, David Miller, Kevin Williams - and the grant holders, Mick Bloor, John Eldridge, Sally Macintyre and Greg Philo - for their contributions to this chapter.

REFERENCES

Beharrell, P. (1993), AIDS and the British Press. In *Getting the Message* edited by Eldridge, J. London: Routledge.

Boffin, T. and Gupta, S. (1990), *Ecstatic Antibodies*. London: Rivers Oram Press.

Brandt, A. M. (1987), *No Magic Bullet*. New York and Oxford: Oxford University Press.

Chippendale P. and Horrie C. (1990), *Stick it up your punter: the rise and fall of 'The Sun'* London: Heinemann.

Chippendale P. and Horrie C. (1990), *Stick it up your punter: the rise and fall of 'The Sun'* London: Heinemann.

Crimp, D. (1992), Portraits of People with AIDS. In *Cultural Studies*, edited by L. Grossberg, C. Nelson and P. Treichler. London: Routledge.

Glasgow University Media Group (1985), *War and Peace News*. Milton Keynes: Open University Press.

Hathaway, D. and Kurtz, I. (1991), 'My Name is Denise I'm HIV positive' Denise Hathaway talks to Irma Kurtz. In *Cosmopolitan* January 1991 pp 68–69.

Kitzinger, J. (1991), Judging By Appearances: Audience Understandings of the Look of Someone with HIV. *Journal of Community & Applied Social Psychology*, **1**, 155–163.

Kitzinger, J. (1993), Understanding AIDS: researching audience perceptions of Acquired Immune Deficiency Syndrome. In *Getting the Message* edited by Eldridge, J. London: Routledge.

Miller, D. and Beharrell, P. (1993), AIDS and Access to Television: how journalists use their sources. Paper given at the BSA annual sociology conference 1993.

McGrath, R. (1990), Dangerous Liaisons. In *Ecstatic Antibodies* edited by T. Boffin and S. Gupta, pp 142–155. London: Rivers Oram Press.

Watney, S. (1987), *Policing Desire: Pornography, AIDS and the Media*. London: Comedia.

Watney, S. and Gupta, S. (1990), The rhetoric of AIDS. In *Ecstatic Antibodies: Resisting the AIDS mythology*, edited by T. Boffin and S. Gupta, pp. 1 –7. London: Rivers Oram Press.

Wellings K. (1988), Perceptions of Risk - Media Treatment of AIDS. In *Social Aspects of AIDS* edited by P. Aggleton and H. Homans, pp 83–105. London: Falmer press.

CHAPTER FOUR

Representations of Learning Disability in the Literature of Charity Campaigns

Caroline B EAYRS, Nick ELLIS, Robert S P JONES and Beth MILLER

Department of Psychology University College of North Wales Bangor, Gwynedd LL57 2DG

Many charities acknowledge that they need to 'tug at the heart strings' if they are to obtain the money they need to help people with disabilities. The distinction between what might be considered an acceptable degree of playing on people's sympathy and using negative imagery is obviously a difficult one to determine. Considerable research and debate will be necessary (Scott-Parker, 1989).

This chapter examines the issues highlighted by Scott-Parker (1989) in the King's Fund discussion paper surrounding media images of people with learning disabilities, and, in particular, those used in charity advertising campaigns. We will begin by looking at past and present public perceptions of and attitudes towards disabled people and how these have been reflected in service developments. We will then describe a series of research studies which have investigated a variety of charity poster campaigns in terms of their impact upon subjects' impressions of people with learning disabilities, their donating intentions, and the implications of these impressions for community care policies. Finally we will conclude by discussing the implications of these preliminary findings for the future direction of charity advertising. The wider context of images of disability used in newspapers will also be touched upon.

Historical Antecedents of Contemporary Attitudes

Prior to the latter part of the nineteenth century, people with learning disabilities lived as an integral (although not necessarily particularly valued) part of the community. However, with the advent of the industrial revolution came the growth of the large Victorian asylums which were located, typically, in the rural surroundings of our large conurbations. These provided segregated places of safety and custody for people with mental illness, learning disabilities and so-called 'moral defectives'. Here they were protected from society but also, more importantly, in the face of Eugenic scare mongering, society was protected from them. It was thought necessary to prevent these people from procreating and thus contributing to the collective gene pool.

Variously labelled throughout the centuries as 'idiots', 'morons', 'simpletons', 'imbeciles', 'cretins', and 'subnormals' their position in society has always been one of low status and separation from the mainstream. The fact that these labels, all of which were once neutral terms, sometimes even medical classifications, have become, nowadays, terms of abuse and derision is testament to this. The issue of terminology has become a major focus of attention in recent years and much energy has been devoted to arguing the relative merits of 'mental handicap', 'learning difficulties' and 'learning disabilities'. The impact of labels on public attitudes has been investigated by Eayrs, Ellis and Jones (1993) who found that some do have more negative associations than others. They concluded that the word 'mental' carries particularly strong negative overtones.

In summary, people with learning disabilities have been seen as a non-productive burden on the rest of society, best kept behind locked doors. It is possible to trace vestiges of this historical legacy in the contradictory mix of attitudes and stereotypes held by people today (Jahoda, Chapter 11).

Stereotypes of Learning Disabilities

Wolfensberger (1972) has described a number of 'social role perceptions' or stereotypes, which can be discerned in communal attitudes to people with learning disabilities. They have been seen as "eternal children", "gifts from God", "holy innocents", "objects of pity" or 'burdens of charity'. Whilst seemingly benign, these views set apart and devalue the person with a disability. Children and people who are dependent upon others are not afforded the equivalent rights, responsibilities and respect accorded to people who are independent. Furthermore, Wolfensberger (1972, pp. 15–16) makes the point, along with other Societal Reaction theorists, that "When a person is perceived as deviant, he is cast into a role that carries with it powerful expectancies.......(which) not only take hold of the perceiver, but also the person as well. It is a well established fact that a person's behaviour tends to be profoundly affected by the role expectations that are placed upon him".

Other more sinister social stereotypes which still crop up include the person with learning disabilities being seen as "an object of dread", "a menace", or "a sub-human freak". Even as late as the early 20th century people with learning disabilities were paraded as exhibits in circuses.

Sometimes these stereotypes of people with learning disabilities are quite contradictory, for example, 'a gift from God' and 'punishment for the sins of the parents'. Surveys of public opinion show that the public continues to be confused even today. Despite people's best intentions to be tolerant there are still the remnants of a fear of the 'mentally deranged' and the 'child molester' and it is these stereotypes that can so easily surface and be reinforced by charity advertising images and copy. We will return to this point later.

Changes in Social Services

Within the development of the social services there has been a slow but dramatic change over the last three decades and a major force in the design and development of these services has been the principle of normalisation as developed by Bank-Mikkelson (1969), and Nirje (1969; 1970) among others. The most influential proponent in the UK and the USA has been Wolfensberger (1972; 1975; 1980; 1983; 1985). He has subsequently dropped the term 'normalisation' in favour of 'social role valorisation' in an attempt to prevent its misleading interpretation as 'making people normal'. Social role valorisation is defined as "the use of culturally valued means in order to enable people to live culturally valued lives" (Wolfensberger, 1980 p. 80).

In reality this means people with learning disabilities should become more visible, assuming their rightful place in the community, as neighbours and friends. It means less segregation into 'specialist' units such as schools and hospitals where everyone is similarly labelled. It means an opportunity to participate in everyday mainstream life and to enjoy the same dignity, respect and basic human rights as any other member of society. Wolfensberger emphasises that normalisation does *not* refer to trying to make people normal or denying their unique needs, but rather making available the specialist help and support necessary to enable them to have as normal a lifestyle as possible.

This change in perspective has gradually been reflected in government legislation promoting the closure of large institutions in favour of policies which concentrate on community care. Many statutory services have embraced the principle of normalisation as their guiding philosophy and have frequently adopted high profile mission statements along these lines in their service plans. However, achieving a better quality of life for people with learning disabilities makes a huge demand on resources and, with increasing competition, from other sectors of the health and social services for limited funds, there is no doubt that reliance on charity-based resourcing will remain a significant aspect of care provision.

The Role of Charities in Service Provision

The charities, therefore, are not simply icing on a cake, but rather, fundamental pieces in a complex jigsaw of service provision. They are also big business in which the marketing and promotion of the product is an important issue. "The 18 top spending disability-related charities obtained media coverage worth £4.25 million in the 12 months ending June 1988" (Scott-Parker, 1989 p. 1). In a survey by Susan Scott-Parker in 1989 which questioned a group of charities about the purposes behind their advertising campaigns the main rationale given was to 'promote a brand 'image' of the charity and to pave the way for increasing public donations. Raising awareness, educating the public and influencing attitudes were also cited as aims though these were secondary to fundraising. With 150,000 charities competing for the attention of potential donors there is tremendous pressure on charities to use any means available for promoting their own particular 'product', or in this case, 'disability'. Furthermore in recent years the pressure has been increasing; figures from the Charities Aid Foundation suggest that since 1987 charitable donations from individual donors have been consistently dropping. However an anomaly has been highlighted by Thomas and Wolfensberger (1982). Whereas in business and industry products are promoted in the best possible light, this does not necessarily follow in the human services. Here, there seems to have been an assumption that the most effective ways of getting people to part with their money is to play upon their feelings of guilt and pity. Traditionally then, we see poster images which convey sadness, dependency, impoverishment, and pessimism. Figure 4.1 shows a poster used by Mencap which exemplifies these points. The child has a bleak future. The associations with Christmas and the crucifixion add to the pathos and also echoes other stereotypes such as 'holy innocent', 'eternal

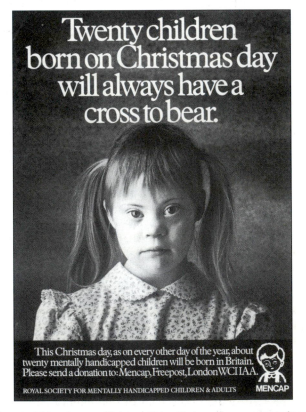

Figure 4.1   Twenty children born on Christmas Day will always have a cross to bear.

child' or 'object of pity'. Not only is there competition between charities for public generosity but also between the media carrying the appeals. It is arguable that the medium likely to have the widest and most significant impact is television, particularly such major events as Live Aid and Comic Relief. With the ability to project dramatic and poignant images directly into people's homes, in the context of a programme of entertainment together with the facility for telephone pledges and credit card donations it forms a powerful recipe for promoting a cause.

It has been argued that the very existence of charity is devaluing for those who are its beneficiaries (McCormack, 1988) and confirmation that people on the receiving end are an 'out group'; in other words outcasts from mainstream society. This is further compounded by the use of negative imagery in poster campaigns, emblems such as logos and other publicity material.

The Role of Images in Advertising

The powerful role played by symbols and imagery in the development of positive and negative value judgements is stressed by Wolfensberger and Thomas (1983). They suggest that "...a transfer phenomenon exists whereby the meanings, sentiments, values, etc. attached to one place, person, idea, or symbol can become attached to another entity which is juxtaposed to it." (p.31) This is the mechanism commonly used in commercial advertising, for example, cigarettes have been associated with cool mountain streams, attractive women, blocks of gold and enviable lifestyles. However, the transfer phenomenon works equally in the formation of negative associations.

Take, for example, some of the stereotypes mentioned above; the disabled person as subhuman, animal, or even vegetable. A poster published some time ago by Barnado well illustrates this point. It features a happy family grouping with an attractive young boy in the foreground. The caption reads "Our son was like a caged animal. Barnado's turned him into a little boy". Although this poster unarguably has high impact value the phrase used juxtaposes the client with images of an animal, the stereotype of that which is sub-human and of incarceration. The whole effect echoes a zoo which, as we know, contains wild, dangerous animals kept separate for people to stare at. Another example is the poster "Jane is wanted by the police" (Figure 4.2). Here we have the juxtaposition of a person with learning disabilities and the police together with a confusing double entendre. The small print explains that "people with mental handicap are presently employed as uniform attendants". Again, we see the possibility of reinforcing a negative stereotype. In this case it is an object of menace with criminal associations.

One consequence of these poster campaigns is the frequent appearance in the media of images of people with disabilities which stress their difference from others and which create a negative representation. This is a crucially important issue in the light of community care policies where the success or failure of community integration is dependent, to a large

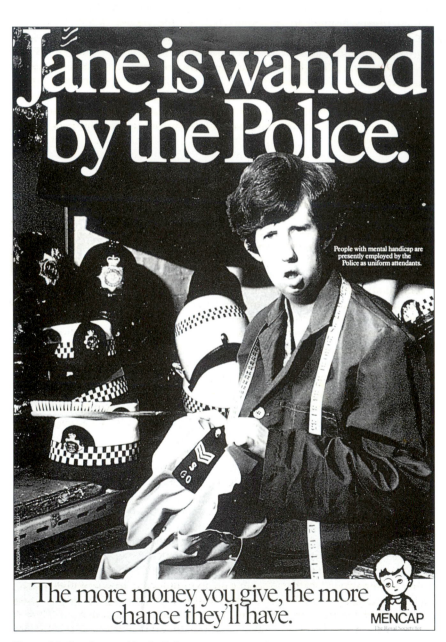

Figure 4.2   Jane is wanted by the Police.

extent, on the acceptance and support of people with learning disabilities by local communities.

The work of Moscovici (Farr, 1987) has stressed the importance of analysing the contribution of images which exist in the mass media. The media both reflect dominant social representations and also may in turn modify them. In the case of charity posters, the viewer stands the chance of having his or her individual stereotypes challenged but also of having them reinforced. If the stereotype of handicap which the onlooker brings to the situation is one of insufficiency, affliction, restriction and alienation (see Stockdale, Chapter 2) many posters will convey a message which conforms with this view. Indeed, there is a widespread belief that if a poster were to be too successful in challenging such a stereotype it would lose its impact as a means of stimulating donations. There is then a fundamental conflict between the aim of raising funds in the most effective manner possible and the use of publicity material which may inadvertently promote and reinforce images of people with disabilities as being different, less valued members of society who need our pity rather than command our respect.

EXPERIMENTAL STUDIES

Whereas the French research on social representations emphasises the importance of sampling both public opinion and the contents of the mass media, these are generally separate exercises. In the series of studies described below, conducted by the present authors and colleagues, the object of study was the interaction between samples of media material and the people viewing them. Enquiry was made along two specific lines. These are (a) the impact the material makes on the viewer's impression of people with learning disability and (b) their donating intentions as a consequence of their impressions. We wanted to discover whether it is possible for charity advertising campaigns to stimulate donations successfully whilst representing people with disabilities as valued human beings.

In the initial study by two of the present authors (Eayrs and Ellis, 1990), 38 subjects were asked to rank ten Mencap posters (see Figure 4.3) along 15 bipolar constructs. For example, for the construct 'guilt' the two poles were labelled "this poster makes me feel guilty" and "this poster does not make me feel guilty". These phrases were written on cards and placed at opposite ends of a line. Subjects then had to sort through the posters, which were mounted on separate cards, and place them between the two poles according to their views. This process was repeated for the 14 other constructs. These covered a wide range of attitudes and included pity, sympathy, comfort, liking and avoidance; it asked which posters portrayed people with learning disabilities as having the same rights, value, and feelings as every one else. Finally, we asked which posters would be most likely to prompt them to give active help, and also monetary donations to Mencap.

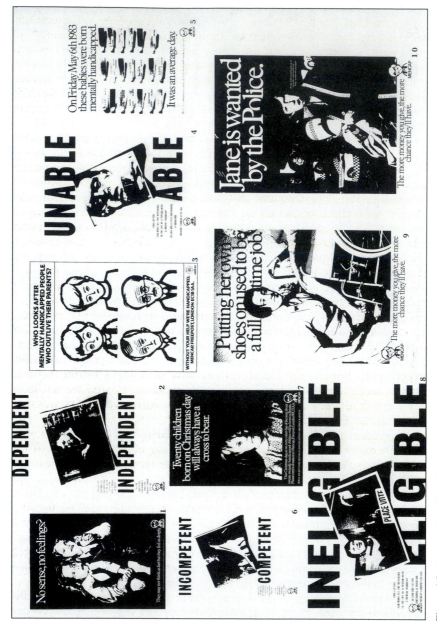

Figure 4.3   A composite of ten Mencap posters.

The results from this study showed that on average subjects said they would be most likely to donate money to Mencap on seeing posters 1 ("No sense, no feelings?") and 7 ("Twenty children born on Christmas Day"). These two also prompted the highest levels of sympathy, guilt and pity and they were also, perhaps significantly, the only posters which featured pictures of children. Conversely they would be *least* likely to give money in response to posters 8 (Ineligible/eligible) and 10 (Jane is wanted by the police). Furthermore, these were the very posters which evoked the lowest levels of sympathy, pity and guilt, but they were both rated highly on rights, value and capability.

Thus the present study confirmed the hypothesis that a conflict does indeed exist for charities in choosing their advertising campaigns; namely that images which are good at raising funds are not good at promoting more positive attitudes and vice versa. We must, however, sound a cautionary note. It is debatable just how far we can generalise from the findings with these particular posters which are, of course, campaigns which have long passed now, to other poster campaigns. Furthermore, there are a number of issues regarding the method used in the research which may cast some doubt over the validity of the findings. *Firstly,* we were asking people to tell us which posters they thought would provoke them to donate. It is a well known phenomenon that people are poor predictors of their own behaviour. *Secondly,* we were putting them in an artificial situation which bore little resemblance to real life. For example, they had a prolonged look at the posters whereas in real life it would probably be more of a fleeting glance. *Thirdly,* the method forced subjects to assign, perhaps falsely, a different position to each poster and thus encouraged them to find differences which perhaps under natural circumstances they would not have been aware of. *Lastly,* the subjects may have had very different previous exposures to the posters in naturalistic settings.

In a second project (Cochrane, unpublished research report), which involved experimentally designed positive and negative posters for a bogus charity, an attempt was made to get one step closer to measuring genuine donating behaviour by asking the subjects to distribute actual money between different charities on the basis of the posters. A much larger sample of subjects participated; a total of 120 (58 male, 62 female) university undergraduates between the ages of 18 and 30 (mean 20.1 years). An independent subjects design was used whereby there were six separate groups of 20 subjects and each group was given one of six posters to look at. This was an attempt to avoid priming subjects to respond to the posters differentialy.

Each poster contained the same picture of a group of adults with learning disabilities standing against a neutral background. Each poster had a different form of words, three negative and three positive in tone. The positive wording of the posters was taken from Schearer (1984). The negative posters highlighted need, dependency, and lack of progress in life, while the positive posters highlighted training for employment, rights, and developmental progress just like other people.

This study found no significant differences between the posters which portrayed people negatively and those which portrayed them positively on either the attitude measures or in the amount donated. A number of possible explanations for the conflicting findings between these two studies are possible. There were procedural differences; a same subjects repeated measures design was used by Eayrs and Ellis and an independent subjects design by Cochrane. The subject groups differed; members of the general public versus undergraduates. Finally, the poster selection was much more uniform in the second study, the differences between them being in the captions. It is arguable that visual images have a far greater impact than the text. An interesting next step would be to vary the images in a series of posters while holding the wording constant. This aspect has yet to be investigated.

However, in a subsequent study by three of the present authors (Miller, Jones and Ellis, 1993), the response differences between various groups of subjects were investigated. Five separate groups were questioned about their responses to two posters. These were university students, 13 – 14 year old school children, parents of children with Down's syndrome, staff employed in caring roles and a group of the general public. The two posters, used in the study, 'Kevin' and 'David', are shown in Figure 4.4. These two were chosen because both displayed small boys with Down's syndrome, both were in black and white, and both were aimed at raising money by stressing that the future opportunities for development of Kevin and David depended on it. The 'Kevin' poster was produced by Mencap and depicts two boys sitting together. One has Down's syndrome (Kevin) and the other, Matthew, does not. Matthew has his arm round Kevin's shoulders and both boys look serious. The caption reads 'When Matthew's 18 he's going to College. When Kevin's 18 he's going nowhere'.

The 'David' poster shows a happy looking boy with Down's syndrome sitting under a tree. The slogan runs: "You say Mongol. We say Down's Syndrome. His mates call him David." This was produced by the Down's Syndrome Association. The 'David' poster, while not beyond criticism from a normalisation perspective, was judged to be the more positive of the two because the subject is smiling and reference to his mates implies normality…he has friends just like any other kid. This contrasts with the 'Kevin' poster which portrays a rather resigned looking lad who is in a position of dependency depicted by the caring attitude of the other child's embrace. The wording confirms this by predicting such a negative outlook for Kevin by contrast with Matthew.

This study employed an independent subjects design. Half of each group of subjects were shown one of the two posters and asked to complete a questionnaire which examined subject's stated propensity to donate, their feelings of comfort on meeting people with Down's syndrome after viewing the poster and their perceptions of the capabilities and characteristics of those portrayed.

Two issues were explored. Firstly, when asked how likely they would be to donate to the charity there was no overall difference between the way subjects responded to the 'Kevin' and 'David' posters. In other words, the

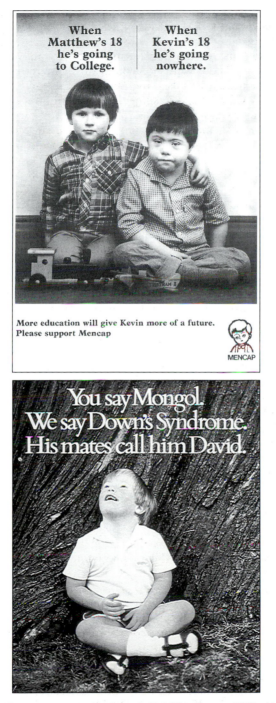

Figure 4.4   The two posters used in the study by Miller, Jones and Ellis, 1993.

more negative poster in this case did not seem to be more successful for the purposes of fund-raising. However, when we compared the different groups of subjects, we found that there was a difference in their stated propensity to donate. As seen in the histogram in Figure 4.5, those most likely to donate were University students, followed by school children and then by parents. Care staff and members of the general public were least likely to say they would donate. However, there was an interesting, though non-significant, trend in these last two groups to donate more to the negative 'Kevin' poster than to the positive 'David' one. This trend reflects the findings of our first two studies. The first used a general population sample and found a difference between positive and negative posters; the second used university students and found no such difference.

Secondly, we examined the effect of the posters on feelings about meeting someone with Down's syndrome. This is important because it gives us some index of the effect of posters on community acceptance of people with learning disabilities. We assume that the more comfortable people say they feel the more they will accept them as neighbours, work mates, etc. For most subjects the 'David' poster engendered greater feelings of comfort on next meeting a person with Down's syndrome. This does flag up the impact of poster campaigns on other areas of interest than fund-raising and shows that they may indeed hinder or facilitate public acceptance of community integration.

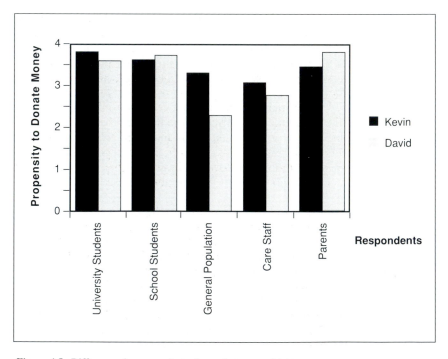

Figure 4.5   Differences in propensity to donate between subject groups.

Finally, although there was no difference between posters as to the capability of people with learning disabilities, there was a significant difference on how their general personal characteristics were perceived. David was seen more positively with adjectives such as 'nice', 'strong', 'attractive' and 'knowledgeable' being applied to this poster more frequently than to Kevin. Again this is important because the image we want to project would include 'nice to know', 'good to have around' even if not particularly capable.

Subjects in all these studies are being asked to respond to a gestalt. There are numerous differences between the posters such as the fact that Kevin was not alone, an invidious comparison is made between Kevin and Matthew, different charities are named, etc. Therefore without further component analysis, as suggested in relation to Cochrane's study, it would be impossible to say which features of the posters accounted for David being viewed more positively. It would certainly be interesting to subject the recommendations suggested in the various guidelines (see below) to systematic empirical investigation.

Many of the posters discussed above are from campaigns which, although contemporaneous with the study, have long since been dropped so it is worthwhile spending some time considering some more recent poster material. In 1991 a series of posters emerged which departed from the previous style in two main ways. They used colour rather than monochrome and omitted images of the disabled people. One of these posters, shown in Figure 4.6, uses the every day image of a football match scene. The overt message is that people with learning disabilities share the same feelings, appreciation of beauty, and excitement. The poster is very positive in the sense that it emphasises sameness rather than difference. As such it makes an interesting contrast with the earlier poster series 'No sense, no feelings?' which uses the format of a rhetorical question to convey the same message. (see Figure 4.3, poster 1). The gloomy appearance of the former image stands in stark contrast to the cheerful and colourful football match and a transition in the thinking behind the poster images is obvious. However some caution is indicated from the findings of Eayrs and Ellis (1990) in that posters which portrayed people with learning disabilities as having the same feelings as other people are not consistently associated with donating and might actually be avoided by respondents.

The decision to omit people with learning disabilities from this series of posters is perhaps best understood as an attempt to overcome the representational problems referred to by Farr (this volume) in relation to people whose disability frequently is not visually obvious. However, although dealing with the representational problem, there is a risk of conveying a more sinister message, namely, that people with learning disabilities are so insignificant, voiceless, or horrible to look at that it is preferable to omit them from public view. Furthermore the results of the Eayrs and Ellis (1990) study showed that the single poster in that study which omitted any human form was ranked lowest on "actively wanting to help" and "spending time with".

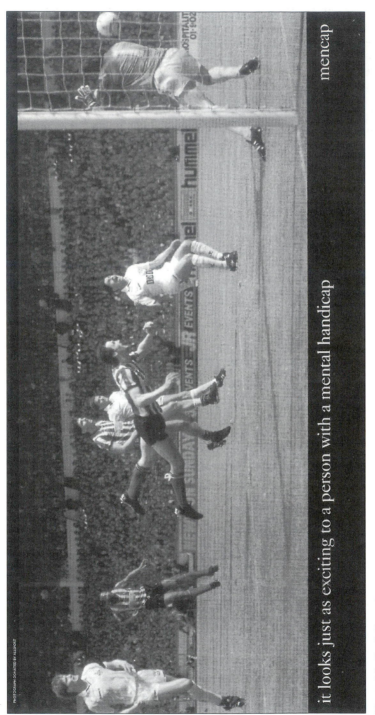

Figure 4.6 Football match.

Mencap underwent a major relaunch in 1992 with the aim to "totally revolutionise and update the Society's image" and subsequent promotional material appears to have addressed many of the negative aspects found in its previous public image. In response to pressure from user representation and other quarters of public opinion the 'Little Stephen' logo has been dropped in favour of five photographic images of real people which will appear on letters, posters and other promotional material. (see Figure 4.7). These represent the wide range of Mencap's beneficiaries in terms of age, race and gender and portray people enjoying life singly and together. They appear to be positive and inviting images which make no direct appeal to pity or guilt in the onlooker and it would be interesting to repeat an empirical investigation into their impact on people's attitude and donating intention.

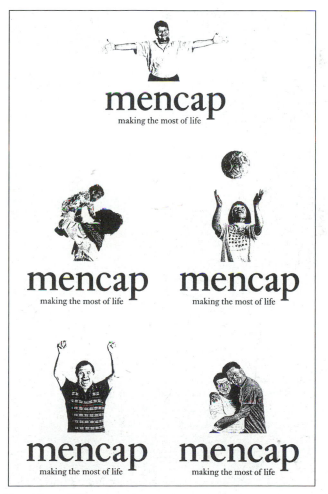

Figure 4.7   Mencap logos 1992.

STEREOTYPES IN THE MEDIA

The issue of media representation of disability is far wider than charity poster campaigns. The creation, reinforcement and modification of public attitudes to people with learning disabilities is continually being affected by the messages people receive in all kinds of contexts including the newspapers, television and radio. McCormack and Fitzpatrick (1987) surveyed different kinds of promotional material distributed by disability agencies in Ireland by applying the United Nations guidelines for the positive portrayal of people with disabilities. These emphasise that people with a disability should be depicted in ordinary settings at work or at leisure, as part of the general population, in a multi-dimensional manner without the use of demeaning stereotypes and language. They found that two-thirds of the material presented people negatively within the terms of the guidelines. Wertheimer (1988a) found that many job advertisements for posts within social and health services and the voluntary sector still used devaluing terminology. She also looked more widely at the portrayal of people with learning disabilities in a wide selection of local and national newspapers and again found distorted coverage and frequent negative stereotyping (Wertheimer, 1988b). In a six week survey period a total of 1,489 press cuttings featuring the words "mental handicap" or "mentally handicapped" were available for analysis. During the survey period two major stories featured heavily and occasioned sensational headlines in some newspapers. These concerned the legal process in reaching a decision on the sterilisation of a young woman with learning disabilities, "Jeanette", and the disclosure that members of the Queen Mother's family had been placed in a mental handicap hospital. These stories completely dominated all other coverage relating to people with learning disabilities and, Wertheimer suggests, distorts the image of people with learning disabilities which is given out to the public. The majority of stories portrayed people with learning disabilities as victims and there was still much confusion between mental illness and mental handicap (learning disabilities).

It would be optimistic to think that by raising awareness and through education that journalists could be persuaded to adopt a more enlightened approach in reporting on issues concerning people with learning disabilities. Guidelines to journalists do exist but it is debatable how well these are known to specialist medical or social services correspondents let alone to their non-specialist colleagues. In a pilot study in North Wales it was decided to attempt to influence 'what the papers say' by monitoring local press coverage and making a direct intervention at the level of the editorial office of a local weekly newspaper. In this study two of the present researchers, Jones and Eayrs, monitored two local papers for a 6 month period and recorded the number of articles published on learning disability, the use of quotations by people with learning disabilities, the percentage of articles which included photographs of people with learning disabilities as active participants and the percentage of articles which were about fund-raising. The aim was to increase the number of articles which showed people with learning disabilities as active, positive members of local communities and decrease the number of articles which reported fund-raising events or other 'special' activities. We therefore hoped to increase the numbers of quotations, and active photographs while reducing the type of coverage which shows one non-disabled adult handing over a large cheque to another non-disabled adult. Following the 6-month monitoring period each newspaper received a different form of intervention. Newspaper A was sent a letter summarising the findings of the monitoring exercise and enclosing a copy of the NUJ guidelines (Campaign for Real People). The editor of newspaper B also received written feedback from the monitoring exercise and a copy of the NUJ guidelines but was also visited personally and interviewed by a person with a learning difficulty who explained the findings of the monitoring exercise and made a number of recommendations for the future coverage of 'learning disabilities' in addition to the NUJ guidelines.

The monitoring exercise continued over the next six months but neither newspaper was informed of this. Following this second monitoring exercise the following results emerged (Tables 4.1 and 4.2). Newspaper B which had received the personal appeal had reduced its overall coverage of learning disability by 27 percent and the coverage of fund-raising events by 8 percent. 'Active' photographs of people with learning disabilities had increased by 41 percent and articles with quotations had increased by 8 percent. Thus the overall coverage of learning disabilities had decreased while the quality of that coverage had significantly increased. Newspaper A, on the other hand, had also decreased its overall coverage of learning disabilities (down by 47 percent) but had improved its coverage of fundraising events by 87 percent while at the same time decreasing the number of active photographs by 33 percent. This study suggests that media presentation can be successfully manipulated and that the best advocates for change are the individual stakeholders involved. It is notable that guidelines on their own were not as effective.

Table 4.1 – Results from Newspaper A

Newspaper A	Percent of articles on disability which refers to learning disability	Percent of articles about learning disability which includes quotes	Percent of photos about learning disability which shows person as passive	Percent of photos about learning disability which shows person as active	Percent of articles about learning disability which is about fund-raising
Pre-Baseline	53%	0%	67%	33%	12%
Post-Baseline	6%	0%	0%	0%	100%
Difference following visit	Down by 47%	No change	Down by 67%	Down by 33%	Up to 88%

Table 4.2 – Results from Newspaper B

Newspaper B	Percent of articles on disability which refers to learning disability	Percent of articles about learning disability which includes quotes	Percent of photos about learning disability which shows person as passive	Percent of photos about learning disability which shows person as active	Percent of articles about learning disability which is about fund-raising
Pre-Baseline	54%	4%	60%	30%	26%
Post-Baseline	26%	9%	71%	71%	18%
Difference following visit	Down by 28%	Up by 5%	Up by 11%	Up by 41%	Down by 8%

CONCLUSIONS

The Need for New Images

There is some, although by no means conclusive, evidence that the twin objectives of raising funds and positively influencing public attitudes may be incompatible. However, we have only looked at a very small proportion of charity advertisements and it is apparent that some posters do a better job than others in achieving both objectives. Nevertheless the challenge remains to come up with new images and slogans which attain high impact, stir the public out of its complacency and challenge existing negative stereotypes whilst presenting people with learning disabilities in ways that preserve their dignity and value as human beings and command our respect. There is some evidence (Stockdale and Farr, 1987) that people will give money to causes which challenge their prejudices and ignorance with a positive message.

Guidelines

There are various guidelines available suggesting appropriate ways of portraying people with learning disabilities in the media (e.g. Schearer, 1984; N.U.J.(undated); Scott-Parker, 1989). For example, presenting people with learning disabilities as active rather than passive; in situations that are ordinary or typical for their community; in situations that are typical for their age; enjoying the company of others who include people without disabilities. Charities and the advertising agencies which take on their brief need to be aware of the available advice. Some of these qualities are illustrated in a poster published by the Down's Syndrome Association (Figure 4.8) which shows three young people doing normal, valued activities and looking as though they are enjoying themselves. The caption is a message of hope, that it would be really worthwhile to donate to such a positive end. This contrasts sharply with "Kevin's going

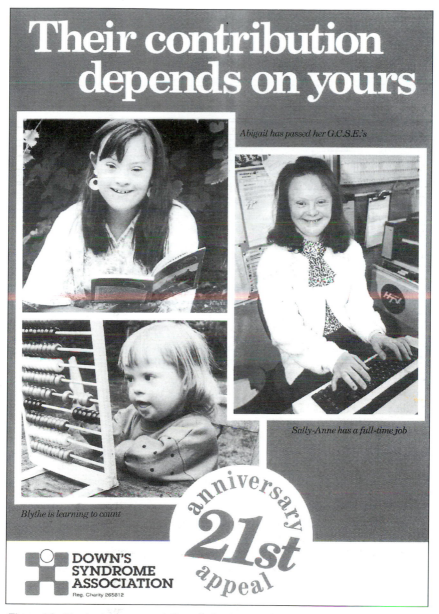

Figure 4.8   21st Anniversary appeal (Down's Syndrome Association).

nowhere". It would be interesting to investigate the impact of these two images on the willingness of potential employers of people with learning disabilities to take on a new employee who needs perhaps rather more help than the average.

As noted above, the issue is wider than charity posters and attempts need to be made to influence media representations within this wider context. Guidelines are only useful if key people are aware of them and act on them.

Targeting

The evidence that posters have a varying impact on different subject groups raises the possibility of greater selective targeting by charities. This could be in terms of the segment of the public at which the poster is aimed or the objectives (educational or fund-raising) of the poster campaign itself. An example of the former is the recent poster campaign from the Terence Higgins Trust, (Chapter 2) aimed at promoting safer sex and aimed specifically at the homosexual population. The Spastics Society's educational campaign- 'Our biggest handicap is other people's attitude'– on the other hand is a good example of a campaign with an educational objective.

Market research into patterns of donating, for example between different age or socio-economic groups, could be linked to more fine grained experimental research into which images or approaches make the greatest impact. At this detailed level of analysis it becomes clear that posters differ in so many respects such as cartoon versus photographic representation, inclusion or omission of images of people with disability, presence or absence of children and so forth that it is difficult to know which are the elements that account for a poster's success. Research is needed with much larger samples of posters before these details can be evaluated. It is also likely that these factors will not be simply additive but rather they will interact in complex ways. Such information may also inform setting the objectives for any particular campaign. For example, it is probable that children are not substantial donors. However they may be important to target for educational campaigns as their attitudes will be affecting people with disabilities for years to come. Children are also the donors of tomorrow. In the study by Miller, Jones and Ellis reported above it was significant that school children were much more positively affected by the posters in terms of their reported feelings of comfort at the prospect of meeting a person with Down's syndrome.

A fascinating study by Radley and Kennedy (1992) compared the views about charitable giving of three different groups based on economic and educational status. These were business, manual and professional people. Their findings revealed that there were significant differences in the preferences for donating to various charities between the groups and the groups talked about very different concerns. The 'less advantaged group' were moved by posters which evoked feelings of pity but also by those which touched a personal chord such as by identifying their own experience with a relative or acquaintance with a disability. On the other hand respondents in the professional group were scathing about images which seemed to deliberately set about evoking pity and made comments which denoted more influence from current ideological change in relation to disability. The professional group were also far more inclined to take a 'universalist' position in which the focus of their concern was seen to be attacking the cause and not the symptoms of social disadvantage. It may be interesting to see how far over the coming decade the ideology of normalisation filters through to influence the social representations of disability in the wider society. The arguments presented to these two different groups in order to create the greatest impact on their donating intentions would arguably be quite different; appealing to personal identification on the one hand and the promotion of equal rights for everyone on the other.

Whilst financial gain is a major preoccupation of the charities, other objectives include both public acceptance of people with disabilities and also the community's active involvement in supporting people with disabilities. Some attempts have been made to include people with disabilities in the general media. A number of commercials on American television include people with disabilities in ordinary television adverts such as those for McDonald's hamburgers and Levis. These examples are targeted primarily at young people and are aimed at promoting the person with disability as an ordinary friend whom it is good to have around. Several years ago in the UK a young girl with Down's Syndrome, Nina, was included in the soap Crossroads, which not only educated the viewer about Down's syndrome in general but also had the effect of raising the profile of children with learning disabilities in the public arena.

Self-advocacy

Lastly we return to Scott-Parker's observations: "Advertising agencies and charities have a unique relationship, part business, part philanthropy and part mutual aid. While their way of working together is superficially modelled on the usual commercial relationship of agency and advertiser, there are important differences in the way things are done, why they are done, and how the participants view each other. The major differences arise because the commercial framework has no room in it for a human product: Fiesta cars do not complain that their job prospects are damaged by Ford advertisements.........The commercial model leaves disabled people out in the cold......They are not clients, not audience, not product, not customer.........Although people with disabilities are the ones who stand to suffer or benefit, the standard commercial model for managing advertising leaves them out in the cold. 'They aren't in the brief'" (Scott-Parker, 1989, p. 1). This quotation highlights a further aspect of charity advertising; that of the enfranchisement of the person with disability him or herself. Involving people with disabilities in the running of the charitable organisation is already becoming a reality and must be regarded as a positive step forward.

In this chapter we have attempted to bring an empirical approach to bear on an ideological issue. However, whilst there are various arguments based on empirical evidence for the avoidance of posters bearing negative images appearing in the public domain, perhaps the most convincing challenge comes from people with learning disabilities themselves. As Gary Bourlet, past president of People First, a pressure group representing people with learning disabilities, writes about one of Mencap's earlier campaigns "We think that these posters discriminate against people with learning disabilities....... We find them in very bad taste. The posters make it look as if Mencap wants to make money out of pity. We don't want people to feel sorry for us." (Letter to Sir Brian Rix, Secretary-General, Mencap 25.6.86).

REFERENCES

Bank-Mikkelson, N. E. (1969), A metropolitan area in Denmark (Copenhagen). In *Changing Patterns in Residential Services for the Mentally Retarded.* edited by R. Kugel and W. Wolfensberger. Washington, DC: Government Printing Office.

Cochrane, V. (1990), *Positive and negative imagery in posters: The effect on attitudes towards people with mental handicap.* Unpublished research report.

Doddington, K. (1992), *Charity advertising: Its effects on attitudes towards people with learning difficulties.* Unpublished research report.

Eayrs, C. B., and Ellis, N. (1990), *Charity advertising: For or against people with a mental handicap? British Journal of Social Psycholgy*, **29**, 349–360.

Eayrs, C. B., and Ellis, N., and Jones, R.S.P. (1993), Which label? An investigation into the effects of terminology on public perceptions of and attitudes towards people with learning difficulties. *Disability, Handicap and Society*, **8**, 2, 111–127.

Farr, R. M. (1987), Social representations: A French tradition of research. *Journal for the Theory of Social Behaviour*, **17**, 4, 343–369.

McCormack, B. (1988), Voluntary fund-raising - a disservice to people with severe learning difficulties? In *Concepts and Controversies in Services for People with Severe Learning Disabilities* edited by R. McConkey and P. McGinley, pp. 83–103. Galway: Bros. of Charity and St Michael's House Research Trust.

McCormack, B. and Fitzpatrick, A. (1987), *The projection of client needs by service agencies: A survey of disability agencies in Ireland. In Health For All: Meeting the Challenge.* Proceedings of the 12th World Conference on Health Education. Dublin: Health Education Bureau. Vol.2, 921–924.

Miller, B. Y. Jones, R. S. P. and Ellis, N. (1993), Group differences in response to charity images of children with Down's syndrome. *Down's Syndrome: Research and Practice*, **1**, (3), 118–122.

National Union of Journalists (undated) *Campaign for Real People.* Pamphlet available from: Equality Council, the NUJ, 314, Grays Inn Road, London WC1X 8DP.

Nirje, B. (1969), The normalisation principle and its human management implications. In *Changing Patterns in Residential Services for the Mentally Retarded.* edited by R. Kugel and W. Wolfensberger. Washington, DC: Government Printing Office.

Nirje, B. (1970), The normalisation principle - implications and comments. *Journal of Mental Subnormality*, **16**, 62–70.

Radley, A. and Kennedy, M. (1992), Reflections upon charitable giving: A comparison of individuals from business, 'manual' and professional backgrounds. *Journal of Community & Applied Social Psychology*, **2**, 113–129.

Schearer, A. (1984), *Think Positive! Advice on presenting people with mental handicap*. Brussels: International League of Societies for Persons with Mental Handicap.

Scott-Parker, S. (1989), *They Aren't in the Brief*. London: King's Fund Centre.

Stockdale, J. E. and Farr, R. M. Social representation of handicap in poster campaigns. Paper presented at the London Conference of the British Psychological Society, December, 1987.

Thomas, S. and Wolfensberger, W. (1982), The importance of social imagery in interpreting societally devalued people to the public. *Rehabilitation Literature*, **43**, 11–12, 356–358.

Wertheimer, A. (1988a), *Images by Appointment: A review of advertising for staff in services for people with learning difficulties*. London: Campaign for Mentally Handicapped.

Wertheimer, A. (1988b), *According to the Papers: Press reporting on people with learning difficulties*. London: Campaign for Mentally Handicapped.

Wolfensberger, W. (1972), *The Principle of Normalization in Human Services*. Toronto: National Institute on Mental Retardation.

Wolfensberger, W. (1975), *The Origin and Nature of Our Institutional Models*. New York: Human Policy Press.

Wolfensberger, W. (1980), The definition of normalisation: Update, problems, disagreements and misunderstandings. In *Normalisation, Social Integration and Community Services* edited by R. J. Flynn and K. E. Nitsch. Baltimore: University Park Press.

Wolfensberger, W. (1983), Social role valorization: A proposed new term for the principle of normalisation. *Mental Retardation*, **21**, 234–239

Wolfensberger, W. (1985), Social role valorization: A new insight and a new term for normalisation. *Australian Association for the Mentally Retarded Journal*, **9**, 4–11

Wolfensberger, W and Thomas, S (1983), *PASSING: Program Analysis of Service Systems' Implementation of Normalization Goals: A method of evaluating the quality of human services according to the principle of normalization. Normalisation Criteria and Ratings Manual* (2nd Edition) Canadian National Institute on Mental Retardation.

Part II — Professional and Lay Representation of Health, Illness and Handicap

FIVE   Professional and Lay Representations of Health, Illness
            and Handicap: A Theoretical Overview   93
            Robert M. Farr and Ivana Marková

SIX   The Self and the Other: Perception of the Risk of
            HIV/AIDS in Scottish Prisons   111
            Ivana Marková, Kevin J. McKee, Kevin G. Power and
            Eleanor Moodie

SEVEN   Clinical Diagnosis and the Joint Construction of a
            Medical Voice   131
            Karin Aronsson, Ullabeth Sätterland Larsson and Roger Säljö

EIGHT   The Mentally Ill Person and the Others: Social
            Representations and Interactive Strategies   145
            Bruna Zani

NINE   Lay Explanations of the Causes of Diabetes in India and
            the UK   163
            Mary Sissons Joshi

CHAPTER FIVE

Professional and Lay Representations of Health, Illness and Handicap: A Theoretical Overview

Robert M FARR[1] and Ivana MARKOVÁ[2]

[1]*Department of Social Psychology, The London School of Economics and Political Science, Houghton Street, London, WC2A 2AE.* [2]*Department of Psychology, University of Stirling, Stirling, FK9 4LA*

THE FORM AND NATURE OF REPRESENTATIONS

The representations of health, illness and handicap which we explored in Part I were to be found, mainly, in the mass media of communication. They are publicly available for analysis and comment. The images, soundtracks, texts, etc. are there to be viewed, listened to and read. They comprise part of our material culture and, as such, are available as objects of critical comment in much the same way as advertisements can be read as the folklore of an industrial society (McLuhan, 1951). The views and opinions of cultural critics on how health, illness and handicap are represented in the media are just as apposite for our purposes as those of psychologists or of other social scientists.

The representations of health, illness and handicap which are the objects of interest to us in Part II are located elsewhere. They are embedded in the minds of individuals or expressed in custom and ritual; as, for example, in various forms of institutional care. They are manifest in a spoken word or a deed rather than in print or on film. They are expressed inter-personally rather than in the form of a cultural product. They are much more difficult to isolate and to examine than the representations studied in Part I. In large measure this is because the actors themselves are unaware of the messages they convey. Much of what they communicate is inadvertent. Representations may be expressed in a highly ephemeral or even casual manner, as in various forms of talk. Unless these representations are captured and recorded at the time they just disappear, quite literally, into thin air. Alternatively they may be so mundane and obvious as to be virtually invisible (Ichheiser, 1949). This occurs, for example, in the routine care of the elderly, the sick and the handicapped. The obvious is no longer noticed, except, perhaps, by outsiders. To locate and to isolate these representations requires all of the skills and some of the guile of the social scientist.

The term 'representation' is used here very broadly. It highlights the fact that it is not the actual causes, objects or events which exist independently of human beings that are of interest to us here. We are concerned, rather, with how these causes, objects and events are perceived and interpreted by individuals and groups of individuals, and with how these perceptions and interpretations are reflected in their thinking, imagining, talking, accounting and acting. We are particularly interested in how people perceive the causes of illness and of handicap and how they assess the risks involved both for themselves and for others. The term 'representation' is most commonly associated, by many social psychologists, with Moscovici's theory of social representations. However, this term is also meaningful in other theoretical contexts, e.g. in anthropology (Sperber, 1985); in attribution theory (King, 1983) and in social constructivist approaches to health and illness (Stainton-Rogers, 1991). We prefer the term 'representations' to such other terms as 'accounts' (Stainton-Rogers, 1991) or 'schemata' because representations, whether conscious or unconscious, are a necessary precondition of verbal accounts, of particular ways of thinking about events and people, of certain fears, motives and actions.

The historical dimension is important in regard to both language and institutions. Common sense is characterised by the co-existence of representations many of which are incompatible with each other. Old representations co-exist alongside new ones. This is a state of affairs that lay people tolerate better than scientists. In the field of health care and of law and order new priorities must be realised within a context that still reflects how the problem was previously represented. Former representations of deviants, of handicap and of illness are enshrined in the bricks and mortar and layouts of our prisons, institutes and hospitals. These structures cannot be dismantled overnight to make way for the embodiment of new representations of deviance, handicap and illness. Many representations in our everyday vocabularies are quite archaic. A cloakroom, for example, is a place where cloaks are left even though few of us, today, wear cloaks. We continue to talk of sunrise and sunset to refer to dawn and dusk, respectively, even though we know it is the earth that spins and rotates around the sun and not vice-versa. It is not only at the level of individual words that we retain outmoded representations and express contradictory viewpoints. Language as a whole reflects the collective experience of the community whose language it is. It continues to evolve as native speakers of that language utter new thoughts and express themselves in ways that differ from their forebears.

Representations are also reflected in what people do not say (because they take it for granted) and in what is implied by what they do. For example, the villagers studied by Jodelet (1991) did not include the clothes of their lodgers with family clothes in the same washtub or spin dryer because of primitive beliefs about the contagious nature of mental illness.

The villagers were unable to articulate the theories which underlay their daily routines until they were questioned by Jodelet who had first observed these practices before seeking to explain them. The research technique best suited to identifying and isolating these forms of representation is participant observation. This is the technique used by Jodelet and also by Goffman in his studies of institutional life.

SCIENTIFIC AND LAY REPRESENTATIONS

In this overview we are concerned not so much with the construction of scientific knowledge *per se* (as, for example, in scientific research) as with its application to particular problems in the fields of health, illness and handicap. We are concerned with the interface between those who are experts and those who are not. The experts with whom we are principally concerned here are health care professionals rather than medical scientists through the term, which we borrow from Schutz (1966), applies to both groups. Schutz distinguishes between the 'expert', the "well-informed citizen" and the 'man in the street' as ideal types, each having different kinds of knowledge. Knowledge, within the context of the sociology of knowledge, is "whatever passes for 'knowledge' in a society, regardless of the ultimate validity or invalidity (by whatever criteria) of such 'knowledge'" (Berger and Luckmann, 1966, p.15). The health care professional, by virtue of his or her professional training, and the research scientist are both 'experts' in terms of Schutz's classification. There are important differences amongst experts, however, in this uses of knowledge. Wolpert (1992), whose work we discuss below, warns of the dangers of confusing science and technology. The latter is more concerned with the application of knowledge rather than with its discovery. Whilst we do not necessarily accept Wolpert's distinction between these two rather broad fields we would argue that the physician is closer to the technologist than to the scientist. The interface with which we are concerned is not that between the medical scientist and the man or woman in the street – or even the 'well-informed citizen'. We are concerned with the interface between the health care professional and the man or woman who has stepped in from the street to such a medical consultation. We are concerned with the application of medical knowledge and technology to particular cases. The health care professional acts as a broker between the world of medical science and lay men and women who are anxious to know if this knowledge applies to them.

Although we are here concerned primarily with professional and lay representations something should first be said about the differences between scientific and lay representations. Scientific explanations and knowledge are concerned with the study of objects and events which exist quite independently of human individuals. The virologist, for example, seeking to establish the nature of the HIV believes that a virus exists quite independently of his or her current representation of it. Scientific knowledge is supposed to be impartial and unaffected by either societal values or the cognitive biases of individual scientists. It is based on intellectual rigour and empirical evidence. This does not mean, however, that when a scientific discovery is made there is a smooth transition from the unknown to the known. As Kuhn (1962) maintained, scientific explanations themselves are liable to biases that are related to particular philosophical positions and world-views that determine what is foregrounded in the perception of reality and what remains as background. Scientific knowledge is concerned with the 'reified universe' (Moscovici, 1984). Moscovici believes there is little or no relation between common sense and science. They comprise two quite discrete universes of discourse and follow two quite different kinds of logic. While the logic of science is grounded in established evidence and proceeds from premise to conclusion by demolishing, en route, prejudices, opinions and unjustified beliefs, the logic of common sense relies on convention and consensus 'the verdict has priority over the trial' (Moscovici, 1984).

Wolpert (1992), in *The Unnatural Nature of Science*, also distinguishes sharply between science and common sense. For Moscovici social representations circulate within the consensual universes where lay people discuss scientific, medical and other matters. There may be little or no relation between a scientific theory and how that theory is represented in such lay discourse. In Part I, for example, we had occasion to note there was little or no relation between the representation of HIV as some sort of gay plague and basic research on the virus (Farr, 1993). The distinction between social representations of AIDS and research on the virus is akin to the distinction between appearances and reality. Lay men and women are more accepting of appearances than are scientists and may also prefer to deal with social representations of reality rather than with reality itself. Scientists, on the other hand, are more at home when wrestling with reality and when dealing with entities such as viruses and genes. Scientists and laity alike, however, accept that while they may inhabit quite different worlds, it is desirable to establish some links between the two, however tenuous those links may be (Marková, 1992). Lay people, as well as scientists, like to understand the world in which they live. Lay people are, as Moscovici and Hewstone (1983) noted, amateur scientists.

There is an important difference between natural scientists, like Wolpert, and social scientists, like Moscovici, when it comes to the study of lay representations of science. Natural scientists wish to correct these erroneous lay representations and thus advance the public's understanding of science. Social scientists, however, believe that lay representations are worthy of study in their own right.

PROFESSIONAL AND LAY REPRESENTATIONS

In medical circles the contact is rarely direct between lay people (i.e. patients), on the one hand, and research scientists, on the other. The world of the research scientist is a highly decontextualised one. It is far removed from the life-world of ordinary men and women. The relationship between the two is usually mediated by a physician or a consultant or some other kind of health care professional who is clinically responsible for the patient.

In Part II we explore the representations of health, illness and handicap both of health care professionals and of lay people. These two communities of people differ from each other not only in their representations of the world but also in their manner of thinking, their methods of argumentation and even in their vocabularies. The physician is closer to the world of science than are his or her lay clients.

Professional representations of illness are quite wide-ranging and lie somewhere along a continuum between purely scientific explanations at one end and lay explanations at the other. At the scientific end of the continuum are medical explanations of illness based upon scientific discoveries. They are equivalent, more or less, to scientific explanations. At the other end of the continuum are the representations of health, illness and handicap held by various paramedical professionals and by health educators. These representations usually involve fewer scientific details. The explanations of health-related issues given by some professionals may be very similar to those of an educated lay-person, e.g. the explanations of HIV/AIDS given by prison officers in the study by Marková et al. in this volume.

Such paramedical professionals, in order to deal with health-related issues, may be given a short course during their training designed to improve their understanding of scientific findings. Such training, for example, is given to prison officers in order to equip them to take appropriate action to protect themselves and those in their charge from the risks of infection by HIV. In addition, professional and lay representations may interact with and affect each other. The closer health care professionals are to intelligent lay people the greater the degree of overlap between their respective representations. In other respects scientific knowledge about diseases and public knowledge about vulnerability to such diseases are not easily reconciled since they are two quite distinct forms of knowledge and have quite different aims (Marková, 1992).

The clinician or health care professional is usually closer to the patient's life-world than is the research scientist. In the course of a medical consultation, for example, the results of scientific laboratory tests need to be interpreted in terms of the life-circumstances of the individual patient and their significance needs to be explained in lay terms. It is the clinician who acts as the interpreter. Aronsson, Sätterland Larsson and Säljö, in their contribution, distinguish between the voice of medicine and the voice of the life-world. The former, the voice of science, is highly decontextualised. The latter is highly contextualised. Sometimes, however, the patient may actively adopt the professional voice. Due to her own extensive medical history, Lisa, the patient described by Aronsson et al., has become proficient at speaking in the medical voice. She insists on conducting the consultation in the medical voice and the physician, in this particular interview, remains insensitive to the life-world of his patient.

Joshi, in her contribution, identifies some difficulties in how her English and her Indian informants conceive of heredity in relation to diabetes. She deals with the treatment of diabetes in both an English and an Indian context. Since diabetes is a chronic condition it exemplifies many of the characteristics of a handicap. There are no differences between the medical staffs of the hospitals in the two countries in regard to their scientific understanding of this condition. The differences occur in the clinical contexts in which the physicians advise their patients and in the cultural contexts in which those same patients monitor and treat their own diabetes. Clinicians in both countries are sensitive to the cultural context. Indeed the notion of a handicap only makes sense in the context of a cultural setting. The medical condition may be the same in both countries (i.e. in the decontextualised world of medical science) but the nature of the handicap will differ as between the two cultures. Culture is important in the context of diabetes because this is a medical condition in which patients treat themselves often over the period of a lifetime.

So far we have described representations as being lay in contradistinction to representations which are either scientific or professional. Their nature can be understood in terms of what they are not as well as in terms of what they are. We shall now consider representations that lay people have of each other. One can only understand other in relation to self and self in relation to other. From the perspective of someone who is ill and who has a handicap the representations that others have of self are scarcely neutral. Here, in Part II, we are concerned to identify the co-existence in society, of different representations of illness and of handicap. The implications of these differing representations for the selves of those of whom they are a representation is a major theme in the overview to Part III.

Such representations depend upon individuals' own idiosyncrasies as well as on the images that circulate in society (cf. for example, Skelton and Croyle, 1991; Bishop and Converse, 1986; Bolton and Singer, 1992). These idiosyncrasies have been widely studied in recent years and they include variables such as individuals' membership of particular stigmatised groups (e.g. Power et al., 1992; Marková and Power, 1992); whether or not they are concerned about a particular illness (Ditto, Jemmott III and Darley, 1988); whether they had experienced the disease in question (e.g. Jemmot III, Croyle and Ditto, 1988); how they categorise themselves in relation to others (Stockdale et al., 1989; Marková et al., this section) and so on.

Zani, in her contribution to Part II, traces the representation of the mentally ill as 'other' or different. While Jodelet (1991) studied the consequences of this powerful representation in a rural setting in France, Zani demonstrates its operation in an urban setting in Italy. It is a representation that sets the mentally ill apart from other categories of persons who are ill. When the representations of an illness or a handicap are unfavourable, as they are in the case of mental illness and of mental handicap, they are the source of the sense of stigma experienced by those suffering from the illness or displaying the handicap. Goffman (1963) considered stigma in relation to various forms of physical handicap. Lay representations of various forms of illness and of handicap can themselves constitute a further source of handicap. 'Our biggest handicap is other people's attitude' was one of the themes of a poster campaign, considered in Part I, on behalf of The Spastics Society. Zani discusses the importance of how the other is represented in relation to such everyday interactions as those between the mentally ill and a range of lay people such as shopkeepers and service personnel in the local community where the mentally ill live. Health care professionals and those for whom they care should jointly be concerned to change representations that are unfavourable. Many of these social representations of illness and of handicap are also responsible for some of the unintented consequences of social reforms which we discuss later in this overview.

PROFESSIONAL AND LAY EPISTEMOLOGIES OF HEALTH, ILLNESS AND HANDICAP

We pointed out above that professional and lay representations of health and illness are cultural phenomena which, to some extent, determine the kinds of explanations of illness and handicap within a particular culture at a particular point in time. In some cultural – historical periods professional and lay explanations may be in greater accord than in others. For example, until the eighteenth century medical knowledge was relatively limited. Intelligent lay people quite easily grasped descriptions of symptoms and the various diagnostic criteria that were of different illnesses (Ackerknecht, 1982; Schober and Lacroix, 1991). Not only the vocabulary of illnesses but also their causes and explanations were common to laypersons and medical professionals alike. However, the situation radically changed in the nineteenth and twentieth centuries when medical science and technology led to significant advances in the knowledge of illnesses and their treatment. While lay explanations of illnesses have remained relatively unchanged, research and medical science have made dramatic changes with respect to its explanatory frameworks (Ackerknecht, 1982). The gap between professional and lay explanations has widened.

The aim of science is to provide knowledge. When there has been something to explain scientists, ever since Aristotle, have referred to causes and their effects. Both causes and effects have been understood as invariants and their observed regularities have contributed to the certainty of scientific knowledge. Most explanations of causality have been in terms of discrete events which are linked in causal chains (Hanson, 1958). For example, if we ignore cases of genetic mutation, the scientific explanation for the cause of haemophilia (a congenital disorder of blood clotting) is in terms of the transmission of a defective gene to the next generation in a sex-linked recessive fashion. This means that, in accordance with the law of Mendelian inheritance, all daughters of a man with haemophilia will become carriers, i.e. they will inherit a defective gene from their fathers. Each son and each daughter of a woman who is a carrier will have a fifty-fifty chance of inheriting the defective gene. The haemophilia will be manifested in affected sons. Affected daughters will usually show no symptoms of the disease but they will transmit the gene to the next generation in the same fashion as their mothers. Similarly, adult polycystic disease of the kidney is *caused* by a defective gene, transmitted in an autosomal dominant fashion to the offspring of those who carry the gene. This means that each offspring of an affected parent has a fifty-fifty chance of inheriting the defective gene. In the case of both haemophilia and adult polycystic disease of the kidney, the cause-effect relationship is unambiguously defined: the manifestation of the disease is always *the effect* of the presence of a defective gene.

In contrast to causes that have been identified scientifically, lay (and, occasionally, professional) representations of causes are socially and culturally constructed. These are not invariant across time and culture. Thus, in recent decades, social scientists have identified a limited number of causal factors that lay persons use in their causal explanations. For example, in Herzlich's original study environmental factors seemed to play a causal role in regard to illness (Herzlich, 1973). It was essentially a germ theory of illness that emerged from many of the protocols in the Herzlich study. These are 'causes' as they appear in the context of representations, i.e. they are perceived rather than actual causes (Farr, 1977). Other causal elements frequently used in lay explanations of illnesses are, for example, stress, dieting, food and drink, aging, etc. (e.g. Williams, 1983; Lau and Hartmann, 1983; Joshi (Chapter 9); Schober and Lacroix, 1991). Even if the public and those at risk of a particular disease understand its true cause, they may not think, for one reason or another, that it applies to themselves as individuals. For example, individuals at risk of a specific genetic disorder may understand the law of Mendelian inheritance and its application to genetic diseases in general, yet they may fail to apply it to themselves. Instead, they may construct a model of heredity that has little or nothing to do with scientific knowledge and they may even provide good reasons for thinking as they do.

In many kinds of illness and of disability causality cannot be stated as clearly and unambiguously as it can in those cases that follow the law of Mendelian inheritance. In some families a disposition to angina, or mental illness or diabetes (Chapter 9) may run for several generations. No exact cause, e.g. a defective gene, has been identified in these cases. The same behaviour on the part of two different individuals may or may not lead to a particular disease. Smoking, for example, does not always lead to lung cancer. In these cases the relationship between cause and effect is contingent, rather than necessary. Other factors, such as the individual's high level of immunity, could override the effect of what is considered to be a major contributor to the occurrence of lung cancer, i.e. smoking. This is the sort of situation that poses particular problems for health education. Since the relationship between cause and effect is contingent rather than necessary, the individual as an agent adopts strategies of coping that are based on the belief that he or she is less vulnerable than others and has greater power to affect his or her own destiny. Although many patients in Joshi's sample (Chapter 9) knew that diabetes was genetically co-determined in their families they sought to explain their illness in other ways. Her data show that while medical science offers the familial diabetic patient a probabilistic explanation of their disease, the patients, not being satisfied with probabilities, actively sought a different kind of explanation. Although they understood the idea of heredity, it was difficult for them to grasp its probabilistic nature.

The explanation of causality in terms of causal powers (Foster, 1935; Harré and Madden, 1975), of liabilities (Sayer, 1984) and of a dialectic interaction between an active and changing organism and its environment, 'with causes and consequences closely interwoven' (Hinde, 1990, p.162), have all been proposed as alternatives to the traditional positivist view of causality that has prevailed for decades in the natural sciences. For the anti-positivist, the nature of an object, whether a physical object or a living organism, and its causal powers are *internally* related (Sayer, 1984; Marková, 1990a). This means that an object, for example dynamite, has a disposition, e.g. an unstable chemical structure, to explode if particular conditions obtain; that people can change their health behaviour strategies because of their ability to monitor their own life-styles; and so on. For an object to have a causal power assumes that it only has a *potentiality* for causing something rather than that this potentiality will always be realised. Thus a person who smokes may never develop lung cancer; a promiscuous person may not catch HIV; and so on.

People seek causes when there is something to explain. They do not ask about causes when events run smoothly and activities follow their expected course. They take health for granted but try to explain the causes of illness or disability (Herzlich, 1973). Explanations of phenomena in terms of causal powers and of liabilities are better suited to human agents who try to control and to predict the world in which they live than are the traditional cause-effect accounts of causality. The perception of causes is part and parcel of attribution theory which has been a vigorous topic of research in social psychology for the past three decades. In his seminal volume on *The Psychology of Interpersonal Relations*, Heider (1958) took stock of what he called 'naive psychology'. He argued that the relation between common sense and science is different in psychology to what it is in other sciences:

> *'Intuitive' knowledge may be remarkably penetrating and can go a long way toward the understanding of human behaviour, whereas in the physical sciences such common-sense knowledge is relatively primitive*

> (Heider, 1958, p.2)

A fundamental aspect of this common sense knowledge is that the individual is an agent who tries to control and to predict his or her own world. For Heider, the perception of causes by a naive person is a matter of immediate apprehension rather than a matter of cogitation. However, our common sense itself is socially or collectively constructed (Moscovici, 1984), and, therefore, what appears to be immediate, such as an intuition or common sense, is often the result of socio-cultural processes in which the individual participates.

In the light of this discussion, while a scientist searches for causal explanations by means of scientific research, lay people perceive, rather than seek, causes. In justifying their own actions or questioning those of others, they often have a stock of ready answers and standard queries. People can also act deliberately so as to thwart the predictions of others as to how they will act. Prophesies can also easily become self-fulfilling. Lay people are often satisfied with apparent causes of health and illness.

RISK AND THE PERCEPTION OF RISK IN RELATION TO ILLNESS AND HANDICAP:PROFESSIONAL AND LAY EPISTEMOLOGIES

Searching for the causes of events means inquiring into *why* something has taken the course it has. It thus implies finding out something about the *past*. Indeed, as Russell (quoted by Hanson, 1958 p.50) argued, 'the chain of causation can be traced by the inquiring mind from any given point backward to the creation of the world'. In contrast to events for which causes are sought in the past, risk is associated with the *future*, with events that could happen. The representation of the future is different from the representation of the past. This is true conceptually and as well as linguistically. In the traditional theory of causality, causes are conceived of as the necessary origins of events, and so there is a degree of certainty about them; risk, by way of contrast, is only a probable occurrence. It was already maintained by the seventeenth century mathematician Bernoulli that while causes relate to things in the world, risks relate to things in the human mind (Gigerenzer et al., 1989).

In the history of science the concepts of cause and of risk have been inter-related. Two of the classic proponents of the theories of mathematical probabilities, such as Bernoulli (1738/1954) and Laplace (1774), maintained that probability is a measure of human ignorance. They believed that with an increase in knowledge, the underlying hidden causes of events will be discovered. Therefore, in the absence of such knowledge underlying causes must always be assumed (Gigerenzer et al., 1989). Mathematical models concerning the statistical frequencies of events in gambling and insurance were first developed in the sixteenth and seventeenth centuries. Originally, in the work of Pascal (1963) and of Huygens (1657/1920) the notion of mathematical probability was based on the idea of fair play, i.e. equal expectancy of profit by the involved parties (cf. Gigerenzer et al., 1989, p.21). The client and the assurance company were supposed to have an equal expectation of gain, i.e. expectation "worked to one's disadvantage' (Huygens, 1657/1920, p.60). Douglas (1992) maintains that in the seventeenth century when, in English, the term 'risk' was probably coined, it meant no more than *chance*. 'Risk' was used to express the probability of the occurrence of an event and it involved a calculation of both gains and losses. Thus it was *neutral* with respect to outcomes. Nowadays, however, risk only refers to *negative* outcomes and means danger from future hazards. The term 'risk' has now acquired a similar meaning to that of 'danger'. However, Douglas (1992, p. 4) points out that, in contrast to 'risk', "danger does not have the aura of science or provide the pretension of a possible precise calculation".

Today, theories of risk still imply a close relationship between cause and risk. In the area of health it is usually assumed that with increasing knowledge a greater number of causal pathways can be used to make even more accurate predictions about risk relations (Backett et al., 1984; Spasoff and McDowell, 1987; Hayes, 1992). Hayes, however, challenges this view arguing that knowing a causal pathway does not necessarily lead to a better prediction. For example, chance always remains chance. It is not affected by any change with respect to areas delineating known and unknown causal pathways. For instance, even if couples, who are at risk of producing a child with a genetic disorder are given more accurate information about the risks, and so decide not to have children, the genetic disorder will not necessarily be eliminated due to the proportion of new cases which appear as a result of mutation. Moreover, while better predictions may relate to the population as a whole, they are never predictions about particular individuals (see below). Additional ethical problems may arise if health care professionals and health educators attempt to identify individuals at risk with the intention of informing them about their situation and thus reducing their own and their offsprings' risk (e.g. Thomas, 1982; Marková, 1990b; also Part III of this volume).

The perception of risk appears at present to be one of the most commonly explored variables in health-related research and one of the most salient psychological characteristics in existing models of health behaviour. As Prohaska et al. (1990) maintain, risk perception features in the health belief model (Becker, 1974) and also in Leventhal et al.'s (1980) common sense representation of illness. These authors argue that risk perception is an important component of the coping process and of adaptation (Leventhal, Meyer and Nerenz, 1980). The concept of risk is also fundamental to lay and professional explanations of genetic disorders, and its understanding is an essential part of genetic counselling. No doubt the importance of the concept of risk and of risk perception will increase as our knowledge of genetic disorders is enhanced and more and more disorders are found to be genetically and environmentally co-determined. Finally, health education campaigns are based on the assumption that people's perceptions of their risk of contracting a disease are essential in any attempt to change their health-related behaviour (Marková and Power, 1992).

Despite the prolific use of the concept of risk and its variations in research into professional and lay explanations of health, illness and handicap, the concept, as used at present, is neither coherent nor clearly defined (Hayes, 1992). In professional terminology, terms such as 'precursor', 'risk factor', 'risk indicator', 'probability' and so on are ambiguous and are often used without formal definition by those 'who communicate about health risk assessment methods' (DeFriese, 1987, p.585). In lay terminology, terms such as 'perceived vulnerability', 'perceived susceptibility', 'perceived risk', 'concern', 'perceived danger' and others, are used without any proper conceptual distinctions (Calnan and Johnson, 1985). Moreover, a particular notion, say, 'risk', may in lay terminology, underlie quite different concepts, e.g. statistical, cognitive or cognitive–emotional concepts of risk. Let us consider, for example, the statistical concept of risk. While the scientific concept of risk is based on calculating probabilities, research into lay perceptions of risk shows that people find it difficult to use knowledge to calculate low-probability events (Prohaska et al., 1990). Moreover, they simply may not calculate at all the probability that they are at risk (Slovic, 1987). The literature has shown that the interpretation of statistical probability is highly idiosyncratic (Pearn, 1973; Kessler, 1979). Perceptions of the risk of illness differ from one individual to another and may be unrelated to epidemiological evidence of the real degree of risk. What is a high risk for one person, may be a low risk for another. For example, if a person expects the risk of the occurrence of a genetic disorder for his offspring to be 50% but learns it is only 25%, he or she will probably consider this to be a low risk. On the other hand, if the person thinks in terms of a 10% risk and learns it is 25%, such news will be a disaster. Discussing this issue with respect to a dominant genetic disorder, Hungtington's chorea, Wexler (1979) pointed out that in real life a fifty-fifty risk always means for a particular individual a 100 percent certainty that he or she will either develop or not develop the condition. However, such a certainty changes from moment to moment and from day to day, depending on the individual's mood, mental state and other circumstances. In health-related research the notion of risk perception is commonly conceived of as a unidimensional variable, which ignores the fact that its meaning could be different at different stages of an individual's coping with the threat of illness.

The meaning of risk for the particular individual is likely to be co-determined by the individuals' own experience of that illness, by his or her beliefs and values. The actions of the individual provide a feeling of control. Some of these issues are taken up by Marková et al. in their contribution to Part II focusing on the perception of risk of HIV/AIDS by prison staff and prisoners. These authors explore the participants' concern, as distinct from their perceptions of risk. Their contribution shows the importance of the individual's feeling of control with respect to how they conceptualise the risk of HIV/AIDS both for themselves and for others. The notion of risk implies several distinct issues, such as threat to the individual's well-being, an increased danger of developing complications with respect to his or her health (Hayes, 1992), and uncertainty about the individual's future (Prohaska et al., 1990, p.385). Some of these issues overlap with each other, others are part of quite different conceptual frameworks and are in much need of clarification.

These components of risk perception are, themselves, social constructions, and they are co-determined by moralities, ideologies and political fashions. As Douglas (1992) puts it:

> *Although ordinary persons undoubtedly scan frequencies and assess*
> *them in their everyday decisions, the way they think is not like*
> *causal theory before the advent of probability, nor like probability*
> *theory either...Cultural theory brings us somewhat nearer to*
> *understanding the risk perception of lay persons by providing a*

systematic view of the widest range of goals that the person is seeking to achieve. Instead of isolating the risk as a technical problem we should formulate it so as to include…its moral and political implications   (Douglas, 1992, p.51).

Since risk is a social and a cultural construct, its interpretation by the individual depends on social norms and on social expectations. The perception of risk is based on moral values and beliefs and disease is often viewed as a punishment (Douglas, 1985; Marková and Wilkie, 1987; Herzlich, 1973, Sontag, 1979). What is perceived as immoral behaviour and the resulting punishment threatens the integrity of the self. Punishing events that degrade the self cannot easily be incorporated into a positive picture of the self that the individual is usually motivated to preserve. People with HIV/AIDS are often judged in these terms. Thus people avoid admitting risk for an event associated in their moral code with shame or deviation (Weinstein, 1988; Prohaska et al., 1990).

SOME UNINTENDED CONSEQUENCES OF SOCIAL REPRESENTATIONS

Goffman (1961) used participant observation to study what he called "the underlife" of total institutions such as prisons and old-style psychiatric hospitals. He described prisons and psychiatric hospitals as "total institutions". This is what they are from the perspective of their inmates. The inmates, but not the staff who look after them, spend twenty-four hours a day within the confines of the institution. They are not as free as their custodians are to come and go as they please. They have been deprived, by virtue of their crimes or their illnesses, of any entitlement to a separate, more private, life at home apart from their life within the institution. This creates a tension between custodians and inmates because for the latter, but not for the former, the prison or the hospital is a total institution (Goffman, 1961; Perrow, 1965).

The 'total institution', as revealed by Goffman, has a number of undesirable consequences. It isolates certain categories of people, e.g. prisoners, the mentally ill or the mentally handicapped, from the rest of the community. A category is always a nascent representation. The institution gives form to the representation. The building of such an institution increases the visibility of its inmates as social outcasts in the eyes of the local community and fosters the development of negative stereotypes concerning this category of person. This is the view from outside of the institution. The representations from this perspective are mainly lay representations. The view from inside the institution may be even worse. The categorising of people does not cease at the gates of the institution.

The inmates become institutionalised. This is a process of socialisation that goes on within the walls of the institution. The degree of their institutionalisation depends upon the length of their residence and the totality of the institution in which they reside. A prison is clearly more of a total institution than is a hospital for the mentally handicapped. The old style state psychiatric hospital probably lies somewhere in between these two extremes. The longer the period of residence and the more total the institution the less likely is it that a particular resident will be able to survive on his or her own within the community beyond the institution. They have become socialised to life within the institution. Many modern reformers now wish to reverse this whole process.

The social reformers who created asylums were enlightened people by the standards of their day. They had the welfare of their clients at heart. Good intentions, alone, however, are never enough. We saw in Part I, for example, how certain charities, in their zeal to raise funds, inadvertently perpetuated, rather than challenged, negative stereotypes concerning the handicaps of their clients. The founders of asylums did not intend to institutionalise their patients yet they set in train a series of reforms that, a century or two later, resulted in just that. The unintended consequences of their reforms are dealt with at some length in Part III. A reform, at the outset, is a blueprint or representation in the mind of the reformer of what the future might be like. Once it ceases to be a blueprint or a plan and becomes, for example, a building or a social programme, it becomes a representation in reality, i.e. some thing of which others can now form their own representations. It acquires a life of its own. The consequences may be quite different to those envisaged in the original reform.

Chombart de Lauwe (1971/1978) has spent a lifetime analysing social representations of childhood. She has explained changes in the representation of the child in the course of the last century. Most of these are the representations that adults form of children. She has also interviewed town planners and architects concerning their representations of childhood (Chombart de Lauwe, 1984). Her argument is that adults create the worlds in which children grow up. We wish to argue in similar vein, that representations of illness and of handicap are translated into health care facilities and programmes. Modern reformers face similar problems. In the field of mental illness and mental handicap the most commonly preferred alternative to the total institution is some form of care in the community. Yet this, too, can lead to some unintended consequences as Jodelet (1991) vividly demonstrates in her study of Ainay-le Château. Villagers, there, have been living with the mentally ill as their lodgers for almost a century now. At first the practice was strongly disapproved of, especially by the agricultural unions. This was because the lodgers became a source of cheap labour on local farms. There was also opposition to having the mentally ill as neighbours. Providing accommodation in Ainay-le-Château and surrounding villages soon became an important part of the local economy. The villagers now no longer notice the mentally ill. Psychiatric patients and the mentally handicapped have been living amongst them for several generations. What was initially strange and threatening, on closer and longer acquaintance, becomes familiar and obvious and, hence, no longer remarkable. The enlightened policy on the part of the state of boarding out psychiatric patients in rural homes would appear, from those criteria, to be a success. This, however, is not the full story.

In the villages studied by Jodelet the mentally ill are still treated as outcasts (the local word is "bredins") even though they dwell under the same roofs as the villagers. Often their accommodation is segregated, physically, from that of other members of the family. They typically eat separately from the rest of the family. Jodelet used participant observation to study the underlife of these villages in much the same way as Goffman (1961), earlier, had studied the underlife of total institutions. Psychiatric patients at Ainay-le-Chateau are no longer inmates of a total institution. They are, however, prisoners of the social representations of madness held by those amongst whom they dwell. The social representations have all the coercive force of a Durkheimian 'social fact'. They place constraints on the freedom and independence of the actor in that particular social setting. If those representations were to become too oppressive, then an asylum might, once again, become a place of refuge.

Reforms can assume a number of different forms. Reform need not lead to the creation of a new institution, like the asylum, or a new programme, like care in the community. It could be a change in the legal status of certain categories of person. In his analysis of the ideology of success and failure Ichheiser (1949) argued that a representation of the individual as responsible lies at the heart of the legal code in many Western cultures (Farr, 1991). When a person is found guilty of committing a criminal act then the full force of the law will take effect and he or she will be punished. Reformers wished, for highly laudable motives, to treat certain persons as being ill rather than criminal. Should this murderer be sent to hospital or to prison? This was the basis for the plea of insanity in Victorian murder trials (Smith, 1989). A set of rules were established following the case of Regina vs. McNaughton (1843) whereby legal proof of insanity in the commission of a crime hinges on establishing that:

> .... *at the time of committing the act, the party accused was labouring under such a defect of reason, from disease of the mind, as not to know the nature and quality of the act he was doing or, if he did know it, that he did not know he was doing what was wrong. (The English Reports, Volume 8, p. 718)*

Under these special circumstances a person may no longer be held to be fully responsible for his or her actions. This merciful provision, however, creates a legal precedent for categorising certain people as being mentally ill. The McNaughton rules enshrine a particular representation of mental illness. This same representation of mental illness can also be used to commit a person to hospital against his or her own will.

While the original motive for this provision may have been humanitarian it can also be used to deprive citizens of their civil liberties. Its consequences, then, may be far from benign. Goffman himself campaigned against the use of such provisions. Committing people to hospital involuntarily makes the institution more like a prison than like a hospital. It also makes the mental hospital more of a total institution than the general hospital. A similar court case in France in 1835 in which Pierre Rivière murdered his mother, sister and brother initiated a comparable sequence of events in France (Foucault, 1978). The representations of mental illness that are enshrined in legal codes are an important part of the culture of a particular society. Such representations are central to our interests in Part II of the present volume.

Representations are, indeed, historical and cultural phenomena. They often continue to operate even when they are no longer appropriate. When it comes to reversing some of the unintended consequences of earlier reforms it may also be necessary to reform the law. The freedom and autonomy of the individual, both in society and in law, is an important topic in Part III of the present volume.

REFERENCES

Ackerknecht, E. H. (1982), *A Short History of Medicine*, Baltimore: Johns Hopkins.

Backett, E. M., Davies, A. M. and Petros-Barvazian A. (1984), The risk approach in health care. *Public Health Papers* # 76, World Health Organisation, Geneva.

Becker M. H. (1974), The health belief model and personal health behaviour. *Health Education Monographs*, **2**, 326–473.

Berger, P. and Luckmann, T. (1966), *The Social Construction of Reality*. Harmondsworth, Middlesex: Penguin Books.

Bernoulli D (1738/1954), Specimen theoriae novae de mensure sortis, *Commentarii academiae scientarum imperialis Petropolitanae*, 5, 175–92 (English trans. by L. Sommer, Exposition of a New Theory on the Measurement of Risk, *Econometrica*, **22**, 23–36.

Bishop, G. D. and Converse, S. A. (1986), Illness representations: A prototype approach, *Health Psychology*, **5**, 95–114.

Bolton, R. and Singer, M. (eds.), (1992), Rethinking AIDS prevention: Cultural approaches, *Medical Anthropology*, **14**, 139–364.

Calnan, M. and Johnson, B. (1985), Health, health risks and inequalities: An exploratory study of women's perceptions. *Sociology of Health and Illness*, **7**, 55–75.

Chombart de Lauwe, M-J (1971), *Un Monde Autre: L'enfance, De ses représentations à son mythe*. Paris:Payot. (Deuxième edition, 1978).

Chombart de Lauwe, M-J (1984), Changes in the representation of the child in the course of social transmission. In R. M. Farr and S Moscovici (eds) *Social Representations*, Cambridge: Cambridge University Press. (pp. 185–209).

DeFriese G. H. (1987), A research agenda for personal health risk assessment, *Health Services Research*, **22**, 581–94.

Ditto, P. H., Jemmott III, J. B. and Darley, J. M. (1988), Appraising the threat of illness: A mental representational approach, *Health Psychology*, **7**, 183–201.

Douglas M. (1985), *Risk Acceptability According to the Social Sciences*, London: Routledge and Kegan Paul.

Douglas M. (1992), *Risk and Blame*, London and New York: Routledge.

English Reports (1900–1932), Edinburgh: W. Green & Son. Volume 8.

Farr, R. M. (1977), Heider, Harré and Herzlich on health and illness: Some observations on the structure of 'représentations collectives'. *European Journal of Social Psychology*, **7**(4), 491–504.

Farr, R. M. (1991), Individualism as a collective representation. In V. Aebischer, J. P. Deconchy & E. M. Lipiansky (Eds.), *Idéologies et Représentations Sociales*. (pp. 129–143). Couset: Delval.

Farr, R. M. (1993), Common sense, science and social representations. *Public Understanding of Science*, **2**, 111–122.

Foster, M. B. (1935), Christian theology and modern science of nature, *Mind*, **44**, 439–466.

Foucault, M. (Ed.). (1978), *I, Pierre Rivère, having slaughtered my mother, my sister, and my brother...* London: Peregrine Books.

Gigerenzer, G., Swijtink, Z., Porter, T., Daston, L., Beatty, J. and Kruger, L. (1989), *The Empire of Chance*, Cambridge and New York: Cambridge University Press.

Goffman, E. (1961), Asylums: Essays on the social situation of mental patients and other inmates. New York: Doubleday/Anchor Books.

Goffman, E. (1963), Stigma: Notes on the management of spoiled identity. Englewood Cliffs, New Jersey: Prentice-Hall.

Hanson, N. R. (1958), *Patterns of Discovery: An inquiry into the conceptual foundations of science*, Cambridge: Cambridge University Press.

Harré, R. and Madden, E. H. (1975), *Causal Powers*, Oxford: Blackwell.

Hayes M. V. (1992), On the epistemology of risk: Language, logic and social science. *Social Science and Medicine*, **35**, 401–7.

Heider, F. (1958), *The Psychology of Interpersonal Relations*, New York: Wiley.

Herzlich, C. (1973), *Health and Illness*, London: Academic Press.

Hinde, R. (1990), Causes of social development from the perspective of an integrated development science. In G. Butterworth and P Bryant (eds), *Causes of Development* New York and London: Harvester Wheatsheaf.

Huygens, C. (1657), *De Ratiociniis in ludo aleae*. In *Oeuvres Completes de Christiaan Huygens*, XIV, Martinus Nijhoff: The Hague, 1920.

Ichheiser, G. (1949), Misunderstandings in Human Relations: A study in false social perception. *American Journal of Sociology*, **LV**(Supplement), 1–72.

Jemmott III, J. B., Croyle, R. T. and Ditto, P. H. (1988), Commonsense epidemiology: self-based judgments from laypersons and physicians, *Health Psychology*, **7**, 55–73.

Jodelet, D. (1991), *Madness and Social Representations*. London: Harvester/Wheatsheaf.

Kessler, S. (1979), The genetic counsellor as psychotherapist. In A. M. Capron, M. Lappe, R. F. Murray, T. M. Powledge, S. B. Twiss and D. Bergsma (eds.), *Genetic Counseling: Facts, values and norms*, New York: A. R. Liss.

King, J. (1983), Attribution theory and the health belief model. In M. Hewstone (Eds.), *Attribution Theory: Social and functional extensions.* (pp. 170–186). Oxford: Blackwell.

Kuhn, T. S. (1962), The Structure of Scientific Revolutions. In *International Encyclopedia of Unified Science*. Volume 2. Chicago: University of Chicago Press.

Lau, R. R. and Hartmann, K. A. (1983), Common sense representations of common illnesses, *Health Psychology*, **2**, 167–185.

Laplace P. S. (1774), Mémoire sur la probabilité des causes par les événements, *Mémoires présentées a l'Académie des Sciences*, **6**, 621–56.

Leventhal, H., Meyer, D., and Nerenz, D. (1980), The common sense representation of illness danger. In S. Rachman (ed.), *Contributions to Medical Psychology* **2**, Oxford:Pergamon.

McLuhan, H. M. (1951), *The Mechanical Bride: Folklore of Industrial Man*. New York: Vanguard Press.

Marková, I. (1990a), Causes and reasons of social development. In: G. Butterworth and P. Bryant (eds), *Causes of Development*, New York and London: Harvester Wheatsheaf.

Marková, I. (1990b), Ethics as a branch of societal psychology: Its particular relevance to the social psychology of medicine. In: H. Himmelweit and G. Gaskell (eds.), *Societal Psychology*, London: Sage.

Marková, I. (1992), Scientific and public knowledge of AIDS: The problem of their integration. In M. Von Cranach, W. Doise & G. Mugny (Eds.), *Social Representations.* (pp. 84–88). Bern: Huber.

Marková I. and Power K. G. (1992), Audience response to AIDS health education messages. In Edgar T, Fitzpatrick M. A. and Freimuth V (eds.) *AIDS: A Communication Perspective*. Hillsdale: Laurence Erlbaum.

Marková, I. and Wilkie, P. A. (1987), Representations, concepts and social change: The phenomenon of AIDS, *Journal for the Theory of Social Behaviour*, **17**, 389–407.

Moscovici, S. (1984), The phenomenon of social representations. In R. M. Farr & S. Moscovici (eds.), *Social Representations*. (pp. 3–69). Cambridge: Cambridge University Press.

Moscovici, S. & Hewstone, M. (1983), Social representations and social explanations: From the 'naive' to the 'amateur' scientist. In M. Hewstone (Eds.), *Attribution Theory: Social and functional extensions*. (pp. 98–125). Oxford: Blackwell.

Pascal, B, (1963), *Oeuvres completes*, ed. by de Louis Lafuma, Paris: Seuil.

Pearn, J. H. (1973), Patients' subjective interpretation of risks offered in genetic counselling, *Journal of Medical Genetics*, **10**, 129–34.

Perrow, C. (1965), Hospitals: Technology, structure and goals. In J. G. March (Eds.), *Handbook of Organisations*. (pp. 910–971). Chicago: Rand McNally.

Power, K. G., Marková, I., Rowlands, A., McKee, K. J., Anslow, P. J. and Kilfedder, C. (1992), Comparison of sexual behaviour and risk of HIV transmission of Scottish inmates with or without a history of intravenous drug use. *AIDS Care*, **4**, 53–67.

Prohaska T. R., Albrecht G, Levy J. A. et al (1990), Determinants of self-perceived risk for AIDS. *Journal of health and Social Behaviour*, **31**, 384–94.

Sayer, A. (1984), *Method in Social Science: A realist approach*, London: Hutchinson.

Schober, R. and Lacroix, M. (1991), Lay illness models in the Enlightenment and the 20th century: some historical lessons. In J. A. Skelton and R. T. Croyle (eds.), *Mental Representation in Health and Illness*, New York: Springer-Verlag.

Schutz, A. (1962–66), *Collected Papers*. Volumes I–II. Den Hagg: Nijhoff.

Skelton, J. A. and Croyle, R. T. (eds.), (1991), *Mental Representation in Health and Illness*, New York: Springer-Verlag.

Slovic, P. (1987), Perception of risk, *Science*, **236**, 208–285.

Smith, R. (1989), Mad or bad? Victorian stories of the criminally insane. *LSE Quarterly*, **3** (1), 1–20.

Sontag, S. (1979), *Illness as Metaphor*, London: Allen Lane.

Spasoff R. A. and McDowell I, (1987), Potential and limitations of data and methods in health risk appraisal: Risk factor selection and measurement, *Health Services Research*, **22**, 467–97.

Sperber, D. (1985), Anthropology and psychology: Towards an epidemiology of representations. *Man (New Series)*, **1**, 73–89.

Stockdale, J. E., Dockrell, J. E. and Wells, A. J. (1989), The self in relation to mass media representations of HIV and AIDS: Match or mismatch? *Health Education Journal*, **48**, 121–130.

Stainton-Rogers, W. (1991), *Explaining Health and Illness: An exploration of diversity*. New York: Harvester/Wheatsheaf.

Thomas, S. (1982), Ethics of a predictive test for Huntington's chorea, *British Medical Journal*, **284**, 1383–85.

Weinstein, N. D. (1988), The precaution adoption process, *Health Psychology*, **7**, 355–386.

Wexler, N. S. (1979), Genetic 'Russian Roulette': The experience of being 'at risk' for Huntington's disease. In S. Kessler (ed.), *Genetic Counseling*, New York and London: Academic Press.

Williams, R. (1983), Concepts of health: An analysis of lay logic, *Sociology*, **17**, 185–205.

Wolpert, L. (1992), *The Unnatural Nature of Science*. London: Faber & Faber.

CHAPTER SIX

The Self and the Other: Perception of the Risk of HIV/AIDS in Scottish Prisons

Ivana MARKOVÁ, Kevin J McKEE, Kevin G POWER and Eleanor MOODIE

Department of Psychology, University of Stirling, Stirling, FK9 4LA

RISK PERCEPTION AND RISK BEHAVIOUR

Perception of risk is socio-culturally established. How people perceive the risk of particular events or whether they evaluate risk positively or negatively is co-determined by their values, their appraisals of costs and gains, and the manner in which they attribute blame, and so on (Douglas, 1992). From the evolutionary point of view, risk-taking endangers survival. Yet, sometimes survival can be better achieved by taking risks. For example, both theoretical models and observations of animal behaviour have shown that risk-aversive choices are favoured by some animals when they are not hungry and they take more risk as their hunger increases (Beardsley, 1983). Images of risk-taking in humans have a rich history. The beginnings of probabilistic thinking can be traced to ancient Greek philosophers and inferences about heredity with respect to genetic disorders, such as haemophilia, appeared in the Talmud. Interest in mathematical calculation of risk for insurance, juristic and commercial purposes started to develop in the sixteenth and seventeenth centuries. More recently, a study of risk and probability related problems has also become part of the natural sciences (Gigerenzer et al., 1989).

Today, risk-prone choices are part of everyday life, from crossing road to gambling and climbing mountains, to car racing and illness-related activities. In fact, most of our daily activities involve some risk and it is often difficult to specify which activities are and which are not risky. Moreover, what is and what is not considered risky is associated with a variety of factors ranging from fashions to the knowledge individuals may have about the event in question. There are professional and lay expectations as to how much risk particular groups of people should take. For example, risk-taking behaviour in people with haemophilia, a genetic disorder of blood clotting, has been described by a number of researchers

(Katz, 1970; Agle, 1975; Marková et al., 1980). They argued that a proportion of men with haemophilia often engage in high risk activities, such as playing football and other games that put strain on their muscles, thus increasing the likelihood of their bleedings. More recently, researchers and the public have focused their attention on risk-taking behaviour of various groups of the population that are particularly prone to HIV infection such as promiscuous heterosexuals, drug users and homosexuals. As Douglas (1992) maintains, risk-taking and risk-avoidance have something to do with the relationship between the self and the community. Individuals may or may not take risks as a result of community pressures and community censorship, blame accusations and so on; and such community values will be drawn from cultural systems of belief.

Risk, Culture, and Illness

The social and cultural components of risk perception related to illness have been mostly studied by sociologists and anthropologists in the context of collectively constructed social knowledge, culturally transmitted beliefs, emotions, fears and threats.

In early societies, disease was perceived to be the work of supernatural forces. It was believed that people who risked violating social taboos were struck down with illness by the spirits and gods who watched over the community. Disease was therefore a social marker of the boundaries of acceptable behaviour (Dubos, 1968). With the advance of science, naturalistic explanations for disease became more prominent, but competed for public acceptance with the religious pronouncements of the day. In the West, the rise of Christianity during the medieval period reinforced the link between sin or moral transgression, punishment, and illness (Lyon and Petrucelli, 1987). This period in history saw Europe ravaged by a series of plagues. In fundamentalist Christian interpretation, plague has always contained a moral resonance, due to the important role allocated to it in Revelations where it preceded the Apocalypse. Just as the signifier tends to take on the attributes of the signified, so plague became indistinguishable from the Apocalypse, and those afflicted with plague became the Damned (Sontag, 1989).

Thus the relationship between sin, punishment, and illness has been well established and beliefs in such relationships have existed in European culture for centuries (Herzlich and Pierret, 1987). As early as in the twelfth century, leprosy, a major disaster in Europe at the time, was connected by the public with immoral activities. Much later, in the sixteenth century Pascal associated the sickness of the body with the sickness of the soul. It was through the pain of the body that the diseased individual should become aware of the sickness of his or her soul. Suffering therefore was seen as the means of redemption of the sinner. Throughout history some diseases signified sin more than others and leprosy and plague were particularly stigmatizing and called for the exclusion of the patient (Herzlich and Pierret, 1987; Douglas, 1992).

The isolation of the afflicted also served to identify the disease with a discrete section of society. Attribution of responsibility for disease has always been part of the social representation of the illness process. Most societies at most times have blamed social 'externals' for the diseases with which they are afflicted: foreigners, travellers, and so forth. However, if a foreign source, and hence attribution of external responsibility, cannot be realised, then society often selects easily identifiable individuals from within its own borders, people usually of low standing and moral worth (Sontag, 1989). Thus, Elford (1987) draws attention to the stigmatization of leprosy in Chinese settlers in Hawaii in the last century. The Chinese were also seen as inferiors and as an economic threat, and were also easily identifiable by facial features. The increase in leprosy was attributed to them, although the records do not support the conclusion that the Chinese were an important source of leprosy.

The cultural nature of such beliefs and practices can be seen by the fact that the exclusion of people with leprosy was not universal across cultures. Diagnoses of leprosy in the East, in the Kingdom of Jerusalem, were made in medieval times and detailed and precise descriptions of leprosy were given. But they were detached from moral judgments and sin was not associated with leprosy. There was an order of leper knights, and no objections existed to crowning a person with leprosy as a king. In his analysis of this case Pegg (1990), cited by Douglas (1992), studied historical, economic and political patterns of the time. He maintained that in contrast to Europe, the political system in the Kindgom of Jerusalem was characterized by egalitarian rather than hierarchical societal patterns.

This century, the cultural link between sin and disease, sanction and isolation, was most powerfully realised during the outbreak of syphilis in the decades leading up to the first World War. As recounted by Brandt (1988), syphilis could produce debility, insanity, paralysis, sterility, and blindness. Occurring during Victorian times, syphilis, being sexually transmitted was a double threat to society since sex itself was a form of 'social death', not spoken of in polite society. The public, and in some cases scientific, perception of syphilis as casually transmitted was prevalent, and this belief was maintained even after the discovery of the causative agent. This belief lead to draconian public health measures, such as the removal of all door knobs from US navy ships. The development, in 1906, of the Wasserman test for asymptomatic syphilis lead to the widespread screening of the population. However, due to a false positive rate of 25%, toxic treatments and social stigma were heaped on many individuals 'innocent' of the double transgression of having indulged in illicit sex and of harbouring the syphilitic spirochaete. During the First World War, radical quarantine programmes were introduced. In the US, 20,000 women were held as suspected 'spreaders' of syphilis, the criteria for their isolation ranging from their occupation (e.g. prostitution) to their ethnic background (e.g. recent immigrants).

In more recent decades, the relationship between sex, sin, and disease has once again been foremost in the public mind, with the advent of AIDS. However, on first encounter, the form of sex most clearly linked with

AIDS was homosexual sex. The initial labelling of AIDS as GRID – Gay Related Immune Disease – lead to an association in the public mind between homosexuality and the syndrome. The early public announcements concerning AIDS did not make clear the distinction between homosexuality *per se*, and a characteristic homosexual lifestyle, and therefore the idea that AIDS afflicts only particular social groups was initiated, and has persisted (Horton and Aggleton, 1989). The data indicating that homosexuals, drug users, and ethnic minorities – socially stigmatised communities – have a higher risk of HIV/AIDS taps the ancient social beliefs in the relationship between disease, immorality and punishment. The perception that AIDS is a disease of discrete social groups also serves to reduce personal anxiety over the possibility of contracting the disease: one's risk of AIDS is perceived as low if one is not a member of one of the 'guilty' social groups (see below for a discussion of 'optimistic bias'). A further belief prevalent in society is that an individual who is HIV seropositive is readily identifiable from physical appearance alone. Such a belief has its roots in early cultural representations of an individual's inner character being reflected in his or her physical manifestation, and also links with the historic perception of disease as an agent of bodily transformation and corruption (Chapter 3). The belief serves the purpose of reducing personal anxiety over risk of infection, since one can avoid contact with HIV seropositives if they can be easily identified. It is socially important that people with HIV/AIDS are identified, either through the magical process of observation, or through the scientific process of screening, since the belief that HIV/AIDS can be spread through casual contact is still widespread. Watney (1989) has indicated that the important scientific distinction between contagious and infectious diseases is collapsed in the public mind. Thus, the ancient process of identification and isolation repeats itself. Calls for the quarantining of people with AIDS do not merely reflect a desire to protect society's physical health, however, but also a desire to cleanse society of moral transgressors, and to see them punished for their acts. Thus, evidence shows a scapegoating process whereby particular minority groups, such as homosexuals are held more responsible for their illness than others (e.g. Triplet and Sugarman, 1987; Kelley et al., 1987; Dowell et al., 1991).

Risk, the Individual and Illness

Although collectively shared representations of illness discussed above shape the individual's perceptions, each individual responds to illness and to its risk in his or her idiosyncratic way. Such individual perceptions are co-determined by cognitive, experiential and emotional factors. For example, the individual may categorize him- or herself as a member of a particular social group and therefore not prone to a particular infection, e.g. HIV. Definitions of social groups usually imply or explicitly state some moral criteria that are culturally determined and these, in turn, become part of the individual's self-categorization.

In the area of health and illness, the social scientific studies of people's perceptions of risk have tended to emphasize *either* the socio-cultural *or* the individual component or risk-perception. Psychologists have commonly focused on individual rather than on socio-cultural components of the risk of illness and disease, having implicitly subsumed risk-perception under the cognitively and rationally based perception processes. This approach can be seen in some of the more influential social cognition models of preventive health behaviour, e.g. in the Health Belief Model (Becker, 1974) and Protection Motivation Theory (Prentice-Dunn and Rogers, 1986). These models emphasise the individual's cognitive processes as mediators of attitudinal and behavioural change. The Health Belief Model and Protection Motivation Theory are both grounded in expectancy-value theory: the tendency to perform a particular act is believed to be a function of the expectancy that the act will be followed by certain consequences and the value of those consequences. When such models are operationalised, risk perception is usually empirically measured as a unidimensional continuum of uncertainty that a given event will occur. In the Health Belief Model, risk perception is operationalised as 'perceived susceptibility'; in Protection Motivation Theory, it is operationalised as 'perceived vulnerability'.

Such a representation of risk perception may not adequately reflect the process of risk appraisal. In ordinary language the notions of risk of, susceptibility to, and concern about illness are used indiscriminately and it is likely that even if asked, people might have difficulty in distinguishing between them. These notions are also used interchangeably in the literature on risk perception. However, psychologically, risk can have very different meanings for a given individual, ranging from a predominantly cognitive-rational evaluation and response, to a predominantly emotional evaluation and response. For example, an individual may cognitively comprehend that he or she is at risk of illness, and yet be emotionally unconcerned. Contrastingly, an individual may feel emotionally disturbed by a particular illness, without judging him- or herself to be at risk of the illness. The possible discreteness of cognitive and emotional evaluation of illness is indicated in research by Calnan and Johnson (1985). In this study of lay health representations, interview respondents distinguished between being 'worried' about a given illness, and actually believing that they might contract that illness. Eagly (1992) reviews work that indicates that unless individuals are motivated to do otherwise, information is processed at a superficial level. It could be argued that the evaluation of information regarding one's personal risk of illness is an elaborate process, which one might be motivated to initiate only after reaching a certain level of emotional arousal.

A further variable mediating the risk appraisal process is perceived control. The importance of controllability in risk perception has been established for some time (e.g. Weinstein, 1984). Taylor (1983) noted that high levels of perceived vulnerability to illness was linked to a decreased sense of personal control over one's health. It has been suggested that a sense of personal vulnerability is also necessary if a person is to adopt risk-reduction behaviours. However, an individual cannot increase or lower the risk to the self of a given event unless he or she can independently effect some control over the event through engaging in appropriate behaviours. If the individual does not believe that an event can be controlled, behavioural avoidance is of little utility. The concept of perceived control can thus be used to explain apparently contradictory findings concerning the relationship between perceived risk and health behaviour.

Whether or not an event is perceived to be controllable has been linked to the evaluation of the level of threat or danger to the individual emanating from the event (Leventhal, Meyer and Nerenz, 1980). Thus, higher levels of uncontrollability are linked to higher levels of threat. It could be anticipated that an illness seen by an individual as predominantly uncontrollable (that is, beyond behavioural influence) might produce a negative psychological response towards the perceived source of the threat. Experimental evidence suggests that this is the case. Mondragón and colleagues (1991) found that as the belief in casual transmission of HIV increases (increasing uncontrollability), so too does hostility towards those afflicted with the disease.

The authors' view is that both perspectives, individual and socio-cultural, contribute to the formation, maintenance and changes in professional and lay perceptions of the risk of illness and disease. A similar view has also been expressed by others who call for the interdisciplinary integration of different perspectives in social science (Landrine and Klonoff, 1992). However, to date, attempts to provide such an integration of approaches are still very rare:

> *With no link between cultural analysis and cognitive science, clashes inevitably occur between theory and evidence. Since the theory is not being radically adjusted, irrationality tends to be invoked to protect the too narrow definition of rationality. So instead of a sociological, cultural, and ethical theory of human judgment, there is an unintended emphasis on perceptual pathology (Douglas, 1986, p.3).*

Risk, the Self, and Others

There is extensive knowledge showing that individuals judge their own activities, circumstances, involvements, and success and failure by different criteria than those of others. Very generally, individuals tend to judge their own activities and so on more favourably than those of others. With respect to health and illness, it appears that individuals perceive themselves as less vulnerable to illness and more in control of their health.

In a series of studies Weinstein (1980, 1984) explored the nature of unrealistic optimism with respect to the self. He found that an 'optimistic bias' with respect to the self is related to a belief that one's actions, lifestyles, and personality have more advantageous characteristics than those of their peers thus making the self less at risk of illness that others.

The individual believes that because of these advantageous characteristics, the self is more in control of its life than others are of theirs. Such beliefs seem to be held by people irrespective of their age, gender, education or occupation. Moreover, even if they suffer illness, they tend to judge it as less severe than do others. For example, research by Marková et al. (1984) has shown that patients with haemophilia assessed their difficulties, such as pain, restricted movements, etc., as less severe than did their mothers and other female relatives. It is true, of course, that the emotional suffering of the mothers, their feeling of responsibility for the transmission of haemophilia and the empathy of their relatives might have affected females' judgements of haemophilia. However, continuing on this line of research, Marková et al. (1990) have also found that people with haemophilia made clear distinctions between their own perceptions of haemophilia and those of 'others'. They believed that other people perceive haemophilia as a more severe illness than they themselves did.

Appraising the risks of illness to self and to other is particularly important in transmissible diseases. The circumstances under which transmission is possible will influence the judgments of risk one ir required to make. For example, Wilkie (1993) found in her research that most people with haemophilia and with adult polycystic disease of the kidney did not perceive their illness as sufficiently severe to decide not to have children even if these children would be affected by these diseases. With regard to HIV/AIDS, much research has been devoted to understanding individual judgements of risk surrounding decisions to have unprotected sex, or to share needles during drug misuse.

Some researchers have argued that risk-perception is a component of the coping process through which individuals adapt to threat and temper emotional response (Leventhal, Meyer, and Nerenz, 1980).

Douglas (1986) maintains, however, that the sense of subjective immunity has a survival value. It is adaptive in the sense that it allows people to keep calm in dangerous situations, to get involved in situations the successful outcome of which is unlikely and to attempt to change the course of events putting themselves, as individuals, at risk. Optimistic bias and subjective immunity gives the agent a feeling of being in control of his or her own fate.

HIV/AIDS IN PRISONS

In this section we shall explore some aspects of the lay representations of HIV/AIDS in prisons. Prisons are, in Goffman's sense, total institutions of which prisoners are part. With respect to HIV/AIDS, prisoners are generally viewed as a high-risk group (see below). When in prison, HIV antibody positive prisoners are often considered to be a potential danger for the spread of HIV to other prisoners and prison officers. After release, such prisoners can be viewed as a potential danger to the general public. This section will examine evidence available for such views and it will explore how prisoners and staff perceive their own and others' risks of contracting HIV; and the relationship between risk-perceptions, behaviour and attitudes towards HIV/AIDS issues.

Prevalence of HIV in Prisons

The weight of evidence supports the idea that amongst prisoners there is a higher than average rate of HIV seroprevalence (McKee and Power, 1992; Gillies and Carballo, 1990). However, such a general conclusion obscures the tremendous variation in HIV/AIDS prevalence rates across different countries. In 1987, a survey conducted on behalf of The Council of Europe reported that out of 17 countries, only two had significant numbers of prisoners with AIDS, with 10 patients in Italy and 22 in Spain (Harding, 1987). Harding also quoted a range of HIV seropositivity rates in various European countries: Spain, 26%; Switzerland, 11%; Netherlands, 11%; Luxemburg, 2.1%; and Belgium, 1.2%. Such variation in prevalence rates may come about partially because of discrepancies in sampling methodologies across the different studies from which the figures are drawn. Nevertheless, the variation in rates suggests that the issue of HIV/AIDS in prison is likely to be linked to the wider culture of the population under study, and that evidence from individual prisons or countries cannot be generalised to others without a careful analysis of the social and cultural contexts of the imprisoned population.

High HIV prevalence rates in prisons have led to concern about HIV transmission rates among prisoners, and the effect on the wider community when prisoners are released (McMillan, 1988). Concerns have been further fuelled by speculation concerning possible high levels of HIV/AIDS high-risk behaviours in prisons, such as the sharing of drug injecting equipment within male and female prison populations, and unprotected sex among male prisoners (Prison Reform Trust, 1988; Dolan et al., 1990). Such high risk behaviours are regarded by some authors as more prevalent whilst prisoners are in custody than when they are at liberty. As a result, prisons have sometimes been viewed as incubators for HIV with especially high rates of seroconversion during imprisonment, which in turn increases the risk for those in the general population once prisoners are released. For example, Brown (1993) has stated that "researchers, AIDS workers and recently released prisoners remain adamant: Prisons are dangerous" (p. 1). Brown goes on to conclude that in England and Wales the 'prison service has not accepted the view of most researchers that prisons are actually riskier environments than the outside world' thus implying that the public must be prepared to expect the worst.

However, the available evidence to date does not wholly substantiate the sentiments expressed by Brown. Data concerning HIV seroconversion rates among imprisoned populations, an index of high-risk behaviours occurring in prisons, are inconclusive. Findings generally point to lower rates of seroconversion than would be anticipated if high-risk behaviours were at rumoured levels. Furthermore, the vast majority of research purporting to measure high-risk sexual activities has used samples of ex-prisoners or temporarily liberated prisoners. This raises doubts as to the validity of the conclusions offered (McKee and Power, 1992). When consideration is given to data drawn from studies using samples of prisoners currently incarcerated, there is some evidence to suggest that the majority of prisoners are at greater risk of HIV/AIDS while at liberty than when imprisoned (Dye and Isaacs, 1991; Power et al., 1992a, 1992b).

Taking into consideration the difficulties facing epidemiological studies, it is even more problematic to assess whether, and if so to what extent, statistical evidence about the prevalence of HIV in prisons reflect lay representations of the risk of HIV in prison. However, the speculation that high levels of both HIV seroconversion and risk behaviours occur in prison is likely to have impact on individuals' perceptions of the risk of HIV in prison.

HIV/AIDS: Self-perceived Risk and Intravenous Drug Misuse (IDM)

It is widely acknowledged that a considerable proportion of IDMs will, during their period of addiction, spend some time in prison (Laurence, 1988). This is not only due to arrest for drug-related offences, but also for crimes perpetrated in order to finance their addiction. IDMs increasingly constitute a significant proportion of the prison population (Adler, 1989). Concern has been expressed that, due to the difficulty involved in smuggling drug injecting equipment into prison, incarcerated IDMs will be at high risk of HIV infection because of the widespread sharing of the limited number of needles and syringes available to them (Prison Reform Trust, 1988).

There is a dearth of studies that have actually investigated the estimation by prisoners of their personal risk of HIV infection both prior to and during imprisonment. However, a number of studies have explored the self-perceived risk of HIV amongst IDMs. The evidence from such studies, regarding the accuracy with which individuals involved in HIV risk behaviours can estimate their personal risk, is conflicting. Coleman and colleagues (1988), in a study of 162 IDMs attending two London clinics, found that those IDMs who perceived themselves to be at risk of HIV had higher levels of both high risk sexual behaviours and equipment sharing than those who did not think themselves at risk. The authors suggests that this finding illustrates that individuals are able to apply their understanding of the risk factors of HIV to themselves, and to decide whether or not they are at risk. However, Stimson and colleagues (1988) reported data from a sample of 387 attenders at syringe exchange schemes in England and Scotland. They found that although most individuals had an accurate knowledge of the risk of HIV infection from sharing syringes, very few considered themselves to be at risk of infection. Despite 36% of the sample having recently shared needles and syringes, only 7% of the sample believed themselves to be at risk of HIV. This illustrates a lack of consistency between knowledge of what constitutes HIV risk behaviour and self-perceived risk. A similar disparity between risk behaviour and self-perceived risk was found by McKeganey et al. (1989) in a study of 102 purchasers of injecting equipment from a Glasgow pharmacy. The authors found that over 1 in 10 of the sample were relatively optimistic about not contracting HIV. McKeganey et al. suggest that the optimism could be related to a reported reduction in the sharing of injecting equipment among the sample, but also notes that risk of sexual transmission among the sample was high due to a failure to practice protected sex.

It has been suggested that prisoners who engage in HIV risk behaviours may have previously had only limited access to AIDS-related information, and so may not be fully aware of the inherent risk of their behaviour both for themselves and for others (World Health Organization, 1987). In addition, it is rarely considered that taking risk can have for some people, or for certain categories of people, a positive and attractive value. For example, gambling has been of interest for a long time, yet gambling applied to health has been little explored.

The present authors, in a series of studies investigating various HIV related issues in Scottish prisons, assessed HIV/AIDS knowledge, and HIV/AIDS self-perceived risk prior to and during imprisonment, in 559 prisoners from eight prisons (Power et al., 1993; Power et al., in press). Overall, prisoners were highly knowledgeable about HIV/AIDS-related issues. They were aware of risk of HIV infection through sexual and drug behaviours, and knew that HIV could not be transmitted by routine social contact. However, a substantial number of prisoners were uncertain about the risk of HIV involved in certain aspects of IDM, such as the use of cooking-up spoons and the use of bleach solution as a sterilising agent. Fighting with an HIV seropositive prisoner was also thought risky. Few prisoners perceived their risk of HIV as high during imprisonment. In fact, they reported a reduction in high-risk intravenous drug misuse and almost non-existent high-risk sexual behaviour during periods in custody. Prisoners who perceived their risk of HIV prior to imprisonment as high, had higher levels of both sexual and drug-related HIV risk behaviour than those who perceived lower levels of risk. When outside prison, prisoners did not report adopting sexual risk reduction strategies, such as the regular use of condoms. Taken together, these findings suggest that most prisoners are able to apply their understanding of the risk factors for HIV infection to themselves, and to state whether or not they had been at risk prior to and during imprisonment. However, an accurate assessment of personal risk was not necessarily related to the adoption of protective strategies with regard to sexual behaviour.

Perceived Risk of HIV/AIDS to Self and to Others

The prison environment involves the sharing of toilet and eating facilities, the communal use of prison clothing and bedding, and can involve multiple cell occupancy (Curran, McHugh, and Nooney, 1989). Such conditions could be incorrectly perceived as high-risk for HIV transmission through casual contact. The perception of personal risk of HIV as a result of the belief in casual transmission has been associated with negative attitudes towards those with HIV/AIDS including support for restrictive practices such as compulsory HIV screening and segregation

(Herlitz and Brorsson, 1990). Such negative attitudes, if held by prisoners, could result in serious management problems for prison staff. In the American penal system, prisoners demanding compulsory HIV testing and segregation of those prisoners suspected of, or known to be HIV seropositive, have filed lawsuits against the Correctional Authorities (Hammett, 1988).

Prison staff and prisoners are in different situations with respect to HIV/AIDS. The common representation of prisoners as an HIV/AIDS high-risk group may affect staff's perception of their own risk of HIV infection as deriving from the prisoners, and prisoners' risk behaviours. Prison officers may perceive their HIV risk as emanating from others rather than from self. The prisoners' situation is even more complex. Prisoners involved in HIV high-risk behaviours may perceive their main risk of HIV as originating in their own behaviours, a 'self' source. However, prisoners not involved in HIV high-risk behaviours may see other prisoners as the main source of their own HIV risk, or may see the existing institutional arrangements as the primary cause of any risk they perceive for themselves.

Research into perceived risk for self and for others has been carried out by the present authors (McKee et al., submitted for publication). A random stratified sample of 500 male staff and 480 male prisoners drawn from 7 Scottish prisons participated in a semi-structured interview exploring aspects of HIV/AIDS risk perception. All participants were asked to estimate their risk of HIV/AIDS outside of prison, and the risk to an average member of the general public. Prison staff were also asked to estimate their risk of HIV/AIDS inside prison, and the risk to an average prison officer. Prisoners were asked to estimate their risk of HIV/AIDS inside prison, and the risk to an average prisoner. Data are presented in Table 6.1.

Table 6.1 – Prisoner and prison staff perceived risk and concern towards HIV/AIDS in self and others, inside and outside prison

	Prisoners (mean) N=559	Prison staff (mean) N=591
(a) Risk		
Outside (self)	2.42	1.62
Outside (other)	2.72	2.18
Inside (self)	1.86	2.53
Inside (other)	2.62	2.68
(b) Concern		
Outside	2.30	1.99
Inside	2.46	2.68
General health	3.31	2.67

Note: Mean scores presented are responses on five-point scales measuring perceived risk and perceived concern. Response range for Risk: 'No risk' = 1 to 'Very high risk' = 5. Response range for Concern: 'Not at all concerned'= 1 to 'Extremely concerned' = 5.

It can be seen in the table that both staff and prisoners rated others' risk of HIV as greater than the risk to self, both inside and outside the prison (all p<.001). Prisoners' self-perceived risk of HIV/AIDS inside prison was lower than self-perceived risk of HIV/AIDS outside prison (p<.001). In contrast, staff self-perceived risk of HIV/AIDS inside prison was higher than their self-perceived risk outside prison (p<.001). Similarly, staff rating of an average officer's risk of HIV/AIDS was higher than their rating of an average member of the general public's risk of HIV/AIDS (p<.001). There was no significant difference between prisoners' perceived risk of HIV/AIDS for an average member of the public, and their perceived risk of HIV/AIDS for an average prisoner. Comparing staff with prisoners, staff perceived a higher personal risk of HIV/AIDS inside prison than did prisoners, while prisoners perceived a higher personal risk of HIV/AIDS outside prison, and perceived an average member of the public to be at higher risk than did staff (all p<.001).

The existence of optimistic bias, as evidenced in these findings, has also been found in other HIV/AIDS high risk groups. Joseph and colleagues (1987), in a study of homosexual men, found that perceived risk of HIV/AIDS for the self was significantly lower than the perception of risk for other homosexual men. The difference between the perception of self and other risk of contracting HIV/AIDS also depends on the individual's group self-categorization. Stockdale et al. (1989) found that their sample of homosexuals perceived themselves as being in stable relationships and thus less at risk than heterosexuals who were not in stable relationships. Their sample of heterosexuals, however, stereotyped homosexuals, bisexuals, and IDMs as all being at high risk of HIV infection. The authors pointed out that despite the fact that only about half of her heterosexual respondents were in stable relationships, they identified with heterosexuals in such relationships, distancing themselves from those whom they perceived to be at risk for HIV/AIDS.

Risk and Concern

As part of their study of HIV/AIDS in Scottish prisons, the present authors explored whether prison staff and prisoners distinguish between personal concern about HIV/AIDS and risk. They asked prisoners and prison staff to rate their *concern* about HIV/AIDS for both inside and outside of prison, and their concern about their general health. The responses to these questions are also presented in Table 6.1.

For both staff and prisoners, concern about HIV/AIDS inside prison was higher than their self-perceived risk of HIV/AIDS inside prison (both p<.001). For staff concern about HIV/AIDS outside prison was greater than self-perceived risk of HIV/AIDS outside prison (p<.001). There was no significant difference between prisoners' concern about HIV/AIDS outside prison, and their self-perceived risk. Prisoners were more concerned about their general health, and more concerned about HIV/AIDS as a problem to their health outside prison, than were staff (both p<.001). Staff were more concerned about HIV/AIDS inside prison as a problem to their health, than were prisoners (p<.01).

Thus, for three out of four comparisons, concern about HIV/AIDS was found to be higher than perceived personal risk. The McKeganey et al. (1989) study reported earlier, of the purchasers of injecting equipment from a Glasgow pharmacy, also found that despite their sample's optimism about their risks of contracting HIV, they were highly concerned about HIV/AIDS. Taken together, such findings support the idea that risk appraisal may contain more than one evaluative process, with both cognitive and emotional evaluations of information. Such evaluations may be separately influenced by cultural, social, and psychological factors, and have different effects on behavioural and attitudinal responses.

Further research is required to ascertain why in certain circumstances reported concern and self-perceived risk do not differ, as in prisoners' evaluations of HIV/AIDS outside prison in the present authors' study. One possible explanation is that, for prisoners, evaluation of risk and concern outside of prison is a retrospective exercise when currently incarcerated. Past behaviours retain 'signal value' for individuals' current risk assessments (Slovic, 1987), and therefore the cognitive evaluation of risk behaviours might be expected to remain stable over time, the provision of new information not withstanding. However, the emotional impact of the same behaviours might diminish over time, thus altering the emotional evaluation. The result of time span on risk appraisal might therefore be to reduce levels of concern to that of self-perceived risk.

Risk, Attitudes, and Control

The present authors have carried out a study to explore the relationship between high and low personal HIV/AIDS risk perception, and attitudes towards HIV/AIDS issues. The study sample consisted of 448 prisoners and 294 prison staff drawn from eight Scottish prisons. Prison staff were asked to rate their personal risk of HIV/AIDS inside prison, while prisoners were asked to rate their personal risk of HIV/AIDS outside prison. Selection of these risk environments was made on the basis of findings reported above, indicating such environments to be perceived as the source of greatest HIV/AIDS risk by the respective groups. Participants evaluated their own risk on a 5 point scale, from "no risk at all" to "very high risk". The distribution of the participants' response to the risk question is presented in Table 6.2.

Table 6.2 – Perception of personal risk of HIV/AIDS amongst prisoners and prison staff

Risk	Prisoners (%) N = 448	Prison staff (%) N = 294
None	17.7	3.4
Low	34.9	39.3
Medium	26.9	38.6
High	12.1	17.6
Very high	7.3	0.7

Note: (1) Due to non-completion of some questionnaires, percentages shown may not total 100%.
  (2) The risk to prisoners relates to life outside prison; the risk to prison staff relates to life inside prisons.

Subsequently, participants evaluating their risk as 'none' or 'low' were grouped together as 'low risk perceivers' while participants evaluating their risk as 'medium', 'high', and 'very high' were grouped together as 'high risk perceivers'. Their attitudes towards HIV/AIDS were assessed on the basis of their responses to five attitude statements concerning the following issues: objections to using shared facilities at work when it is found that a workmate is HIV antibody positive; prisoners should be allowed to refuse to wear clothing previously used by an HIV antibody positive prisoner; the government would be justified in creating a centralized file containing the names of all people known to be HIV antibody positive; homosexuals in the general public should be provided with free condoms; people who have contracted HIV through intravenous drug use do not deserve medical care. These particular statements were selected because they represented key HIV/AIDS issues as found in previous research by the present authors in Scottish prisons (McKee et al., submitted for publication). An analysis of variance of the participants' responses to the attitude items found a significant effect for participant status (staff vs. prisoner; $p<.01$) but not for risk status (high vs. low perceivers). Thus, prisoners' attitudes towards HIV/AIDS issues were more positive than staff's. However, an interaction effect (participant status vs. risk status; $p<.001$) was also found: staff high risk perceivers had more negative attitudes towards HIV/AIDS issues than staff low risk perceivers, whereas prisoners high risk perceivers had more positive attitudes than prisoner low risk perceivers. The interaction effect is presented in Figure 6.1.

Let us first consider the difference between prisoners' and staff's attitudes towards HIV/AIDS issues. It is the difference between those who are on different sides of the law. Therefore, it is not surprising that prisoners have more sympathy with those who, just as themselves, are on the 'blame side'. To use Goffman's distinction, there is a difference between those who are in a total institution and those who are outside.

More specifically, for staff, the perceived source of risk is the prison environment, and in particular prisoners, a group of 'others' relative to staff who can be perceived negatively without any damage to the self. In addition, prison staff may perceive little control over their risk of HIV inside prison as a result of this group of 'others'. HIV seropositive prisoners in Scotland are not segregated, and so are not clearly demarcated. Many HIV seropositive prisoners' HIV status will be unknown to staff. Thus, the virus will remain unseen, and the situation remain uncertain. In contrast, prisoners as a whole are already a marginalised sub-group of the population and their relatively more positive attitudes to those who are HIV seropositive could be an expression of sympathy for another marginalized sub-group. In addition, with regard to IDMs, the risk of HIV arises clearly from 'self' behaviours and therefore they are members of the very sub-group at risk.

The importance for risk perception of perceived control and the self – other distinction is also demonstrated in the interaction between participant status and risk status. Among prison staff, low risk perceivers had more

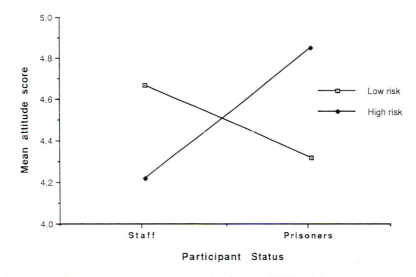

Figure 6.1 – Interaction between participant status, risk perception, and attitude to HIV/AIDS.

positive HIV/AIDS attitudes; in contrast, it is the low risk perceivers among prisoners who have the more negative attitudes towards HIV/AIDS.

Let us now consider the interaction effect. Amongst the staff, the low-risk perceivers had more positive attitudes towards HIV/AIDS issues. It is likely that they perceive less threat of HIV to themselves and therefore their attitudes towards those whom they perceive as responsible for the spread of HIV is more tolerant. However, high-risk perceivers amongst staff have more negative attitudes towards HIV/AIDS issues. It is likely that they feel threatened by those who spread HIV which is outwith their control.

In contrast, amongst the prisoners low-risk perceivers have, in relative terms, more negative attitudes towards HIV. Amongst this group of prisoners, there were very few IDMs. It is likely that IDMs will be viewed by prisoner low-risk perceivers as their main source of HIV/AIDS threat, and also as an 'other' sub-group within prisoners as a whole, thus allowing negative attitudes towards this group without damage to the self. Finally, of the four sub-groups, the prisoner high-risk perceivers had the most positive attitudes towards those with HIV/AIDS. Many of these high risk perceivers are past, present, and possibly future intravenous drug misusers. As mentioned before, they will have a fairly accurate understanding of their risk of HIV. As such, it is likely that they will identify with people with AIDS, making their attitudes more tolerant.

CONCLUSIONS

Throughout history and across many cultures, social representations of illness have been associated with notions of morality and social transgression. When a serious disease strikes society, the social response has frequently involved the identification and vilification of discrete groups prone to that disease. Such groups are often outside society or, if within society, stigmatized sub-groups. By this process, an easily identifiable and conspicuous external or minority 'other' can be blamed for society's ills, and the internal or majority 'self' protected from perceived danger from, and social responsibility for, the illness.

At the individual level, the self-other distinction is also important in risk perception. Individuals have an 'optimistic bias' in the perception of risk to the self relative to others, such bias giving the individual a feeling of being in control of his or her own fate. Social cognition models of health behaviour have allocated an important role to risk perception in influencing an individual's response to a health threat. However, such models usually conceptualize risk perception in simplistic terms. The appraisal of risk can occur on both a cognitive – rational level, and an emotional level. In addition, an individual's perception of control over the risk event will mediate the risk appraisal process, and thereby influence the individual's behavioural and attitudinal response. Furthermore, an individual's perception of risk is interdependent with his or her group self-categorization and, therefore, any analysis of risk perception must include an attempt to relate the observed phenomena to its appropriate social and cultural contexts.

The present authors' work on HIV/AIDS in prison illustrates some of the above issues. An optimistic bias in risk perception was found, as both prisoners' and prison staff's rating of personal risk of HIV/AIDS was lower than their rating of others' risk for both inside and outside of prison. For most comparisons, levels of concern about HIV/AIDS were greater than levels of perceived personal risk, supporting the idea that both cognitive – rational and emotional evaluations of risk are involved in the risk appraisal process. Finally, attitudes towards HIV/AIDS were found to be influenced by an interplay of cognitive and emotional evaluations of risk, perceived control, and group self-categorization by prisoners and prison staff.

REFERENCES

Adler, M. (1989), *Prisoners' rights and prison conditions in Scotland*. Paper presented to the seminar on 'Imprisonment today and tomorrow – new perspectives on prisoners' rights and prison condition', 19–23 September, Freiburg im Bresgau.

Agle, D. (1975), Psychological factors in haemophilia - the concept of self-care, *Annals of the New York Academy of Sciences*, 240, 221–225.

Beardsley, T. (1983), Animals as gamblers. In G. Ferry (ed.), *The Understanding of Animals*, Oxford: Blackwell and New Scientist.

Becker M. H. (1974), The health belief model and personal health behaviour. *Health education Monographs*, **2**, 326–473.

Brandt, A. M. (1988), AIDS in historical perspective: four lessons from the history of sexually transmitted diseases. *American Journal of Public Health*, **78**, 367–371.

Brown, P. (1993), HIV: high risk behind bars, *Answer*, (AIDS new supplement, CDS Weekly Report), 12 March, 1–2.

Calnan, M. and Johnson, B. (1985), Health, health risks and inequalities: An exploratory study of women's perceptions. *Sociology of Health and Illness*, **7**, 55–75.

Coleman, R. M., Curtis, D. and Feinmann, C. (1988), Perception of risk of HIV infection by injecting drug users and effects on medical clinic attendance. *British Journal of Addiction*, **83**, 1325–1329.

Curran, L., McHugh, M., Nooney, K. (1989), HIV Counselling in prisons, *AIDS CARE*, **1**, 11–25.

Dolan, K. A., Donoghue, M. C. and Stimson G. V. (1990), Drug injecting and syringe sharing in custody and in the community: an exploratory survey of HIV risk behaviour, *The Howard Journal of Criminal Justice*, **29**, 177–186.

Douglas, M. (1986), *Risk Acceptability According to the Social Sciences*, London: Routledge and Kegan Paul.

Douglas, M. (1992), *Risk and Blame*, Routledge: London and New York.

Dowell, K. A., Lo Presto, C. T. and Sherman, M. F. (1991), When are AIDS patients to blame for their disease? Effects of patients' sexual orientation and mode of transmission, *Psychological Reports*, **69**, 211–19.

Dubos, R. (1968), *Man, Medicine and Environment*, London : Pall Mall.

Dye, S. and Isaacs, C. (1991), Intravenous drug misuse among prison inmates: implication for spread of HIV, *British Medical Journal*, **302**, 1506.

Eagly, A. H. (1992), Uneven progress: Social psychology and the study of attitudes, *Journal of Personality and Social Psychology*, **62**, 693–710.

Elford, J. (1987), Moral and social aspects of AIDS: a medical students' project, *Social Science and Medicine*, **24**, 543–49.

Gigerenzer, G., Swijtink, Z., Porter, T., Daston, L., Beatty, J. and Kruger, L. (1989), *The Empire of Chance*, Cambridge and New York: Cambridge University Press.

Gillies, P. and Carballo, M. (1990), Adult perception of risk, risk behaviour and HIV/AIDS: a focus for intervention and research, *AIDS*, **4**, 943–951.

Hammet, T. M. (1988), *AIDS in Correctional Facilities: Issues and Options*. 3rd Edn. US Department of Justice, National Institute of Justice.

Harding, T. W. (1987), AIDS in prisons, *British Medical Journal*, **297**, 873–874.

Herzlich, C, and Pierret, J. (1987), *Illness and Self in Society*. Baltimore: The Johns Hopkins University Press, (French original, 1984).

Herlitz, C. and Brorsson, B. (1990), AIDS in the minds of the Swedish people: 1986–1989, *AIDS*, **4**, 1011–1018.

Horton, M, and Aggleton, P. (1989), Perverts, inverts and experts: the cultural production of an AIDS research paradigm. In P. Aggleton, G. Hart and P. Davies, (eds), *AIDS:Social Representation and Social Practices* London: Falmer Press.

Joseph, J. G. Montgomery, S. B., Emmons, C, Kirscht, J. P., Kessler, R. C., Ostrow, D. G., Wortman, C. B. and O'Brian, K. (1987), Perceived risk of AIDS: assessing the behavioural and psychosocial consequences in a cohort of gay men, *Journal of Applied Social psychology*, **17**, 231–250.

Katz, A, H. (1970), *Haemophilia. A Study in Hope and Reality*. Springfield: Charles. C. Thomas.

Kelley, J., Lawrence, J. Smith, S., Hoop, H. and Cook, D. (1987), Medical students' attitudes toward AIDS and homosexual patients, *Journal of School Health*, **62**, 549–56.

Landrine, H. and Klonoff, E. A. (1992), Culture and health–related schemas: a review and proposal for interdisciplinary integration, *Health Psychology*, **11**, 267–276.

Laurence, J. (1988), Condom issue in jails to beat AIDS, *New Society*, **22**, 5.

Leventhal, H., Meyer, D., and Nerenz, D. (1980), The common sense representation of illness danger. In S. Rachman (ed.), *Contributions to Medical Psychology* **2**, Oxford: Pergamon.

Lyon A. S. and Petrucelli R. I. (1987), *Medicine. The Illustrated History*, New York: Abradale Press.

Marková, I., Forbes, C. and Inwood, M. (1984), Consumers' views of genetic counselling in haemophilia. *The American Journal of Medical Genetics*, **17**, 741–752.

Marková, I., Lockyer, R. and Forbes, C. (1980), Self–perception of employed and unemployed haemophiliacs, *Psychological Medicine*, **10**, 559–565.

Marková, I., et al (1990), Self–and other–awareness of the risk of HIV/AIDS in people with haemophilia and implications for behavioural change, *Social Science and Medicine*, **31**, 73–79.

McKee K. J, Marková I, and Power K. G., (Submitted for publication). Concern, perceived risk and attitudes towards HIV/AIDS in Scottish prisons.

McKee, K. J., and Power, K. G. (1992), HIV/AIDS in prisons, *Scottish Medical Journal*, **37**, 132–137.

McKeganey, N., Barnard, M. and Watson, H. (1989), HIV–related risk behaviour among a non–clinic sample of injecting drug users, *British Journal of Addiction*, **84**, 1481–1490.

McMillan, A. (1988), HIV in prisons, *British Medical Journal*, **297**, 873–874.

Mondragón, D., Kirkman–Liff, B. and Schneller, E. S. (1991), Hostility to people with AIDS: risk perception and demographic factors. *Social Science Medicine*, **32**, 1137–1142.

Pegg, M. G. (1990), Le corps et l'autorité: le lèpre de Badouin IV, *Annales ESC*, mars–avril, **2**, 265–87.

Power, K. G., Marková, I., Rowlands, A., McKee, K. J., Anslow, P. J. and Kilfedder, C. (1992a), Intravenous drug use and HIV transmission amongst prisoners in Scottish prisons, *British Journal of Addiction*, **87**, 35–45.

Power, K. G., Marková, I., Rowlands, A., McKee, K. J., Anslow, P. J. and Kilfedder, C. (1992b), Comparison of sexual behaviour and risk of HIV transmission of Scottish inmates with or without a history of intravenous drug use, *AIDS Care*, **4**, 53–67.

Power, K. G., Marková, I., Rowlands, A., McKee K. J. and Kilfedder, C. (1994), Inmate self–perceived risk of HIV injection inside and outside Scottish prisons, *Health Education Research*, **9**, 47–55.

Power, K. G., Marková, I., Rowlands, A., McKee, K. J. and Kilfedder C. (1993), HIV and AIDS–related knowledge amongst inmates of Scottish prisons, *Health Education Journal*, **52**, 13–18.

Prentice–Dunn, S. and Rogers, R. W. (1986), Protection Motivation Theory and preventive health: beyond the Health Belief Model, *Health Education Research*, **1**, 153–61.

Prison Reform Trust, (1988), *HIV, AIDS and prisons*. Prison Reform Trust, London.

Slovic, P. Perception of risk, (1987), *Science*, **236**, 208–285.

Sontag S. (1989), *AIDS and its Metaphors*, Harmondworth: Penguin.

Stimson G. V., Donoghue, M. Alldritt, L., Dolan, K. (1988), HIV transmission risk behaviour of clients attending syringe exchange schemes in England and Scotland, *British Journal of Addiction*, **83**, 1449–1455.

Stockdale, J. E. Dockrell, J. E., and Wells, A. J. (1989), The self in relation to mass media representations of HIV and AIDS – match or mismatch? *Health Education Journal* **48**, 121–130.

Taylor, S., (1983), Adjustment to threatening events: a theory of cognitive adaptation. *American Psychologist*, **38** (11), 1161–1173.

Triplet, R. and Sugarman, D. (1987), Undergraduate and graduate students' attitudes toward AIDS, *Psychological Reports*, **60**, 1185–86.

Watney, S., (1989), The subject of AIDS, In P. Aggleton, G. Hart, and P. Davies, (eds), *AIDS: Social representation and social practices*, London: Falmer press.

Weinstein, N. D. (1980), Unrealistic optimism about future life events, *Journal of Personality and Social Psychology*, **39**, 806–820.

Weinstein, N. D. (1984), Why it won't happen to me: perceptions of risk factors and illness suspectibility, *Health Psychology*, **3**, 431–457.

Wilkie, P. A. (1993), *Genetic counselling and adult polycystic kidney disease: patients' knowledge, perceptions and understanding*, Unpublished PhD thesis, Department of Psychology, University of Stirling.

World Health Organisation (1987), *Special Programme on AIDS. Statement from the consultation on prevention and control of AIDS in prison*, Geneva: W.H.O.

CHAPTER SEVEN

Clinical Diagnosis and the Joint Construction of a Medical Voice

Karin ARONSSON[1], Ullabeth SÄTTERLUND LARSSON[2] and
Roger SÄLJÖ[2]*

[1]*Department of Child Studies, Linköping University,
S-581 83 Linköping, Sweden*
[2]*Department of Communication Studies, Linköping University,
S-581 83 Linköping, Sweden*

INTRODUCTION

According to the dominant perspective on human communication, linguistic signs derive their meaning from the fact that they refer to objects and events in the world. Words 'point to' an extra-linguistic reality, and sentences uttered or written contain 'propositional content' that makes claims about states of affairs in the world. This assumption of a correspondence between the sign and what is signified is part of a pervasive attitude to communication in lay, as well as scholarly, discourse. When people communicate, they use 'concepts' to 'transport content' to another individual, who, in turn, 'decodes' the 'concepts' to create an inner image of what is 'meant'. This 'conduit metaphor' of communication, described by Reddy (1979; cf. Linell, 1988), is so much part and parcel of our understanding that it may indeed be difficult to see what is problematic about it.

In this paper, we try to avoid some of the hidden assumptions that follow from such a mechanistic perspective on human communication. One of the most problematic aspects of this attitude, and of the rationalist, Cartesian, conception of language, thought and human action as a whole (cf. Marková, 1982), is that "the interplay of signs is not treated as a reality in its own right." (Silverman and Torode, 1980, p.3). Human communication is thus construed as a second-order phenomenon, as merely an abstract version of the 'objective' world in which people have their 'real' interests, projects and commitments.

In our perspective, communication is *per se* a significant form of social action. It is through the use of language and other means of

---

* Roger Säljö presented a first version of this paper at the "International Conference of Applied Psychology" in Kyoto, July 22–27, 1990. The authors appear in alphabetical order.

communicating that it is possible to coordinate social activities, to recreate and to maintain social order. The world in which we live and act is thus embedded in language and we know it as nothing else. That linguistic expressions have referential meaning, i.e., that they 'point to' an external reality, does not imply that the world is independent of our way of naming it and talking about it; words exist "only from within a form of social life already constituted by the ways of talking in which such words are used." (Shotter, 1987, p. 11; cf. Rommetveit, 1973). To study human communication in this perspective is not to study a separate and enclosed realm of reality that can be captured in a language devoid of reference to what people do in 'real' life. When we communicate, we act in the world by creating contexts in which relationships and commitments are developed and maintained and in which concrete and abstract projects are jointly pursued.

LINGUISTIC COMPLEXITY AND MODERN SOCIETY

From a social constructivist point of view, professional interviewing can be seen as a type of recycling of 'facts' into accounts that make sense in, for instance, medical or legal bureaucracies (Aronsson, 1991). Accounts of the past are inherently contestable in that all narration is perspectivized and evaluative (Volosinov, 1973). Different interviewers therefore may generate different accounts of the past (Mishler, 1986). In medical consultations doctors interview patients about their medical histories and their plans or hopes for the future (pregnancies, operations, recovery, etc.). In interviewing patients, doctors become intimately familiar with patients' biographies and life projects.

The particular issue which interests us here is interaction in medical settings. Such interaction can be viewed as an instance of institutional discourse (Agar, 1985), where specific forms of understanding and of explaining the world have evolved to fit the needs of actors operating in specialized "provinces of meaning" (Schutz, 1962; Berger and Luckmann, 1966) in complex societies. As is obvious from the literature, interaction in such settings is generally asymmetrical in terms of power, expertise and the distribution of interactional space. The professionals, i.e. the physicians, ask more questions and they control topics and topic boundaries, to mention just a few of the differences in communicative roles and responsibilities that appear in the literature (cf. Aronsson and Larsson, 1987; Fisher, 1984; Larsson, 1989; Todd, 1983). Communication in institutional settings builds on a different set of assumptions than does everyday interaction. The specific ways of describing the world that develops are part of what Habermas (1970) refers to as rational-purposive communication, i.e., interactional patterns that serve certain ends and that form part of the domain of work in society. The encounter between the patient and the physician is motivated by the fact that the former needs the assistance of the professional, and the unequal distribution of conversational power is linked to this dependency of the layman on the expertise of the interlocutor. This interaction is furthermore subordinated to the exchange of economic resources in society. Salient features of interaction in specific provinces of meaning, however, do not merely concern who talks and how much each interlocutor is privileged to talk. The specific modes of referring to and understanding reality-the "ways of world-making" (Goodman, 1978)-also change as professional languages develop. Mishler (1984), in an in-depth study of medical discourse, has illustrated the conflict between what he refers to as the "voice of medicine" and the "voice of the life world", "representing, respectively, the technical -scientific assumptions of medicine and the natural attitude of everyday life" (p. 14). The voice of medicine is part of what Habermas (1970) refers to as "technocratic consciousness"; the scientific, bio-medical frame of reference, within which problems are understood and interpreted. Significant discursive features of this voice are "affectively neutral, functionally specific, context-stripping questions and responses by physicians" (p. 164), and focus on "objective parameters" of the situation that isolate "symptoms from patients' more general problems and life-world experiences." (loc. cit.). Mishler (1984) illustrates how such context-stripping, objective features of situations are used to appropriate patients' accounts into the voice of medicine. In one instance, a patient introduces her heavy drinking into the conversation with her physician, and in the following quotation one can see how the physician in a very concrete sense decontextualizes this problem from the patient's life-world circumstances (from Mishler, 1984, p. 165).

Dr   ...How long have you been drinking that heavily?

P   ...Since I've been married.

Dr   ...How long is that?

P   (giggle...) Four years.

By requiring the patient to specify how long she has been drinking, the physician achieves several things. He indicates that the answer in socio-biographical terms, "since I've been married", does not count as an adequate response. By insisting on the exact number of years as the required quantification, the physician invokes the voice of medicine by asserting "universalistic criteria for the adequacy of a response" (p. 165). He also decontextualizes the problems of drinking from the life-world concerns and worries of the patient by not responding to her invitation to see the connection between her marriage and her health problems. In his study, Mishler also illustrates in a sensitive account how a physician can move beyond the technological language of the voice of medicine by addressing patient issues and concerns in life-world terms. In the present article we want to add to Mishler's analysis and to illustrate what is, in some sense, the opposite case; how patients sometimes appropriate perspectives on themselves and their health problems characteristic of the voice of medicine, and how they actively contribute to maintaining a dialogue within that voice.

THE CASE OF LISA

The problem of conflicting voices in dialogues in professional settings is generally approached by supposing that the dominant party controls the dialogue by invoking a technical voice and selectively attending to what patients say to fit the technological-rational interests of the biomedical model. Mishler (1984, p. 182) summarizes his findings by saying that "what we found in typical medical interviews (was that) the lifeworld was "absorbed" into the technocratic consciousness expressed in the voice of medicine." (cf. Todd, 1983; Larsson, 1989). However, all dialogues presuppose mutuality in terms of the perspectives employed by the interlocutors and in the following we shall attempt to illustrate, by means of a case study, how patients' contributions to interaction may in subtle ways evoke or reinforce the use of the technical-scientific language characteristic of the voice of medicine.

The patient we will focus on is Lisa, 28 years of age, who has a long and complex medical history. This case is drawn from a larger study of patient-doctor interaction that has been reported in detail elsewhere (Aronsson and Larsson, 1987; Larsson, Säljö and Aronsson, 1987). In the present analysis we shall draw on data from the transcribed consultation with a specialist in a hospital clinic of internal medicine, as well as from two post-consultation interviews, one with Lisa and one with the physician. These interviews were carried out immediately after the consultation. The consultation lasted 35 minutes. On this occasion, Lisa is on referral to the clinic for internal medicine for further examinations of possible causes of her obesity. Initially, the physician misconstrues the situation as having to do with her recent menstrual problems and with the fact that her breasts have lactated. Lisa, however, has already received treatment for these problems and she is at present under medication to which she, in her own judgement, has responded favourably. Almost three years prior to this consultation, Lisa had a breast reduction at a clinic for plastic surgery and she suspects that this is connected with the milk coming from her breasts, although she has received no support for this suspicion from the physicians she has consulted.

According to Lisa's own description, her health problems began when she was 19 when she began to suffer from "psychological problems". She was constantly "feeling sick" and eventually she developed "phobias and such stuff" and she found it difficult to use public transport and go by train and tram. She underwent psychiatric treatment, and extensive investigations of the possible causes of her "feeling sick" were carried out, but as the present physician expresses it-in the voice of medicine-in his summary of her description; "they couldn't find anything, could they...". About a year later "this weight increase began", Lisa states in the consultation, "and my legs started to get swollen." In a relatively short time Lisa doubled her weight. Following this Lisa has been a frequent visitor to hospitals and she has undergone extensive examinations by several specialists in different clinics. Her metabolism and her kidney functions have been checked and rechecked and she has visited several clinics for her obesity. She is still under surveillance by the gynaecologist for her menstrual problems. In recent years, she has also developed eczema for which she is receiving treatment from a dermatologist. Her psychiatric problems developed into depressions and when the consultation takes place Lisa has been on sick leave for a lengthy period. She is also undergoing further examinations for her depressions. She is using different kinds of medication; sedatives, anti-depressants as well as drugs for her menstrual problems and the milk in her breasts and for her sickness feelings.

THE EXAMINATION AND PATIENT-DOCTOR RAPPORT

The interaction in the consultation setting runs smoothly with few or no overt signs of misunderstandings on the part of Lisa. In fact, Lisa displays a high degree of expertise in the discussion and she is able to provide fairly exact details about her previous and present test results in different respects. In one passage, where an abnormal value of a hormone test is discussed, Lisa knows her normal values and she can also tell that the value shown in her test must be wrong, since lately it has been consistently going down.

They jointly decide that there must be something wrong with the test and the doctor adds that they "have started using a new computer" which has produced some "strange results". Lisa is also knowledgeable about the different kinds of medication she has been using over the years and she provides exact information on their side-effects.

Excerpt 1		(medical consultation)
11	Dr[*]	Have you noticed any improvement in that connection?
12	L	Well, the menstruation has come back.
13	Dr	Yeah.
14	L	And now, I have increased the dosage to three pills a day, and then the milk has decreased, but that's only a month ago.

As can be seen, Lisa uses medical jargon ('dosage') and she talks about medication in quite a detailed way.

Excerpt 2		(medical consultation)
242	Dr	...have you had any trouble, have you, for instance been constipated or had stomach problems?
243	L	Well, that has been the last few years, but I think that depends on those Anaframil and Semil
244	Dr	Anaframil, Semil...
245	L	Well, I don't know.
246	Dr	Yeah, that's right, that may cause constipation, well, that's quite right.

---

[*] Legends: I = Interviewer (Ullabeth Sätterlund Larsson); Dr = Doctor; L = Lisa

Lisa consistently responds to the doctor's questions in an efficient way (as acknowledged above, turn 246, "well, that's quite right"). In all, she epitomizes the competent patient. In the post-consultation interview, the physician spontaneously talks about Lisa as someone who knows her way around the hospital and who is "easy to inform".

Excerpt 3		(post-consultation interview with physician)
2	I	Do you think she was a normal patient or was she different in any way?
3	Dr	No, she was…what I mean is that she was young and…which always simplifies understanding (...) and, also, she had a certain routine of health care if you put it like that…during the last 10 years. And this made her sort of easy to inform, partially due to her age and partially because she was, sort of used to the environment.

Yet, looking at the encounter from Lisa's point of view, the outcome is very negative and she shows strong emotional reactions during the post-consultation interview, reactions she had evidently suppressed during the dialogue with the doctor.

Excerpt 4		(post-consultation interview with Lisa)
32	L	(...) I felt disappointed when I left…here sort of, I did.
33	I	Why?
34	L	Well I wanted something radical to happen sort of…
35	I	Something should happen with…
36	L	my weight (starts crying)
37	I	You don't think you could say what you really felt, or…
38	L	(shakes her head, cries)

Moreover, Lisa complains that she feels that she is "at a disadvantage".

Excerpt 5		(post-consultation interview with Lisa)
104	L	Yes, I am at a disadvantage, sort of all the time,.
105	I	In what sense?
106	L	In terms of knowledge in some way. I can, I have nothing to oppose (the doctor) with…that would be sort of concrete (...)
108	L	Yes, I can't do anything when he, sort of, says 'no' I can't.

VOICING AND THE CO-ORDINATION OF TALK

To understand this mismatch between a competent patient (who "is easy to inform") and the reactions of disappointment and despair afterwards, one has to scrutinize the consultation and the interview with Lisa to see how Lisa's situation is construed and talked about.

The message Lisa has received in the consultation is that there is nothing medically wrong with her. On repeated occasions the physician explains in detail that all the tests have been negative and that there is nothing else in her symptoms that indicates that there is anything abnormal with her metabolic functions.

> **Excerpt 6**   (medical consultation)
> 328 Dr   (...) Well, Lisa,...as I said, at first one suspects that you
>   could have too low a metabolism. That I haven't sort of...
>   there is nothing that indicates that, neither in the way you
>   feel nor in how you look nor...Also, the laboratory tests
>   indicate that there would not be such a..., let's say cause,
>   that one could easily remedy...

What seems to contribute to Lisa's feeling of despair, and what makes her argue that she is "at a disadvantage" and can do or say nothing when "he says no", is that she is denied a medical explanation of her condition. The therapeutic measures that the physician suggests on repeated occasions are to "reduce your intake of calories", to consult a dietician at the clinic and to increase physical exercise. All of these lifestyle measures are unacceptable to Lisa, who explains that she cannot manage to keep to a diet, nor to do physical exercise.

In Mishler's study, the issue of how the patient relates and responds to discourse in the the two voices is summarized by saying that the patient "tries to stay in touch with the voice of medicine by connecting her statements in response to the physician's questions." (1984, p. 124). However, "at the same time, she adds other information, often in the voice of the life-world. Thus, she attempts to retain her meaning of her problem in its experienced context and, thereby, keep her own perspective alive in the discourse" (loc. cit.).

Yet it is obvious that it would be too simplistic to attribute the tendency to talk in terms of the voice of medicine to the physician alone. In fact, in scrutinizing Lisa's contributions to the discourse it becomes evident that she actively attempts to keep the conversation within that voice. She also makes this clear to the physician by stating in response to one of his lengthy explanations of her negative test results that she had hoped for a biomedical explanation of her condition that would point to a specific disease that could be cured through medication.

> **Excerpt 7**   (medical consultation)
> 261 Dr   (...) if one looks at you here, it doesn't look, you don't
>   look as if you had too low a metabolism...and we've
>   taken tests too, a couple of blood tests that give quite a
>   good picture of that. And they're normal as far as the
>   function of your thyroid gland is concerned, so there...
> 262 L   Mmm, mm...
> 263 Dr   ... no reason to suspect that, there isn't, which sort of
>   many may feel to be unfortunate since it would have been
>   easier to just give, take a pill...
> 264 L   Mm, exactly.

265	Dr	...and increase the metabolism and take away a few kilos...
266	L	Mmm.
267	Dr	...but...
268	L	that's what I had hoped for here, mm,...
269	Dr	That doesn't seem to be the case. Of course, we've only checked this once, we're going to do it once more, but they really look good...and also your other tests appear quite excellent. You've got a sedimentation rate of 5, and your blood value is perfect, about 100%, that is 146.
270	L	Mmm.
271	Dr	...completely normal...and liver and kidney functions are normal, blood sugar and blood fats are normal too (goes on to explain further test results).

It is easy to see that most of the dialogue in the present consultation is kept within the voice of medicine. When the doctor gives his suggestions to reduce the calorie intake and to increase physical exercise, for instance, these measures are not contextualized in the wider circumstances of Lisa's life and work. Both lifestyle issues are addressed within the confines of a strictly biomedical model of man and as involving nothing apart from the technicalities of the intake and burning of calories.

On no fewer than five occasions during the consultation, the physician introduces the dietician as the most suitable person to deal with Lisa's problems. The advice he gives is for Lisa to come and "talk to" the dietician if "she is interested". The relationship with the dietician is, however, consistently referred to against the background that medically there is nothing really wrong with Lisa. To these repeated suggestions of contacting a dietician, Lisa responds either by silent opposition (Aronsson and Larsson, 1987) or by stating that she cannot manage diets. The third time the doctor introduces the dietician, Lisa manages to summon up the communicative energy and courage to go against the doctor's line of thinking by introducing the issue of medication, hence reinstating the voice of medicine as it were, changing the topic from that of lifestyles to that of medicine.

Excerpt 8   (medical consultation)

351	Dr	(...) And moreover I'll write a note on our referral to the dietician.
353	L	Mmm.
354	Dr	You could come here and talk to her some time, couldn't you?
355	L	There are no pills that one can get that would reduce these hunger feelings in the meantime?
356	D	Well, I don't know. Have you tried Novalucid, one could sort of prescribe acid neutralising medication (...)

At the same time as he complies with Lisa's wish to talk about medication, it is obvious that he does this in a way that shows that he does not perceive these pills as an effective means of dealing with Lisa's consistent feelings of being hungry. This is evident, among other things, by his using expressions such as "one could try" these pills and the fact that they are meant for other symptoms than Lisa's. Lisa also knows this since she is familiar with this particular medicine. It is also interesting to see how Lisa temporarily accommodates to the doctor's treatment plan by asking for a pill that reduces "the hunger feelings in the meantime", i.e before she gets to see the dietician. At this stage she has given up hope of getting a 'real' medical treatment of the kind for which she has been hoping.

Even though the physician does what he is supposed to do as an ideal and sensitive clinician, by devoting a lot of time to Lisa and by being eager to provide detailed and repeated information on test results and other aspects of the situation, it is not difficult to see how his argumentation demoralizes Lisa by placing her problems outside the medical sphere. The alternative of referring her to a dietician becomes something that you do since there is "nothing tangibly…medically wrong" as he puts it.

Excerpt 9   (medical consultation)
374   Dr   (…) And then I'll write a note to our dietician and she'll get in touch with you…
375   L   Mmm ..
376   Dr   And then, of course, it's a poor consolation since we have found nothing tangibly…
377   L   Yes, I think so too (laughs).
378   Dr   …medically wrong that one could put one's finger on and say: "Take this medicine and you'll get well." We haven't done that, sort of.

In Lisa's analysis of her own situation, solving the problems of her over-weight should be done through 'real' medical treatment. Such treatment should imply no other consequences for her life than that of reducing her weight. In the post-consultation interview, she presents what she had wanted, but did not dare, to introduce seriously into the discussion with the doctor.

Excerpt 10   (post-consultation interview with Lisa)
45   I   No…but don't you think that the dietician can help you to get a programme that will enable you to manage (a diet)?
46   L   No, honestly speaking, I don't think so. I felt disappointed when I left there (inaudible).
47   I   You want something else to happen?
48   L   Mmnnn…
49   I   What did you, what had you…What did you think would happen?
50   L   Well, not that they would perform an operation but that there was some kind of pill that could be used then, sort of. I had hoped that there would be something wrong with those other tests, the hormone tests then…

Later in the interview, Lisa returns to this issue, and by listening to her, one can see that she has done a lot of thinking on possible medical treatments that she could not find the courage to introduce and to discuss with the doctor.

Excerpt 11   (post-consultation interview with Lisa)
88   L   (...) I feel disappointed anyway, I had expected something more from this.
89   I   (...) What did you think would happen really?
90   L   Well, either I thought like this; He has found something with hormones or whatever these tests were about that they'd taken sort of...and that it would be possible to prescribe something since I have problems with the prolactin (a hormone), and then I thought that or I thought that I wanted sort of to go through an operation then.
91   I   Yes, in what way do you mean?
92   L   Well, have my stomach reduced or the intestines or one of those things you have (inaudible). That's what I wanted to do. Still, I sit in there and agree...
93   I   Why did you do that?
94   L   I don't know. I am like that when I go to places like this. It's like that everywhere.

Lisa's reactions of disappointment are rooted in the fact that she did not dare to discuss these suggestions seriously during the interview. The physician's long and detailed presentation on repeated occasions of all the test results that show that there is nothing wrong with her in a biomedical sense makes it difficult for her to argue her case and ask the critical question as to whether she could have a pill or surgery that would make her lose weight. Metaphorically speaking she loses the battle about the possible causes of her obesity within the medical voice in which she wants to keep it. In her own view, she does this since she has "nothing with which to oppose" the doctor who has the expertise and the power to make authorized statements in this domain.

LISA'S SITUATION AND THE VOICE OF MEDICINE

The point of our analysis so far is that the physician and Lisa form an alliance, as it were, maintaining the conversation within the voice of medicine, and that Lisa is active in maintaining this voice. The attempts by the physician to get her to agree to see a dietician can be read as an attempt to invoke the voice of the life-world by pointing to factors that concern Lisa's lifestyle such as her eating habits, physical exercise and so on; factors that the doctor believes to be essential for explaining her present situation. Lisa's constant negative reactions to diets, physical exercise and similar measures can be interpreted as ways of preventing lifeworld and lifestyle issues from entering the picture and being considered in the context of her health situation. She wants to avoid them because of the implications they carry.

Looking at the consultation and the two post-consultation interviews, it is not difficult to discern life-world aspects of Lisa's problems. For one thing, her general social situation appears difficult. She is living alone and works half time in a day care centre. This job is a semi-sheltered position that she got because of her "psychological problems". For the other half of her time she has a permanent sickness pension. Even though she claims that she likes her job, she has not been there for quite some time owing to her sick leave. Now she feels that it is "awfully difficult to go there at all". In commenting on her living alone, Lisa makes a remark that has similarities with the way that the patient in Mishler's study connected her drinking problems with her marriage.

Excerpt 12   (post-consultation interview with Lisa)
173   I   (...) Have you always lived alone?
174   L   No, I've been living with someone for a couple of years
               too. That was before these problems began...

If one considers the hypothesis that Lisa's existential situation is related to her problems, there are several points in the dialogue with the physician where invitations to take up her life-world surface. It is evident that Lisa is well aware of the fact that she eats too much. About her negative reactions to seeing a dietician, for instance, she says that it will be impossible for her to follow "all those pieces of good advice" that she will get. On a couple of occasions, she responds to the suggestion of seeing a dietician by saying "It [a diet] is more than I can manage" (159). On these occasions, the doctor moves to other issues. He does not probe into her articulated pessimism about diets. In one instance, she makes what could be read as a further specification that connects to her life-world when saying "I cannot make it on my own, sort of" (335). When commenting on her eating habits in the post-consultation interview, she makes an interesting remark that is connected to the success of dieting. She says that "I eat in one way there (at the day care centre) sort of, but in a different way when I am alone at home" (170). The point here is that there is a difference in how much she eats when in the company of others as compared to when eating alone and that this is something that could have been expanded on in the consultation.

The idea behind pointing to this life-world interpretation of Lisa's conception of her situation and of the interaction she has with the physician is not to argue that this interpretation is more correct than the biomedical one dominating the discourse. We know very little about her, a situation which we, by the way, share with her physician who has never seen her before and only knows a small part of her medical history. Nor do we want to argue that she is not really ill at all. Instead, our point is merely to illustrate that there appear to be certain options with respect to how her situation could be framed, to use the language of Goffman, options that are not taken up of in the consultation.

Character work in dialogue is intimately linked to mutual ideas about face (Goffman, 1961). In the interactional construction of a health biography during the medical consultation, the doctor does not probe more deeply into the patient's eating practices or her thinking in the area of physical excercise. The patient, in her turn, does not impose her worries on the doctor. When the doctor does not respond to her misgivings about physical exercise or dieting, she neither details her misgivings, nor does she insist on a medical solution to their problems (e.g. in terms of medication or an operation). In a somewhat collusive fashion, both parties thus avoid penetrating topics that may threaten their mutual respect or esteem (face).

Multi-party talk is inherently collusive in that two persons may directly or indirectly cast a third party as an outsider or a less legitimate party (McDermott and Tylbor, 1987). In the present doctor-patient talk the two principal actors at times speak in the voice of medicine, at other times in the voice of the life-world. The very existence of a technocratic voice and a life world voice seems to create a discursive ambiguity that can be exploited for self- and other-oriented facework. Moreover, an actor may speak in a dominant voice or in ways that cast a different voice as subordinate or less legitimate. Similarly, and perhaps more interestingly, it has been seen how one of the two actors may chose to respond in the voice of medicine to a question posed in the voice of the life-world or the other way around. Ultimately, choice of voice must be related to power hierarchies in that it is the person in control, the professional (doctor) who accepts voice switching. On several accounts, doctors and patients may thus switch between medical voices and life-world voices in ways that can be seen as collusive.

CONCLUSION

At one level, Lisa's problem is an objective, biomedical one; she is obese and she is suffering from different diseases and symptoms. Although she is well aware of the fact that she eats too much, she construes her constant "feeling of being hungry" as the immediate and biomedical cause of her eating. On another level, the experiential basis of health conditions is culturally relative and intimately intertwined with the dominant interpretations of what symptoms mean and how they can be explained. Without denying the objective basis, it seems possible to argue that being ill is based on a collective and shared body of knowledge about the specific nature and origin of diseases. As Herzlich (1973) puts it, the "adult learns from society to be ill" (p. 4) in terms of how to experience bodily reactions as well as how to regard the origins and possible cause and effect-relationships underlying a certain condition. There are 'accounting practices' (Shotter, 1987) for such phenomena that provide order to experiences and conditions that in many cases would lend themselves to multiple interpretations.

The fact that Lisa and her doctor never manage to construct a dialogue outside the voice of medicine is thus linked to the distribution of knowledge in society and the dominance of a certain voice in an institutional setting. Both interlocutors operate within discursive boundaries with respect to what accounts of the patient's situation can be presented and defended as appropriate in the particular context of a medical consultation. To transcend these boundaries is to take risks with potentially high costs for the expert as well as the patient. The expert may feel he/she is moving outside his/her area of expertise and the patient may have to change her perspective on her disease.

The attempt to initiate a life-world dialogue by the physician when suggesting that she see a dietician is resisted by Lisa because of the implications it carries with respect to treatment. She has, in a profound sense, learned to view her problem as biomedical in origin and her excessive eating as secondary to that. The fact that she eats more when she is alone and other similar observations are not in the foreground. The doctor does not probe why a diet, in Lisa's words, is "more than I can manage", nor does Lisa persist in articulating her life-world misgivings (in the way that she, in fact, does during the post-consultation interview). Lisa and her doctor form a biomedical alliance, as it were. The adoption of this biomedical perspective illustrates one of the points made by Habermas (1970); how scientific and rational-purposive forms of understanding infiltrate everyday understanding and gain dominance also over descriptions in the world of laymen. In this sense, and in line with our initial claim about communication as action, we would agree with Gergen (1985) that "descriptions and explanations of the world themselves constitute forms of social action." (p. 268). Experiences of health and illness as well as the clinical practice in health care encounters are shaped within discursive boundaries. It is our belief that to deal successfully with the growing spectrum of diseases that are related to our life styles, it is especially important to analyze doctors' and patients' joint constructions of illness biographies in medical contexts. The stories we live-and tell-about medical problems are collective products and they are mediated through language.

REFERENCES

Agar, M. (1985), Institutional discourse, *Text*, 5, 147–168.

Aronsson, K. (1991), Social interaction and the recycling of legal evidence. In N. C. Coupland, H. Giles and J. M. Wiemann (Eds.), *Miscommunication and Problematic Talk.* (pp.215–243). Newbury Park: Sage.

Aronsson, K. and Larsson, U. S. (1987), Politeness strategies and doctor-patient communication. On the social choreography of collaborative thinking. *Journal of Language and Social Psychology,* **6**, 1–27.

Berger, P. and Luckmann, T. (1966), *The Social Construction of Reality.* New York: Doubleday.

Fisher, S. (1984), Institutional authority and the structure of discourse. *Discourse Processes,* **7**, 201–224,

Gergen, K. (1985), The social constructionist movement in social psychology. *American Psychologist,* **40**, 266–275.

Goffman, E. (1961), *Encounters: Two studies in the sociology of interaction.* London: Allen Lane/Penguin Press.

Goodman, N. (1978), *Ways of Worldmaking*. Indianapolis: Hackett.

Habermas, J. (1970), *Toward a Rational Society*. Boston, MA.:Beacon Press.

Herzlich, C. (1973), *Health and Illness. A social psychological analysis*. London: Academic Press.

Larsson, U. S. (1989), *Being Involved: Patient participation in health care*. Linköping: University of Linköping.

Larsson, U. S., Säljö, R. and Aronsson, K. (1987), Patient-doctor communication on smoking and drinking: Lifestyle in medical consultations. *Social Science and Medicine*, **25**, 1129–1137.

Linell, P. (1988), The impact of literacy on the conception of language: The case of linguistics. In R. Säljö (Ed.), *The Written World* (pp. 41–58). Berlin & New York: Springer.

Marková, I. (1982), *Paradigms, Thought, and Language*. Chichester: Wiley.

McDermott, R. P. and Tylbor, H. (1987), On the necessity of collusion in conversation. In L. Kedar (Ed.), *Power through discourse*. Norwood, New Jersey:Ablex.

Mishler, E. (1984), *The Discourse of Medicine: Dialectics of medical interviews*. Norwood, N. J.: Ablex.

Mishler, E. (1986), *Research Interviewing*. Cambridge, Mass: Harvard University Press.

Reddy, M. (1979), The conduit metaphor - a case of frame conflict in our language about language. In A. Ortony (Ed.), *Metaphor and Thought* (pp. 284–324). Cambridge: Cambridge University Press.

Rommetveit, R. (1973), *On Message Structure*. London: Wiley.

Schutz, A. (1962), Collected papers, *I. The Problem of Social Reality*. The Hague: Martinus Nijhoff.

Shotter, J. (1987), Remembering and forgetting as social institutions. *Quarterly Newsletter of the Laboratory of Comparative Human Cognition*, **9**, 11–18.

Silverman, D. and Torode, B. (1980), *The Material Word*. London: Routledge & Kegan Paul.

Todd, A. D. (1983), *A diagnosis of doctor-patient discourse in the prescription of contraception*. In S. Fisher & A. D. Todd (Eds.), *The Social Organization of Doctor-Patient Communication* (pp. 159–187). Washington D. C.: The Center for Applied Linguistics.

Volosinov, V. N. (1973), *Marxism and the Philosophy of Language*. New York: Seminar Press.

CHAPTER EIGHT

The Mentally Ill Person and the Others: Social Representations and Interactive Strategies

Bruna ZANI

Dipartimento di Scienze del l'Educazione, Universita degli Studi di Bologna, Via Zamboni 34, 40126 Bologna, Italy

INTRODUCTION

In all societies illness has a social dimension. From this point of view, mental illness – an individual reality – is a specific example of the link between individual and culture. If we define illness, in an empirical sense, as an 'elementary form of the event', we can see how different systems of knowledge and meaning combine in the interpretation of that event: the nosological knowledge of cultures and of subcultures on the one hand, and that of the medical scientific establishment on the other (Cozzi and Ceschia, 1988). Augé (1986) has already emphasised the *immediate need for meaning* in any given culture, something which is incompatible with the slow, progressive advance of knowledge. This immediate need to establish the meaning of an illness produces a continuum in which different interpretative planes co-exist. The illness-event participates in a biological, a symbolic, an individual and a social continuum.

A comparison with cultural anthropology is interesting and useful in this context since it allows us to contextualise and to relativise the interpretations and forms of knowledge in each culture for the interpretation of the illness-event. From this point of view the culture of the medical professionals and of their institutions represents only one possible reading of the event.

According to Kleinman (1980) in every cultural context a health care system comprises simultaneously interpretations expressed by several sectors. First, a professional sector (specialized medical knowledge, its institutions, its practitioners), second, a folk system (traditional therapeutic knowledge and its practitioners) and finally, a popular sector (the lay knowledge of common sense, non-specialized, the place where – according to cognitive and explicative models – the decisions and strategies for confronting illness originate). Between these sectors there are obviously varying degrees of overlap and points of interaction. It is no accident that some research, which will be presented later, indicates how, in the culture of the health and psychiatric worker, social representations come into play which are extraneous to their professional knowledge and which form part of the popular sector.

Common sense knowledge is in reality a knowledge shared by all and it organizes itself according to its own rules. Even if it is not systematic and, at times, is contradictory, common sense represents a "cultural system", in which as Geertz (1988, p. 116) noted, "there is an order produced by it that can be discovered empirically and formulated conceptually".

Common sense can be made visible through comparison with other systems of knowledge, or, as emerged recently, through the study of social representations. According to Jodelet (1984), "the concept of social representation indicates a specific form of knowledge, i.e. the common sense knowledge, the contents of which reveal the operation of processes that are generative and that serve distinct social purposes. More generally, it indicates a form of social thought. Social representations are practical and communicable ways of thinking that are oriented towards an understanding and mastery of the environment (both social and material). As such, they offer specific distinguishing features in regard to how either the contents, or the mental operations or the logic (of social representations) are organized. The social distinctiveness of either the contents or the process is attributable to: (i) the conditions and contexts in which the representations emerge; (ii) the means by which they circulate; (iii) the functions which they serve in interaction both with the world and with others" (translated by Farr, 1990 p. 48).

Social representations develop in different domains of everyday life where scientific reasoning is neither a necessary nor an economic way of thinking. They are concerned with 'consensual' universes, where conventions and agreements prevail over experiments and demonstrations, and conclusions over premises. Social representations thus play a central role in establishing, at a symbolic level, everyday experiences and in justifying our attitudes and actions: they are essential for a socio-cognitive adaptation to everyday reality (Carugati, 1989).

The current interest of social psychologists is directed toward a detailed analysis of the logic underlying these common sense forms of knowledge, their relationship to the groups that generate and use them, and the conditions under which such knowledge changes. At present a measure of theoretical agreement has been reached between supporters of a social representational approach and cognitive psychologists interested in the acquisition of new knowledge. This agreement basically concerns two aspects of cognitive functioning:

1. Like an expert scientist, the naive subject in the construction of reality would use, in an 'implicit' fashion, real everyday 'lay epistemologies' which involve the use of categories, concepts and causal schemata possessing all the cognitive characteristics and potentiality of a theory 'savante' (Paicheler, 1984).

2. The iconic, figurative and physical representations seem to be central to the cognitive processes at play in the perception and representation of the causes of perceived phenomena. These latter 'acquire meaning' by virtue means of the explanations elicited by figurative and physical models, capable of providing members of a given group with a coherent apperception of different domains of reality. This parallel between lay and scientific epistemologies has given rise to a great deal of research in the diffusion among the general public of theories and scientific knowledge (Moscovici, 1976; Herzlich, 1969). The theories of the experts are the transformational objects which allow a given group to devise for themselves a common sense understanding of the phenomenon in question. These new understandings are coherent with all previous knowledge, values and schemata for interpreting the world and they legitimize social practice and conduct. The case of AIDS is emblematic from this point of view (Paez and Paicheler, 1990).

The transformation of scientific knowledge into common sense knowledge is only one of the possible relationships between these two kinds of knowledge (Marková, 1992). Today there is an increasing interest in considering the role that common sense plays in the construction of scientific knowledge, as Semin (1987) has showed in his inquiry into naive theories which are postulated as the basis of scientific knowledge. This is particularly relevant in the case of medicine, where there is a discrepancy between 'theoretical knowledge' concerning the formal context of the discipline, and 'practical knowledge', concerning the context of its application.

Bosio (1992), in his survey on general practitioners' understanding of physiopathology of nerves shows how complex and articulated is the relationship between science and common sense in medicine. Medicine, like any other science which constructs its own objects of enquiry starting from common experience, refers to scientific knowledge supported by naive notions that have been borrowed from social knowledge. Medicine contains a dual repertoire of knowledge: one is formal and proceeds in a scientific manner; the other is more implicit and is applied in the course of medical interventions. Common sense is involved not only in the processing of scientific knowledge but also in the construction of a second system of knowledge capable of orienting, signifying and justifying professional practice.

In this chapter I shall present the results of some studies concerning similarities and differences in social representations of mental illness held by health care professionals and by members of the lay public. The social representations of mental illness are now highly heterogeneous. They are no longer linked, in an Italian context, to the institutional setting of the insane asylum. These institutions have closed following the law of 1978. A multiplicity of representations now exists, shared by different groups of subjects, according to their specific social positions and their differing experiences of mental illness.

Lay beliefs about mental health do not arise either out of ignorance or from the misinterpretation of official psychiatric knowledge. They are actively constructed in an effort to make sense of the frequently confusing and often contradictory experiences that people have. As Warwick, Aggleton and Homans (1988) have pointed out, lay beliefs about health and illness relate not only to the personal biography of the individual who adheres to them, but also to more enduring cultural and social structures. Lay health beliefs involve an active interplay between dominant and dominated systems of meaning. Moreover, much research has sought to identify the internal structure of numerous modes of analysis widely used in 'making sense' of health-related conditions. Herzlich (1973), for example, has identified 3 different notions of health (as a state of being, as a quality to be achieved, as a state of doing) and 3 different kinds of explanation (illness as destructive, as emancipatory and as an occupation).

In regard to lay beliefs about mental illness, they are generally syncretic in origin, since they are derived from various sources. I shall trace below the story of the many models which people have developed over the centuries to come to terms with mental illness and to enable them to interact with the mentally ill person. Many of these models, as we found in our research, still persist, despite being archaic conceptions of madness. This is scarcely surprising, since the search for meaning, even though it is a cognitive activity, is not necessarily rational. This poses a methodological problem regarding the necessity and utility of employing multi-method approaches to the study of social representations (De Rosa, 1990; Sotirakopoulou and Breakwell, 1992). There is a significant interaction between communicative codes (verbal or non-verbal, linguistic or figurative), activated as a function of various techniques, and the levels of representation (more or less peripheral or central, variant or invariant) elicited (De Rosa, 1984). Such representations are a function not only of the population variables considered (age, sex, social class, area of residence, training, professional role, etc.), but also of the instruments of investigation used.

FROM MADNESS TO MENTAL ILLNESS

De Rosa (1987), in her accurate and interesting analysis of the development of social representations of mental illness, stresses the 'polymorphic' nature of such representations, showing how some representations of madness, belonging to archaic collective imaginings, are revived as central figurative nuclei in the social representations of children and of adults in our modern society. According to De Rosa, if we assume a linear model of historiographic interpretation, we can identify in history several models of madness. First, the 'magic/holy' vision of madness (the madman as a mythological figure or a monster). This vision was transformed into a 'criminalised' vision (the madman as a criminal, a deviant, a drug-addict). This latter representation was then followed by a 'medicalised' conception of psychiatric science (the madman as sick, cerebropathic, handicapped) which was based on the positivist conception of science and the canons of organicism in psychiatry. Finally, and most recently, a 'psychologised'vision of madness was developed (the madman as depressed, emotionally disturbed, etc.).

However, a deeper examination of the dynamic structure of the 'representational field' of madness based on an analysis both of historical material (written documents, iconographical material, literature, etc.) and of figurative material produced by children and adults reveals the co-existence of different models of madness: the various scientific approaches and their 'popularisation' are bound up with the magico-religious vision.

A similar line of investigation was undertaken by Schurmans (1990) who analyzed the social-historical conditions of the origin of the concept of mental illness in the medical field and its passage into the universe of common sense. He demonstrated how a social consensus gradually evolved concerning certain aspects of the concept. For example, how behavioural disorders became the province of the medical field; how the source of these disorders is localized in the brain; how ideas of cure appear, and how the concept of 'mental illness' is constructed to unite, under one label, a multiform reality. Manifestations of madness, originally considered by common sense to be outside the medical field (seen as symptoms of divine retribution, the devil's hand or a diseased soul), slowly became labelled as illnesses of the body, forming the subject matter of a specialized field of psychiatry (i.e. belonging to the 'reified universe' of science and thus separate from the 'consensual universe' of lay discourse).

The concept of mental illness passed into common sense through the mechanisms involved in the creation of a social representation such as objectification and anchoring. According to Schurmans (1990), however, the expression 'mental illness', created originally to designate a type of physiological disease fundamentally different from madness, became, in its common sense understanding, a term which remains linked to madness and detached from physiological illness.

In her research carried out in Geneva the present author shows the existence of a *décalage* between the scientific and the lay beliefs of mental illness held by a group of primary school teachers. What clearly emerges in the responses of these subjects is a shared consensus concerning the concept of mental illness as 'alterity'; despite the attempts of psychiatry to integrate mental illness with physiological illnesses, common sense continues to stigmatize it as an expression of difference and disorder. However, contradictory conceptions are also expressed: some individuals adopt a medical model according to which mental illness is a natural illness whose management and cure is in the hands of doctors. Others, adopting a multicausal conception of mental illness, emphasize its social origins (e.g. conflicts or social problems) and question the scientific nature of the medical approach and its legitimacy.

These two conceptions, both formulated by the teachers interviewed, are the expression of two different modes of knowledge which do not emerge by chance but are a result of either accentuating or diminishing (induced by the investigative tools used) the competitive relationship between teachers and doctors. If the presence of a superordinate category (the non-mentally ill) is evoked, the teachers register a greater proximity to the doctors and adhere to the more widespread and consensual conceptions of society which recognize the 'knowledge' of doctors. If however they are engaged in their role as teachers and thus in a capacity of potential holders of knowledge, then the values of the 'teaching body' as a group prevail. This leads the teachers to express a more 'social' view of mental illness, calling into question medical power once more (cf. Schurmans, 1990).

The role of social representations of mental illness in regulating the relationships of different social groups with the mentally ill is the main theme in a broadly based collaborative research carried out by social psychologists in Belgium, Italy, Spain and Switzerland. The data from the Italian project will now be presented.

PROFESSIONAL AND LAY REPRESENTATIONS OF MENTAL ILLNESS: A COMPARATIVE STUDY

What is peculiar to Italy in comparison to the other countries involved in the study, is the radical process of 'de-psychiatrization' and deinstitutionalization which was imposed by a national law in 1978. This law totally reshaped the psychiatric health system by starting the gradual phasing out of mental hospitals and the opening of a number of health services on a regional basis. This process affected not only the professional roles and skills of mental health workers, but also the traditional views of the general population. This is the context of a wide-ranging national research project carried out by the author in cooperation with colleagues from the Universities of Rome and Naples. The aims of this project were the following: to collect extensive data from practitioners in psychiatric services and from 'non-experts', to elaborate hypotheses regarding the ways in which scientific thought (psychological – psychiatric) is translated into common sense, to form models of the classification and explanation of mental disease, and to evaluate therapeutic objectives and strategies (for a presentation of the whole research see Bellelli, 1993).

There are three basic reasons for carrying out a comparative study of this kind (Di Giacomo, 1993). The first is methodological: only by comparing different sites can convergences and divergences emerge with respect to the phenomenon in question. The second reason is theoretical; focusing on the nature of the psychiatric process in which different participants, the professional and those who are ill, mutually influence each other and negotiate plans for intervention. The third reason is geopolitical; it is linked to the political and socio-cultural differences that mark the various regions of Italy where the research was conducted (Bologna in the North, Rome in the Centre, and Naples in the South).

Our study involved different social groups: mental health professionals (psychologists, psychiatrists and psychiatric nurses); university students from different disciplines (medicine, psychology, nursing and mathematical sciences); children of different ages, their parents and their teachers. The total sample of adults (as regards the developmental study, see below) comprised 264 professionals, including 89 psychiatrists, 90 psychiatric nurses and 85 psychologists; 480 students divided into four groups of 120 students from each discipline; 180 parents and 90 teachers (approximately one third of each group in each city considered).

The main instrument used to explore social representations in these groups was a questionnaire. It included the following themes: the definition of the mentally ill; the identification of the causes of mental illness, the course and the consequences of mental illness; the strategies considered most suitable for the treatment of the mentally ill; types of intervention and places for treatment.

We expected to find a basically *similar structure* in all the social groups considered, with regard to the representational field of mental illness. However, we expected *differences in the content* of such representations, according to the degree of proximity to and involvement with the topic, on the part of the different groups. One specific hypothesis was that we expected to find intra-group variations in the model of mental illness and in the treatment strategies of the mentally ill as a function of social criteria relating to *professional roles* for the practitioners, and to *educational background* in the case of students (see also Zani, 1993). Only some of the more significant findings will be mentioned here (see Bellelli, 1993, for a more detailed presentation of results).

From an analysis of the questionnaire it was possible to identify the dominant models of both mental illness and treatment strategies. Within the *professional world* it clearly emerged that the psychologists, above all others, expressed a socio-relational conception of mental illness. They considered psychotherapy the best treatment for the mentally ill. The group with whom the patient shared an apartment (i.e. an apartment group) or others in the immediate living environment were identified as the most suitable others to be involved in effecting a cure. The psychiatrists on the other hand tended to emphasise the medical-organizational aspects (based on the importance of pharmacological treatment and hospital admission as therapeutic strategies). The psychiatric nurses, in their turn, adopted a different position to both of these groups by showing a greater concern for what might be called 'medical-social' aspects. They underscored the importance of biological-pharmacological factors for the etiology and choice of treatment best suited to the patient (and in this they were very close to the doctors with whom they shared a common experience and had a longstanding relationship dependency). They were also concerned about the role of the social environment and about social control which, perhaps, had something to do with the traditional role of their own professional group.

There were also some interesting findings among the *students*. The psychology students emerged as supporters of a psycho-social conception of mental disease. In order to treat the mentally ill they thought it was necessary to modify the patient's social environment and to provide psychotherapy. They considered the most suitable places for treatment to be apartment groups and local health centres. They thought that the causes of disease are social or related to socialisation within the family. The other three groups of students on the other hand professed a more medical-clinical conception of mental disease: for them, the causes of illness above all lay in an individual's character and biology. They argued that the most efficient form of treatment is pharmacological and that the best place for treatment is the hospital. A more detailed analysis of the data also pointed to differences within the so-called 'health-related' group, i.e. between future doctors and trainee nurses. The training of nurses seemed to be based on a double matrix, the medical-biological and the socio-relational.

Another kind of analysis revealed differences in the perceptions of mental illness by specialists (health workers) and non-specialists (students, parents and teachers). This comparison produced a sophisticated and complex pattern. Even within the same group representations were found which referred to different models of disease and of the mentally ill. The presence both of older representations, based on a model of the criminalization of the mentally ill, and of more modern representations, based on medicalized, anthropomorphic, or sociological models of mental disease, were detected. The former representations were found using a technique of free associations which is less subject to conscious control than the data obtained from questionnaires. These representations were held, above all, by parents and by certain groups of psychiatric nurses. The students, with the exception of medics, and to some extent the teachers, shared a more social model of disease. Finally, the practitioners presented a more psychologized representation of the mentally ill, emphasising primarily the patient's existential condition and the risks associated with labelling. The psychiatrists alternated between a strongly medical model and a psychological one. Of the different professional groups, the psychiatric nurses were concerned, more than others, with defining the disease 'scientifically'. They tried to defend their role as the daily managers of the patients and they were concerned with their social control.

A further interesting point to emerge from this research concerned regional and social differences in representations. For example, the practitioners in Bologna were more homogenous in their representations than those in Naples, apparently because the implementation of the psychiatric reform in the two regions gave rise to different operating practices. A common attitude towards work in local health services in Bologna may have helped to produce greater homogenization among the various practitioners. In the absence of such a common attitude in Naples, substantial differences in the representations of mental illness remained amongst practitioners there. The research detected traces of a medicalized psychiatry in which medical labels replaced criminalising ones. The use of these labels, as in the case of Neapolitan nurses, however, seemed to be functional in terms of their professional identity.

PSYCHIATRIC PATIENTS AND THE COMMUNITY: SHARED BELIEFS AND INTERACTIVE STRATEGIES

What happens when the mentally ill become regular visitors to shops and bars or passers-by whom anyone can bump into on the streets of the neighbourhood or at a bus stop? In Italy, as mentioned before, the law of 1978 closed mental hospitals to new psychiatric patients and left them in the community at large. Daily cohabitation with patients outside of mental institutions thus became a normal thing. And yet, today, the integration of the mentally ill into the community is still a problem. While there has been a profound change with some interesting experiments taking place (cf. Zani and Nicoli, 1991), the debate at a social level has not yet produced a working consensus that would be in harmony with the legislative principles.

Studies in natural contexts where there are opportunities for contact between psychiatric patients and the local population become important in this context. The classic case is the study by Denise Jodelet (1985, 1989) on the family colony in Ainay-le-Château in France. This study above all showed how the population elaborates defence mechanisms to replace the repressive regimes and social control previously exercised by the mental institution. The encounter between the mentally ill and society is full of ambivalence and triggers processes that deserve careful attention if programmes of integration are to be actively promoted.

Jodelet (1985, 1989) demonstrated how the relational and behavioural models adopted by the population towards patients basically reflected a need to defend the population's social identity which was felt to be endangered by the presence of handicapped people on the public scene, as well as reflecting a fear of being assimilated by the patients. This explains the need for distinctive signs, the constitution of a 'partitive order' (separate meals and washing), the constant distinguishing of 'them' from 'us'. Behind these real discriminatory practices and the ban on contact with the mentally ill, which the population had established over time, lay the fear of being contaminated by their madness. These patterns of behaviour and of interaction were justified by their lay theory of madness and by their model of normal and of handicapped persons. The population had in fact developed 'naive' theories of mental disease and its causes (distinguishing, for instance, between diseases of the brain and nervous diseases), where contradictory elements co-existed and fears and beliefs incompatible with scientific progress survived. The importance of taking these lay social representations into account lies in the fact that they tend to become 'self-fulfilling prophecies': i.e. the people act on the basis of their theories.

This is the framework for the research we have been carrying out over the last few years in Bologna in order to explore the relationship between psychiatric patients and the local population in everyday life situations in the community. The aim is to propose hypotheses regarding the way scientific thought (psychiatric – psychological) is translated into common sense, the creation of classification models for psychiatric patients and mental disease, the mechanisms of inference which underlie social judgement and the links between belief systems and actual behaviour.

The general project examines three districts of the city, each characterized by a different quality of contact with the mentally ill, and by a different degree of visibility of the phenomenon of mental illness. The contact is operationalised in terms of two criteria: (a) density (the number of mental patients/clients of the psychiatric services in each district; (b) typicality of the mentally ill (typical mental patient: the madman in the asylum versus the less prototypical patient; those who suffer at present from psychic disturbances versus former patients, now living in normal apartments).

District 1 (where the Psychiatric Hospital of the city is located) has a low density and a high visibility of prototypical mental patients. District 2 is characterized by a high density and a low visibility of less prototypical patients. District 3 (the control group) has a low density and a low visibility of mental patients.

The general design of the research project is implemented in several phases. *Firstly*, an analysis of the context (the socio-economic aspects of the three districts; the development of the psychiatric services located in each district); interviews with some psychiatric patients who are still residents in the asylum but who are free to leave the asylum during the day; a pilot study involving observations in the shops and streets of District 1 to detect everyday interactional strategies between people and mental patients. *Secondly*, the field research phase, in which the focus was on lay perceptions of the mentally ill and the social categorization processes involved in such perceptions (Nicoli, Zani and Arcuri, 1992). An *ad hoc* questionnaire was administered to a sample of 210 adult people (70 in each district). We predicted that the relative absence of contact (District 3) would be associated with negative representations of mental patients (considered as an 'outgroup' with respect to the 'ingroup', i.e. 'normal people'). The 'quality of contact', however, would make some differences in the other two districts. In District 2 we predicted there would be a reduction in negative images and attitudes towards mental patients while in District 1 the contact would not affect the still existing stereotypical images.

We found weak support for our predictions. The only difference was related to images of the 'normal' and 'mentally ill' person (target variable) while no significant interactions emerged between target variables and districts. Our subjects proved to have quite different images of the normal person and of the mentally ill. The former was described as egoist, open, banal, controlled and arrogant; the mentally ill was considered as altruist, closed, original, impulsive and mild (Figure 8.1).

There seems therefore to be a common picture in the three districts independent of the type and quality of contact with the psychiatric patients, a picture that seems to underline the positive aspects of the mentally ill (altruist, mild, original), giving a more negative evaluation of the concept 'normal person'.

The interaction effect (target x district) we had expected to find appeared in the spontaneous taxonomy task. Subjects were given 30 cards

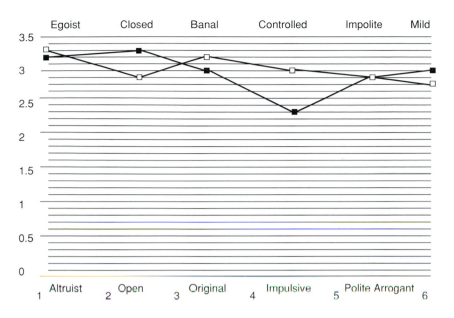

Figure 8.1 – General means of the central tendency index (total sample).

with a single personality trait printed on each (e.g. aggressive, happy, depressed, sincere, isolated, superficial, dangerous, etc.). They were asked to sort the cards into piles in order to create different types of mentally ill persons, and, separately, of a normal person.

Cluster analysis performed on each matrix (traits x targets) for each district revealed differences between districts. Subjects in both District 3 (with no contact) and District 1 (who only had contact with the more prototypical patients) shared the same representation of a mentally ill person. This representation was based on the classic dichotomy extrovert – introvert which, in the case of mentally ill, became the opposition between the madman as 'dangerous', 'unpredictable' and 'aggressive' on the one hand, and the sick person as 'depressed', 'sad', 'isolated' and 'frightened' on the other. The subjects in District 2, who had contact with less prototypical patients, were better able to differentiate the typologies of the mentally ill, and they showed a richer, less stereotyped, representation of the mentally ill (Figures 8.2a and 8.2b).

In the second field study (Nicoli and Zani, 1992) we addressed the professional category of shopkeepers, since the distinctive feature of their work is a daily contact with people. This means that they are particularly involved in contructing and exchanging with others social representations of different groups of people. We interviewed 124 shopkeepers (tobacconists, grocers, butchers, barmen/barmaids, etc.), half men and half women, living in the three districts of Bologna (about a third of the sample

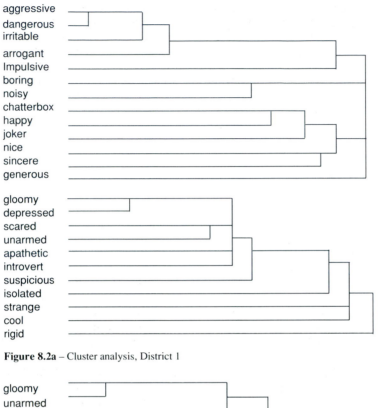

Figure 8.2a – Cluster analysis, District 1

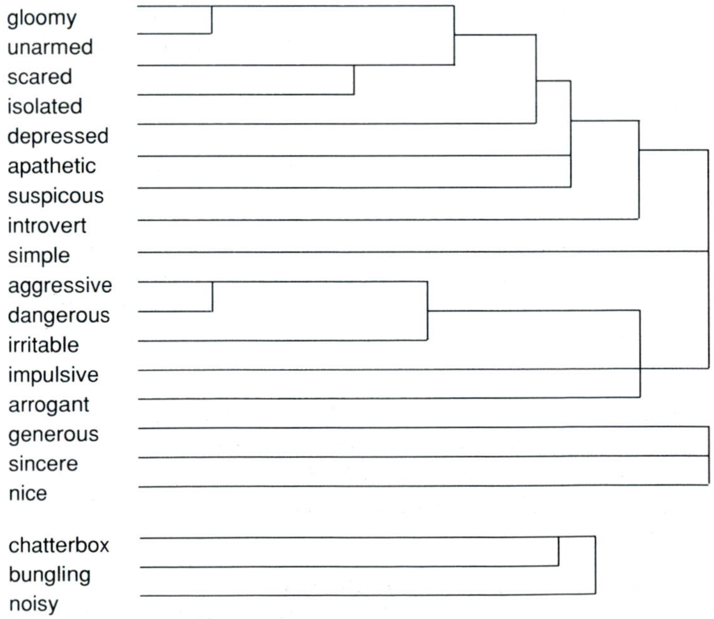

Figure 8.2b – Cluster analysis, District 2

came from each district). In District 1 we chose all the shops located in the streets around the Psychiatric Hospital; then we tried to find similar types of shops in the other two districts. The shopkeepers were individually interviewed during normal working hours on the following topics: the interpersonal relationships with customers (the typology of their customers, behavioural and relational problems linked to the actual or supposed presence of mental patients in their shop); images of mental illness (aetiology, treatment and definition); their opinions concerning the law of the 1978 which closed psychiatric hospitals to new patients; the categorization processes (ways of describing a mental patient to other people; ways of recognizing a mentally ill person).

Content analyses of transcripts of the interviews provided the following findings:

(a) there was a consistency between the subjects' descriptions and identifications of the mentally ill. The subjects searched for the same cues and signs in different groups of 'others'. They sought confirmation of the hypotheses they formed about other people. Hypothesis testing was the most common form of reasoning.

(b) The common nucleus of mental illness concerned its aetiology. In all districts subjects were able to distinguish between the causes of mental illness that we have categorised as exogenous (family, critical events, conditions of life) and endogenous (heredity, illness).

(c) Subjects in all three districts considered the same elements as essential components of their representations of mental illness. However, they attributed different meanings to these components so that the resulting configuration of such elements generated completely different representations. This 'network of meanings' (Moscovici, 1992) is based on the conception of 'seriousness', which is affected by both the knowledge and the emotions of the subjects. Consideration of the seriousness of an illness, in its turn, affects prognosis (positive or negative) and the strategies of action deemed appropriate towards the mentally ill.

In District 1, the shopkeepers made a positive prognosis, and were convinced that the intervention of institutional agents (experts, specialized clinics) was necessary to aid the patients; in particular they considered 'soft' techniques of control and rehabilitation important. For example, a hairdresser said:

> *Since I'm from this district and know the psychiatric hospital, I think it would be a mistake to keep them locked up in the wards when there is a lovely big garden outside. I reckon there should be some nice big gates at the entrance and then let the patients roam round in the garden.*

In District 2 the prognosis was also positive, and the shopkeepers were more inclined to stress the importance of rehabilitation and of other forms of assistance, even at a personal level.

In District 3 the prognosis was negative, e.g. 'the mentally ill will never recover'. The shopkeepers proposed what we called 'hard' techniques of control (institutions, the intervention of the police, etc.).

In conclusion, our findings suggest that in the absence of familiarity with mental illness (i.e. illness as an unknown and somewhat mysterious and troubling object), subjects in District 3 adopted a particular way of coping with mental illness. Although they were used to dealing with a wide range of different people, they adopted an attitude of rejection towards the mentally ill. They incorporated in their representations of mental illness all the more traditional elements of common sense with their clearly negative connotations. The shopkeepers in District 1, on the other hand, who had a degree of familiarity with patients from the psychiatric hospital, adopted an almost technical attitude towards the mentally ill. They learned how to deal with them, and they acquired a kind of practical knowledge. Yet, they maintained a clear distinction between the normals and 'them'. As a bartender told us:

> *Doing this job (barman) you become a psychologist (!): you can tell what they want (the mentally ill) from the way they behave, their facial expressions, especially the eyes. The best thing to do as far as they are concerned is to isolate them, but not in an old-fashioned asylum but in a nice place with a beautiful park round it.*

In District 2 where the psychiatric patients were more numerous but less visible, the shopkeepers were more tolerant and decidedly more humanitarian in their proposals for intervention at both an institutional and a personal level. This demonstrates the interdependence between the elaboration of lay beliefs and the personal experiences of daily life.

CONCLUSIONS

We have shown above that throughout human history mental illness and the treatment of mentally ill people have aroused strong emotions. The beliefs and attitudes towards madness and mental illness have reflected the prevailing conditions of the time, often characterised by a deep ambivalence among both mental health practitioners and members of the lay public. Today we live in a time when the increased presence of mental patients in the community is a reality. The general public more frequently meet mentally ill people in day-to-day life. It is extremely important to know the public response to this new situation. Given the recent emphasis on community care for the mentally ill, knowledge of shared beliefs and attitudes are needed if this care is to succeed (Bhugra, 1989). It is very likely that such responses will vary from one place to another depending on a number of parameters. In this respect, the notion of a social representation is particularly useful in order to understand how people structure their social and relational worlds, give meaning to their daily experience and orient their actions within those social worlds.

In a recent lecture, Moscovici (1993, pp. 162–163) has suggested some lines of reflection on the theory of social representations. *Firstly*, he said that "folk knowledge is grafted onto canonic themata that motivate or compel people in their cognitive search. This is what comes to their minds when some unfamiliar item or information strikes them and what they communicate about". Experience tells us that when an object, for example madness, enters the field of our exchanges, we consult the register of themata to select the one that allows us to represent it to ourselves. Moreover, Moscovici continued, "Once the object is hooked on a thema which is radically unutterable, because its only content is potential, it becomes the actual content of a representation when it gets anchored to a context, a network of meanings. To be anchored means that it has a reference and receives a determinate semantic value".

Secondly, the content of representations appears to us to comprise beliefs which are concentrated and collective since they are set above other beliefs. These other beliefs "are distributed among the members of a group and can be reinvented all the time, growing again like plants as long as their roots have been safeguarded" (Moscovici, 1993, p. 168). The reference here is to the hypothesis of the *central core*, which is autonomous and salient and whose causal role is to produce peripheral meanings and images associated with them. We think that our research findings can be better understood using the frame of reference provided by Moscovici's (1992) lines of reflection.

It is particularly striking that different social groups presented the same structure of the representational field, whether they were professional or lay people, adults or children, people living in different social and economic contexts, or belonging to different social classes. This structure, represented graphically along two axes in two dimensional space, opposes the sphere of normality (normal person, oneself) to that of abnormality (sick person, mentally ill person, madman), and the area of physical illness to that of mental deviance. Moreover, normality and self are described positively. The abnormal/pathological is described negatively, as 'other than self'. The mentally ill person is seen as extremely distant from the self and completely different which gives a quite clear indication of his or her perceived 'otherness'. This concept of otherness (strangeness) could be considered as the thema, which allows us to know and to understand madness. It acquires its meaning in relation to the self and other and according to the need for a categorical differentiation between sanity and insanity, deviance and normalcy.

The different dimensions of the representational field of mental illness constitute the central nucleus characterised by the persistently negative connotations of mental illness versus the positive evaluation of a normal person. Over and above this central core, which is common to the different subgroups, there are differences in the content of social representations, depending on a wide range of variables. We were able to demonstrate the existence of intergroup differences regarding both the models of mental illness and strategies of relating towards the mentally ill in health workers and in groups of lay people. We also identified some intra-group variations with respect to professional roles (in the case of practitioners), educational background (in the case of students), proximity and familiarity (in the case of persons living in different districts of a city). A final remark concerns methodology and the utility of adopting different methodological approaches. It emerged clearly from our data that only by using a variety of instruments (questionnaires, free associations, opened questions, scales of social distance) was it possible to highlight the different dimensions underlying the representations as well as the criteria that help subjects to organize them.

REFERENCES

Augé, M. (1986), L'anthropologie de la maladie. *L'Homme: Revue Francaise d'Anthropologie*, **97–98**, 81–90.

Ayestaran, S. and Paez, D. (1986), *An outline for a cross-cultural research on social representation of 'mental illness': Preliminary discussion of data collected in Spain from a psychogenetic perspective.* Paper presented at the International Congress on Cross-Cultural Psychology, Istanbul.

Bellelli G. (1993), (ed.) *L'altra malattia. Come la società pensa la malattia mentale.* Napoli: Liguori.

Bhugra, D. (1989), Attitudes towards mental illness: A review of the literature. *Acta Psychiatrica Scandinavica*, **80**, 1–12.

Bosio, A.C. (1992), *Science, common sense, medical knowledge: How/why does (doesn't) a nerve work? A survey of General Practitioners' understanding of nerve physiopathology*, Paper presented at the 1st International Conference on Social Representations, Ravello (Italy), 3–5 October.

Carugati, F. (1989), Everyday ideas, theoretical models and social representations: The case of intelligence and its development. In *Everyday Understanding: Social and scientific implications*, edited by G. R. Semin and K. Gergen. London:Sage.

Cozzi, D. and Ceschia, C. (1988), Common sense and the representation of mental illness. *Per la Salute Mentale/For Mental Health*, **4**, 169–179.

De Rosa; A. M. (1984), Psychogenetic aspects in social representations of "mad person" and "madness". In *Psicosociologia de la Enfermedad Mental: Ideologia y representacion social de la enfermedad mental*, edited by S. Ayestaran, pp.219–284. Bilbao: Imprenta Boan.

De Rosa, A. M. (1987), The social representation of mental illness in children and adults. In *Current Issues in Social Psychology*, edited by W. Doise & S. Moscovici, pp.47–138. Cambridge: Cambridge University Press.

De Rosa, A. M. (1990), Per un approccio multi-metodo allo studio delle rappresentazioni sociali. *Rassegna di Psicologia*, **3**, 103–154.

De Rosa, A. M. (1993), Agenzie di socializzazione e rappresentazioni della malattia mentale in et evolutiva. In *L'altra malattia: Come la società pensa la malattia mentale*, edited by G. Bellelli, Napoli: Liguori.

De Rosa, A. M. and Schurmans, M. N. (1990), Madness imagery across two countries. *Rassegna di Psicologia*, **3**, 177–193.

Di Giacomo, J. P. (1993), Aspetti metodologici nello studio delle rappresentazioni sociali. In *L'altra malattia: Come la società pensa la malattia mentale.*, edited by G. Bellelli. Napoli: Liguori.

Farr, R. M. (1990), The social psychology of widespread beliefs, In *The Social Psychology of Widespread Beliefs*, edited by C. Fraser and G. Gaskell, pp.47–64. Oxford: Oxford University Press.

Ferreira Arzac A. (1984), Influencia de las variables informacion y edad sobre las representaciones sociales de la enfermedad mental. In *Psicosociologia de la Enfermedad mental*, edited by S. Ayestaran, pp.55–89. Bilbao: Imprenta Boan.

Flick, U. (1992), Combining methods - Lack of methodology: Discussion on Sotirakopoulou & Breakwell. *Ongoing Production on Social Representations*, **1**, 43–48.

Geertz, G. (1988), *Antropologia Interpretativa*, Bologna: Il Mulino.

Herzlich, C. (1969), *Santé et Maladie*. Paris: Mouton.

Herzlich, C. (1973), *Health and Illness*. New York: Academic Press.

Jodelet, D. (1984), Representations sociales: Phénomènes, concepts et théorie. In *Psychologie Sociale*, edited by S. Moscovici, Paris: Presses Universitàires de France.

Jodelet, D. (1985), *Civils et bredins. Rapport à la folie et représentations sociales de la maladie mentale en milieu rural francais*, Thesè d'Etat, EHESS, Paris.

Jodelet, D. (1989), *Folies et Representations Sociales*. Paris: Presses Universitaires de France.

Linville, P. W. Fischer, G. W. and Salovey, P. (1989), Perceived distributions of the characteristics of ingroup and outgroup members: Empirical evidence and a computer simulation. *Journal of Personality and Social Psychology*, **57**, 165–188.

Kleinman, A. (1980), *Patients and Healers in the Context of Culture*. Berkeley: University of California Press.

Marková, I. (1992), Scientific and public knowledge of AIDS: The problem of their integration. In *Social Representations and the Social Bases of Knowledge.*, edited by M. von Cranach, W. Doise and G. Mugny. Lewistone, New York: Hogrefe & Huber.

Moscovici, S. (1976), *La Psychanalyse: Son image et son public*. Paris: Presses Universitaires de France.

Moscovici, S. (1993), Introduction Address. *Papers in Social Representations*, **2** (3), pp. 160–170.

Nicoli, A. and Zani, B. (1992), *When the customers are mad: The shopkeepers' representations of mental illness*. Paper presented at the First International Conference on Social Representations, Ravello, 3–5 October.

Nicoli, A., Zani, B. and Arcuri, L. (1992), *Lay perceptions of mentally ill persons: Contact, familiarity and social categorization processes*. Paper presented at the XXV International Congress of Psychology, p. 263. Hillsdale: Erlbaum

Paez, D. and Ayestaran, S. (1984), Representaciones sociales de la enfermedad mental y pertenencia a groupos de diferente distancia ante ella. In *Psicosociologia de la Enfermedad Mental: Ideologia y representacion social de la maladie mentale*, edited by S. Ayestaran, pp.7–54. Bilbao: Imprenta Boan.

Paez, D. and Paicheler, H. (1990), Connaissances du sens commun et attitudes vis-à-vis du Sida. In *Santé Publiques et Maladies Transmission Sexuelle*, edited by N. Job-Spira, B. Spencer, J. P. Moatti and E. Bouvet, pp.520–524. Paris: John Libbey Eurotext.

Paicheler, H. (1984), L'épistémologie du sens commun. In *La Psychologie Sociale*, edited by S. Moscovici. Paris: Presses Universitaires de France.

Petrillo, G. (1993), Sapere naif e sapere professionale. In *L'Altra Malattia. Come la società pensa la malattia mentale*, edited by G. Bellelli. Napoli: Liguori.

Schurmans, M. N. (1990), *Maladie Mentale et Sens Commun*. Neuchâtel: Delachaux & Niestle.

Semin, G. R. (1987), On the relationship between representations of theories in psychology and ordinary language. In *Current Issues in European Social Psychology*, vol. 2, edited by W. Doise and S. Moscovici, pp. 307–348. Cambridge: Cambridge University Press.

Sotirakopolou, K. and Breakwell, G. (1992), The use of different methodological approaches in the study of social representations. *Ongoing Production on Social Representations*, **1**, 29–38.

Warwick, I., Aggleton, P. and Homans, H. (1988), Young people's health beliefs and AIDS. In *Social Aspects of AIDS*, edited by P. Aggleton and H. Homans. London: The Falmer Press.

Zani, B. (1987), The psychiatric nurses: A social psychological study of a profession facing institutional changes. *Social Behaviour*, **2**, 87–98.

Zani, B. (1990), Alcune riflessioni sui metodi di studio delle rappresentazioni sociali. In *Il Metodo del Discorso*, edited by G. Bellelli, pp.168–180. Napoli: Liguori.

Zani, B. (1993), Social representations of mental illness: Lay and professional perspectives. In *Empirical Approaches to Social Representations*, edited by G. Breakwell and D. Canter, pp. 315–330. Oxford: Oxford University Press.

Zani, B. and Nicoli, A. (1991), Le communità terapeutiche in psichiatria: Evoluzione di una pratica alternativa. In *Communità di convivenza e crescita della persona*, edited by A. Palmonari, pp.41–105. Bologna: Patron.

CHAPTER NINE

Lay Explanations of the Causes of Diabetes in India and the UK

Mary SISSONS JOSHI

Psychology Unit, Oxford Brookes University, Gipsy Lane, Headington, Oxford, OX3 0BP

BACKGROUND

The purpose of the present study is to compare lay explanations of the causes of illness in Eastern and Western settings. It examines both the content of the explanations as well as the relationship between types of explanation and adjustment.

The starting point for the study is the social psychology of attribution theory which has not only suggested a classification system for explanations but has elucidated the functions of various types of explanation (Heider, 1958; Kelley, 1971; Wortman, 1976). Empirical research has largely concentrated on explanation within the domain of interpersonal events but similar processes are thought to affect people's interpretations of misfortunes such as unemployment (Furnham, 1982) and illness (Watts, 1982; Hewstone, 1985). Following Bulman and Wortman (1977), there have been many studies attempting to relate lay theories of the causes of illness to adjustment (Watts, 1982; Tennen, Affleck and Gershman, 1986; Tennen and Affleck, 1990). In most of these studies (with a few exceptions such as Taylor, Lichtman and Wood, 1984), patients who report an explicit attribution have been found to be better adjusted in a variety of domains than patients who report no attribution (Turnquist, Harvey and Andersen, 1988). The usual explanation offered for the relationship between explanation and adjustment is that having an explanation of a past event preserves the idea that the world is a place in which events have causes and, furthermore, permits the possibility that one can, in future, control outcomes. However, it is likely that a control model of human thinking is a social representation of the human mind and thus only appropriate to the description of individuals in contemporary North American and European cultures. Indeed, amongst his criticisms of attribution theory, Harré (1981) suggests that certain of its propositions are far from universal and reflect instead values and aspects of the social order prevalent not world-wide but amongst middle-class Americans. Lalljee

(1981) also notes that the concern with prediction and control which is so pervasive in the model of human thinking proposed by attribution theorists may only be "a function of a particular sort of religious and social orientation" (p. 134).

Philosophically speaking "the self" cannot be conceptualised without "the other" (Mead, 1934), and the concept of the person cannot be disentangled from that of agency (Taylor, 1985). However, cultures may be contrasted in terms of the views that they have of self, agency and control (Dumont, 1970; Heelas, 1981; Markus and Kitayama, 1991). The importance given in Hindu philosophy to notions of fate and predestination is reflected in local beliefs whereby control over the future is held to be neither possible nor desirable, and equanimity in the face of misfortune is highly valued (Carstairs, 1957). However, as Totman (1982) has usefully commented, the vocabulary of attribution processes is "strictly contingent upon an initial attribution of freedom, or more accurately, unconstrainedness" (p. 48). Such a concept is the hallmark of Western but not Eastern indigenous psychology (Heelas, 1981; Shweder and Bourne, 1982) and for this reason we may expect certain attributional patterns not to be replicated across cultures.

Any attempt to contrast lay cultural theories of the causes of illness is frustrated by the different methodologies employed by researchers of whom some ask their informants about illness in general (Herzlich, 1973; Lewis, 1975; Horton, 1970; Pill and Stott, 1982; Stainton Rogers, 1991) and others ask about particular illnesses (Taylor, Lichtman and Wood, 1984; Williams, 1986; Mull and Mull, 1988). However, the very notion of identifying an illness as the "same" in two different cultural settings assumes a particular perspective on illness. Eisenberg (1977) has made the useful distinction between the concepts "disease" and "illness" suggesting that illness be understood as the "experience" and disease as the Western biomedical "model" of that experience. Western medicine has, however, had such a pervasive influence throughout the world that some have argued that this kind of medicine should be labelled "cosmopolitan" (Dunn, 1976). Urban and rural populations in non-Western societies live amongst a multitude of medical systems (Carstairs and Kapur, 1976; Nichter, 1980; Kakar, 1982) and are well-known for their simultaneous use of all these systems of care (Madan, 1969; Beals, 1976).

The disease Diabetes Mellitus was chosen as the focus for the present study. Diabetes is a metabolic syndrome in which the pancreas fails to produce insulin. Such a deficiency prevents the patient from properly processing carbohydrate foods and results in a raised blood sugar level which if not treated can lead to a variety of short-term and long-term medical problems (Oakley, Pyke and Taylor, 1978; British Diabetic Association, 1980; Patel and Talwalkar, 1966). Between one to three per cent of the general population in affluent societies suffer from diabetes (Hamman, 1983) with similar rates found in urban India (Bennett, 1983). Diabetic services for the urban population in India are not dissimilar to those provided in developing countries (Bollag, 1983) and many diabetic clinics in cities such as Bombay draw patients from a wide socio-economic range including those well below the wage for unskilled labour (Jain and Patel, 1984).

Diabetic patients treated with insulin attempt to control their blood sugar level on a daily basis by matching the injection of insulin with food input and energy output. As part of this enterprise many patients are involved in regular monitoring of their urine and blood sugar levels. The diabetic regime is "intrusive, pervasive and requires life-long self-regulation of behaviour" (p. 208) (Shillitoe and Miles, 1989) and, as Harris, Linn and Pollack (1984) have commented, "the amount of responsibility the diabetic patient must assume is unique among illnesses" (p. 254). Diabetic patients are concerned not only with control at a day to day level but with control issues in the longer term - i.e. diabetic complications and prognosis. While the relationship between the rigorous daily control of blood sugar levels and long-term complications is a complex one, medical research does indicate a connection (Sonksen and West, 1978; Shillitoe and Miles, 1989). Furthermore, as Posner (1977) indicates, clinicians certainly advise their patients as if there were a clear connection between long-term complications and the daily control of blood sugar levels. Surveys reveal that although many patients are anxious about prognosis, they also find the required regimes oppressive (Sanders et al. 1975; Bloom Cerkoney and Hart, 1980; Hopper, 1981) and clinicians are worried by low rates of patient self-care (Watkins, Roberts et al. 1967; Watkins, Williams et al. 1967; Samanta et al. 1987; Shillitoe and Miles, 1989).

Lay explanations of illness are partly, but by no means entirely, formed by professional medical theories of the causes of disease. A range of studies have demonstrated how concerned patients are to know about their condition in general, and about the cause of their condition in particular. Indeed in a study by Greenberg et al. (1984), patients rated the cause of illness as one of the most desired pieces of information. Yet many studies reveal how patients are frequently disappointed with the amount and type of information they receive (Cartwright, 1967; Stimson and Webb, 1975; Waitzkin and Stoeckle, 1976). Helman (1978, 1990) has noted how causal theorising forms part of the doctor-patient dialogue but also notes how medical and lay models may differ in many important respects, including aetiology.

Diabetes (Madhumeha) was well known to the ancient physicians of India (Patel and Talwalkar, 1968) and while the phenomenon of diabetes is well described by cosmopolitan medicine (Oakley, Pyke and Taylor, 1978), the aetiology of the condition is not fully understood (Spencer and Cudworth, 1983). Genetic factors appear to be involved in the causation of diabetes but only for a proportion of patients. Jolly (1977) comments that the ancient Hindu medical scriptures also suggest a hereditary explanation as "madhumeha can also be caused by born sweetness of the body" (p. 101). Thus patients differ with respect to the availability of a medical explanation for their condition. A partial causal explanation can be offered to the diabetic with a family history of diabetes but no such explanation is available for the non-familial diabetic. For this reason, diabetes provided a suitable arena in which to study the interplay between lay and professional ideas about causation.

METHOD

One hundred and eight insulin-involved adult diabetic patients were interviewed to elicit their theories about the causes of diabetes. All patients were asked a series of questions about diabetes including questions about the cause of their diabetes, their attitudes towards the treatment and their adjustment to the condition. Fifty three English patients (26 males, 27 females; mean age 44.7 years; mean number of years on insulin 11.35) were interviewed while they were attending a diabetes out-patient clinic at the Royal Sussex Hospital, Brighton, England. Patients waiting to see the consultant for regular check-ups were interviewed in the waiting room, and of those approached only one person declined to be interviewed. In Bombay, 55 Hindu patients (33 males, 22 females; mean age 50.51 years; mean number of years on insulin 8.83) were interviewed in diabetic out-patient clinics at Bombay Hospital, Jagjivanram Hospital and S L Raheja Hospital. Only three people approached declined to be interviewed. In both cultures, the interviews lasted from 20 minutes to 2 hours 20 minutes. During the interview as full a written record as was possible was taken of the patients' replies and, if the patient agreed (as most did), the interview was taped for later transcription.

In each culture the interviews were conducted by the author and by two female research assistants. The research assistants in England and India were not aware of the author's particular interest in the distinction between familial and non-familial patients or in the relation between patients' causal theories and reported levels of adjustment. All patients interviewed in Brighton were British Caucasian nationals, and were interviewed in English. In Bombay one third of the patients were interviewed in English although in no case was English the mother tongue of any patient. The remaining interviews were conducted in Marathi or Hindi and were transcribed and then translated into English. The translations of the interview schedule and the interviews were checked by an independent Marathi/ Hindi/ English speaker.

Each patient was classified as either a familial or a non-familial diabetic. To be classified as a familial diabetic the patient had to affirm that he or she had a blood relative who was diabetic and for the purpose of the study the kinship group was defined as parents, parents' siblings, grandparents, siblings and first cousins. Forty eight per cent of patients were familial diabetics (45% in India, and 51% in England). The patients' answers to questions concerning the cause of diabetes were coded into categories chosen after an initial reading of the transcripts and therefore reflecting the vocabulary used by the patients (Harré and Secord, 1972; Strauss, 1987). Classifications were checked by an independent researcher, who was unaware of the particular interests of the author, in order to ensure that the coding was reliable. Many of the interview questions involved a yes/no answer, but patients' elaborations of their answers also provided data for interpretation.

LAY EXPLANATIONS OF CAUSES

Heredity and other "physical" causal categories

Fifty five per cent of Indian and 66% of English patients offered a cause for their own diabetes (see Columns 2 & 4, Table 9.1).

Table 9.1 – Patients' use of causal categories

	INDIA				ENGLAND			
	Col 1		Col 2		Col 3		Col 4	
	Diabetes in general		Own diabetes		Diabetes in general		Own diabetes	
Sample	*52		55		53		53	
Don't know	16	31%	25	46%	13	25%	18	34%
Do know	36	69%	30	55%	40	75%	35	67%
Heredity	11	21%	7	13%	27	51%	10	19%
Age	1	2%	0	0	5	9%	1	2%
Other illness	1	2%	8	15%	9	17%	5	9%
Pregnancy	0	0	0	0	1	2%	3	6%
Diet	19	37%	10	18%	13	25%	5	9%
Stress	8	15%	12	22%	4	8%	6	11%
Shock	2	4%	0	0	17	32%	8	15%
Other	0	0	1	2%	0	0	2	4%
Redescribe	4	8%	4	2%	11	21%	1	2%**
Mean N of causes cited (among those who cited a cause)	1.3		1.4		2.2		1.2	

*   3 patients not asked this question
**   Totals can exceed 100% as patients may use more than one causal category.

The main causal categories used were heredity/aanuvaunshik; diet/me jay khat hoto tyamulay (It is because of what I was eating); stress/manasik tras (mental strain); and shock/dhakka. Back-translation to English is given in brackets where there is no exact Marathi-English equivalent. Amongst those who offered causes, Indian patients listed, on average, 1.4 causes, and English patients listed 1.2 causes. However, familial diabetics were no more likely to offer a cause for their diabetes than were non-familial diabetics (see Table 9.2).

Furthermore, only 31% of familial patients (28% in India and 33% in England) used heredity to explain their own diabetes. Although heredity was the most common response, of the 14 Indian familial diabetics who

Table 9.2 – Familial patients' use of causal categories

	INDIA		ENGLAND	
Sample	25		27	
Don't know	11	44%	9	33%
Do know	14	56%	18	67%
Heredity	7	28%	9	33%
Age	0	0	1	3%
Other illness	2	8%	3	11%
Pregnancy	0	0	3	11%
Diet	3	12%	3	11%
Stress	5	20%	3	11%
Shock	0	0	2	7%
Other	0	0	0	0
Redscribe	0	0	0	0
Mean N of cause cited (among those who cited a cause)	1.2		1.3	

gave a causal response, it only accounted for 41% of the causal responses they offered. Similarly, for the 18 English familial patients who gave a causal account, heredity was the most common response but it only accounted for 38% of causal responses given.

Bearing in mind that the classification of the patients as familial or non-familial came from data provided by the patient, it is at first sight surprising that not all familial diabetics cited heredity as at least one cause of their own diabetes. Although there was one English patient who considered cousins on his father's side not to be blood relatives, for most patients their lack of use of heredity related not to a misunderstanding of genetics but to the quest, in their own terms, for a more "satisfactory" explanation of their own diabetes. Patients certainly did not regard their diabetes as inevitable. Only 12% of familial diabetics reported that they had expected to get diabetes (16% in India, 7% in England); and 77% of familial diabetics stated that they were surprised to get diabetes (71% in India, and 82% in England). Familial diabetics were often perplexed by the enigma of why they, rather than for example a sibling, had diabetes. In their explanations they either passed over heredity or cited a variety of other factors which they saw as "bringing out" their "incipient" diabetes.

The predominant metaphor for the English familial patients was physical with, for example, the notion of "bad diets putting a strain on the pancreas" as in the following case:

> *I think it might be the sugary things, the cakes and sweets I used to eat ... I always thought it would be down to what I ate, because I had eaten too much sugar and there wasn't enough insulin there because I had eaten too much sugar... My sister says she doesn't eat sweets so she won't get it. But then that's silly because she is probably one of the people who will get it. It's not just because you*

*don't eat sweets, but it's through potatoes, bread, rice pudding,
milk, things like that that you don't think of. They will bring it out,
they will cause it. (19 year old female, machinist)*

Patients commonly referred to the effects of physical exertion on the body.
A 20 year old male student talked of a swimming competition involving
"hundreds of lengths which brought it out", and a 47 year old manager of a
bakery recounted how his "exacting job and tiring life had brought the
hereditary tendency out". Other illnesses were often held responsible for
the onset of diabetes. Seventy nine per cent of items mentioned by familial
diabetics in England were physical, and only two of the 18 patients, who
offered a cause for their own diabetes, did not have a physical item in their
repertoire of causes.

The most frequently cited cause for the English non-familial patients
was "shock". One patient talked of the "shock to the system" of a riding
accident in childhood, and another patient talked of "a shock" that "stirred
the diabetes up and brought it on". Three women talked of the shock of the
unexpected death of their husbands which caused their diabetes, and one
male university lecturer joked that the shock of getting married had
brought his diabetes on, before proceeding more seriously to attribute his
diabetes to the shock of a near fatal accident involving his young baby.
One man debated but rejected the idea of shock as a causal factor in his
own diabetes but did attribute his mother's diabetes to shock. A 16 year
old male shop assistant reported that his mother attributed his diabetes to
the shock of his bad exam results, although he himself did not think this
was the cause. Shock was identified by the patients as a dramatic and
unexpected occurrence, where the psychological trauma was seen as
constituting a physical assault on the body.

In her now classic study on social representations of health and illness,
Herzlich (1973) has claimed that the language of illness is not a language
of the body, and writes:

*The body, the actual organic condition, gets forgotten and lost
between illness as the result of the "way of life", and the behaviour
of the patient. Images and notions relevant to normal bodily
functioning are rare and feeble; even more rare are images and
notions designed to express organic pathology and the outbreak of
illness. (p. 134)*

The English patients in the present study, in contrast, produced images of
the body and concentrated on images of the pancreas as "over-worked"
and "strained", and the notion of diabetes as triggered through various
"abuses" of the body. It should be noted that Herzlich's informants were
questioned about illness in general, whereas those in the present study
were interviewed about a particular illness. Furthermore, illnesses may
differ in the extent to which patients employ the physical metaphor in their
causal theories, and it could be suggested that diabetes, with its daily
physical routine of injection and dietary monitoring, is particularly likely
to focus the patients' theorising on the physical domain.

Stress as a causal category

More Indian patients cited stress as a causal factor than did English patients. This was the case both for diabetes in general and for their own diabetes. Family obligations and responsibilities were the most common kind of stress cited. For example, one patient said:

> *There was this incident ... my daughter's marriage was arranged but the ceremony was yet to be performed. My own marriage is an intercaste marriage ... so at that time I was very worried and afraid also whether my daughter's wedding takes place or not. What if it breaks? What if the boy's parents refuse the alliance? This was because such a problem did arise at the time of my son's wedding. There was a girl we had seen, the marriage was settled but later on she refused and got married to another person who she was in love with. I always had this in mind and I used to think whether the same thing happens at the time of my daughter's wedding also ... I think all these worries may have led to the cause of my diabetes. (53 year old housewife, married to a teacher turned farmer)*

Stress was used as an explanation by both men and women in India, and family obligations and their financial consequences were of moment to rich and poor alike as these excerpts indicate:

> *My father died long back. I have three sisters and three brothers. To get those sisters married I had to borrow a lot of money. Repaying it took most of my life and energy. Now I realise living in this family worrying so much about the members resulted in me having diabetes. I had lots of worries. Also because of my (handicapped) son. (53 year old, male, railway facory worker)*

A 63 year old retired Lieutenant Colonel in the Indian army spoke of the death of his elder brother 30 years ago due to cancer. He attrributed his diabetes to the acute mental tension he suffered due to his increased family responsibilities resulting from his brother's death.

Leff (1988) has suggested that family life in developing countries has a different quality from that in the West and that in large extended families individuals may spend less time with any one other particular family member so that "emotional relationships tend to be diluted" (p. 171). A rather different model of emotion in the Indian extended family is proposed by other authors (Mehta, 1976; Roland, 1988; Guzder and Krishna, 1991) who indicate the very high levels of emotional demand that may be placed upon individual family members. Experimental social psychologists (Miller, Bersoff and Harwood, 1990) have also stressed the fundamental importance of social responsibilities for the Hindu Indian. A key desire for Indians is the maintenance of the family as a unit (Shah, 1974) and a number of patients in this study attributed the onset of their diabetes to the mental tension induced by their sons or daughters settling overseas. One 69 year old professional man reported that his 30 year old only son's sojourn in the USA ("with a mind not to return") brought on his (the father's) diabetes 20 years ago and, furthermore, reported that the diabetic consultant had successfully persuaded the son to return by writing to him in the following manner:

> *Your father will not write to tell you this. But insulin alone will not help him. Your father needs association with family members. You must return to live in India.*

The preponderance of psychological models amongst the Indian patients is of some relevance to the somatisation debate in psychiatry where it has been suggested that Asian patients present psychological problems in physical terms (Rack, 1982; Littlewood and Lipsedge, 1982). The debate has primarily focused on the phenomenon of depression but similar analyses have been presented for the phenomena of anxiety and it has been variously suggested that Indian patients either do not have a suitable vocabulary with which to express distress or that they are reticent about discussing stress in medical settings. The interview material reported here suggests that these Indian patients had a vivid and rich conceptualisation of "stress" and had, in their reporting of stress as a causative factor in their diabetes, no hesitation about openly discussing psychological problems.

Marathi has a term "dhakka" which is the equivalent of "shock" but there were no instances amongst the Indian patients of the use of "shock" to account for the onset of their diabetes and only two instances of shock were used to account for diabetes in general. Some English patients, however, did use the concept of "stress" as a causal factor in a similar manner to the Indian patients, differentiated by the patients from "shock" in terms of its enduring and cumulative qualities. As we have already seen, stress for the Indian patients was predominantly focused on the fulfilment of family obligations. In contrast, the English patients saw stress as primarily originating in the workplace or in their dealings with bureaucracies.

Diet as a causal category

Diet was nominated as a causal factor in their own diabetes by 18% of Indian and 9% of English patients, and as a general causative factor by 37% of Indian and 25% of English patients (see Table 9.1). The type of food cited by the diabetic patient was the same in both cultures - with a strong emphasis on over-consumption of carbohydrate - starches and sugar - as a causal factor. People nominated the sweets they had eaten or the coca-cola they had drunk in childhood as causal agents in their illness. A 57 year old English male sales office manager attributed the onset of his diabetes at 38 to "the fact of eating too many sweet things for years and years". A 50 year old Indian man talked of how as a child he had accompanied his maternal uncle, who was Governor of Bombay State, from club to club where they had consumed sherbets and other sugary drinks. Most patients who implicated diet talked of "over-indulgence" but one man from a poor Indian family talked of what he had not eaten as contributing to his diabetes:

> *I was half-starved as a child. Coming from a poor family we had no food for several days at a time while I was a school boy. We were not knowing how to have a proper diet. We might have taken whatever we liked. We might have taken that in excess because we like it. We took three times a day rice. All rice. We were not eating anything else. We should have had more wheat, certain vegetables. Out of ignorance. That may be the cause.*

One 69 year old Indian accountant made the joke that as auditor of a large sugar factory he was bound to get diabetes (although in fact he regarded his diabetes as primarily hereditary). A 58 year old Indian housewife, married to a retired civil servant, blamed her diabetes on rich food she had consumed while abroad in USA. People, particularly in India, blamed the irregularity of meals as well as their content.

Medical and Lay Reasoning

It is unlikely that the patients had acquired their causal theories from medical staff, since many patients, particularly in England, complained bitterly that medical staff had not addressed the causal question with them. Indeed patients responded to questions about cause in the interview with evident relief, saying how delighted they were to be given time to discuss their theories of causation and their anxieties about the issue of causation. During the interview, while elaborating a causal theory, patients would frequently lower their voices and glance around anxiously to make sure that medical and anciliary staff were not listening. This accords with Tennen et al.'s (1986) observation that a researcher's line of questioning may give "these individuals permission to acknowledge what they have been pondering, rather than offering new possibilities" (p. 695).

The English patients' physical theories of the causation of insulin-involved diabetes bear little resemblance to professional biomedical theories. Patients implicated one-off events many years previously as causally relevant to the onset of their diabetes. For example, a 23 year old gardener in Brighton blamed the onset of his diabetes, at the age of 13, on operations he had undergone as a baby. Patients sought meaning in family history available to them, for instance:

> *It seemed a coincidence that my parents had eleven girls and two boys, and the only two who have diabetes are two girls who have the same birthday but were born three years apart. (48 year old housewife, married to a groundsman, recently made redundant by the County Council.)*

Many patients presented quite elaborate causal theories which would appear fanciful to their physicians, for example testing a child's urine every seven years on account of a belief that diabetes "comes out in the second or third generations in seven year gaps."

Medical orthodoxy does not implicate stress or diet in the causation of insulin-dependent diabetes. Obesity is, however, regarded as a factor in the aetiology of non-insulin dependent diabetes in those diagnosed over the age of 45 years (Oakley et al. 1978) although there is no strong evidence for an association between sucrose and other highly processed carbohydrates and diabetes. However, once diagnosed as a diabetic, the patient in England and India is subject to a great deal of advice on their subsequent diet in order that their blood sugar may be brought under control (Godbole, 1976; Bradley and Marteau, 1986). In India 95% of the sample said that they had been given special advice on their diet - with 88%, 65% and 35% saying that they should avoid sugar, carbohydrate (often citing rice and chappattis) and fat, respectively. Seventy six per cent of the Indian sample mentioned diet as part of their treatment. In England all the patients said they had been given special advice about diet and 66% said that diet was part of their treatment. At the time of the study physicians in India and England were in fact moving away from advising very limited consumption of all carbohydrates to advising only against refined carbohydrates (Mann, 1984). Shweder (1977) has suggested that lay causal reasoning is powerfully affected by resemblance. Therefore, given the current emphasis on a diabetic calorie-controlled diet balanced in fat, carbohydrate and fibre, and the historic emphasis on a virtual ban for diabetics of all carbohydrate, it is not surprising that patients implicate diet in their causal theories. The greater use of diet as a causal category amongst Indian patients can in part be explained by the emphasis placed on diet as a cause of illness in Aruyvedic medicine (Jaggi, 1973).

We have already seen that 55% of the Indian sample and 66% of the English sample offered a cause for their diabetes. The English figure falls close to the level of explanation found in studies of this kind in western cultures. Turnquist, Harvey and Anderson (1988) comment that "estimates of the number of subjects who report a causal attribution range from 69% to 95%" (p. 56). The Indian sample, in comparison, is distinguished by its lower rate of causal attribution in as much as 45% of the Indian sample in comparison to only 34% of the English sample could not, in answer to this question, offer a cause for their own diabetes. The numbers of Indian patients unable to offer a cause for their own diabetes is even higher (53%) than the comparable English number (36%) if causal answers which merely redescribe the condition are classified as "Don't Knows". When asked not to focus on their own diabetes but to consider the causes of diabetes in general, the number of patients unable to offer a cause falls to 28% and does not vary by culture which suggests that the Indian patients' tendency not to offer a cause for their own diabetes relates not to education or exposure to particular kinds of medical information but to a different orientation to explanation with respect to self.

More striking perhaps than the rate of causal theorising *per se* was the observation that very few of the Indian sample seemed worried by their inability to offer a cause for their condition and tended to expect the interview to proceed directly to the next question. In contrast, in England, not being able to cite a cause was accompanied by statements of "causal search" such as:

> *I don't really know what caused my diabetes because at the time there were no shocks. I wasn't overweight, it does not run in the family. Things were going smoothly for us at the time, I had a good job I enjoyed, my sons were at university. So it didn't fit into any of those. It was rather out-of-the-blue. I have often wondered about why I am a diabetic but have never come up with any answers as to what caused it. (40 year old female, secretary, married to an army officer).*

English patients talked of their distress at the moment of diagnosis as being partly to do with the inexplicability of causation. A 24 year old women employee of British Telecom, married to a Telephone Engineer, commented:

> *I was very upset. Sitting there in tears. Why should it happen to me?*

The obvious question was "What have I done to deserve it?"

Some non-familial patients reported how surprised they had been to get diabetes because up until that time they had thought diabetes was only a hereditary disease.

None of the Hindu patients spontaneously mentioned "karma" when asked about the cause of their own diabetes which suggests that karma does not constitute a key causal category for lay people in their explanation of diabetes. However, there is some suggestion in the data that Hindu patients take some comfort in the concept of "karma". When patients were directly asked about karma, 64% thought that karma was implicated in their diabetes. Many of the patients greeted the question of karma with a wry smile and an upper class female patient laughed and said:

> *Karma ! I believe in that. Having got diabetes, I believe in that. I mean … this is just a palliative for your own mind. Not to feel sorry for yourself. The idea that you are destined to have it; that it will happen. That works as a palliative for your disturbed mind. (65 year old housewife, married to an officer in the Indian Civil Service)*

Analytically, karma can be considered either as a very elaborate theory of personal causation ("I am suffering in this life due to misdeeds in my previous life") or as a much more general theory of predestination. Philosophers studying the Hindu religion suggest that karma is an example of the latter but not the former. For example, Bowes (1977), writes that karmic explanation is not to be understood as an example of an individual theory of personal responsibility and is not a rebirth in the

Western sense of the same person but of the life force itself. One patient juggled with these two aspects of karma commenting:

> *When troubles come for which I can't find a reason, then I put them on karma. When you aren't doing wrong to anybody and wrong comes to you then ... if I haven't done anything wrong in this birth, but then wrong things come to me. Then I put it on my previous birth. You may not know what you have done in your previous karma but you have to pay in this. These calculations are very difficult ... to whom you did, and how you are getting. But that you cannot calculate. Whether the ... the crux of the thing, is whatever comes to you, accept it. (55 year old female accountant)*

The notion of karma as acceptance was quite common with statements such as "Karma is there, you have to suffer" and "What has happened has happened, why think so much about it."

The role of self-blame

In dealing with patients' causal theories I have not attempted to classify their theories according to the conventions of attribution theory - that is to say according to whether the patients make personal or situational attributions or internal/external attributions. It is inadvisable to classify items such as "heredity" or "stress" on an *a priori* basis across patients. As Turnquist et al. (1988) point out "heredity" has been coded as either external or internal by different authors. "Stress" could be interpreted as an external situational factor or as an internal personality factor. Indeed, the social representations of the terms "heredity" and "stress" within various cultures is a subject worthy of study in its own right. Any attempt to classify such concepts would involve a substantial amount of further questioning of each patient and it must be borne in mind that such interviews may serve to cloud rather than to clarify the issue. Watts (1982) has correctly noted that "patients may be able to entertain a varied series of discrete explanations" (p. 137), even though they tend to only present one of these initially. Similarly it would be improper to assume that one understood by the use of a particular causal item whether the patient was engaging in behavioural or characterological self-blame.

Rather than classify the items offered as causes into attributional categories, patients were directly asked whether they thought there was anything they could have done to prevent themselves from getting diabetes and whether they in any way blamed themselves for their diabetes. As we have already seen, English patients were more likely to nominate a cause for their diabetes and they were also more likely to affirm that something happened in their life to bring on the diabetes (see Table 9.3).

Only a minority of Indian and English patients thought they could have prevented the disease, and diet was the most commonly mentioned single item. No patients blamed others, in the sense of holding them culpably responsible, for their disease and this accords with other research on causal attribution in chronic illness (Tennen et al. 1984; Affleck et al. 1987).

Table 9.3 – Further questions on cause

	INDIA		ENGLAND	
Sample	55		53	
Question	N of patients answering "yes"			
Did something happen to bring on your diabetes?	24	44%	3	62%
Do you think you could have prevented your diabetes?	16	29%	11	21%
Do you blame yourself for your diabetes?	18	38%	3	6%

Among the English patients only six per cent blame themselves for their diabetes and the reply below was typical:

Well, of course it was all the Coca-Cola I drank as a child, but no, I don't blame myself ... I wasn't to know, was I? (35 year old female secretary)

In contrast 38% of Indian patients blamed themselves for their diabetes and the explanation for this can be found in their commentary that they should have known better than to consume the wrong diet. Such a statement was offered not as an indication of the patient's particular risk of diabetes but from the point of view that "we all should know better". A 52 year old man who was a foreman in a naval dockyard blamed himself for his diabetes as he used to eat too many sweetmeats saying "none of us should do that". A 56 year old man who was a Central Government Officer in the Ministry of Commerce commented:

Being a South Indian, we used to take in our diet more of the starch. Rice is our staple food. And when at home, we used to take once a day ghee (clarified butter). You know how in Mysore State they take raw ghee. I was taking that but I shouldn't have.

The roots of the excess-restraint dilemma so commonly reported by these patients can be traced to traditional Aruyvedic and folk medicine in India which place great stress on care, balance and restraint of diet (Nichter, 1980; Kakar, 1982; Goody, 1982), while the culture simultaneously places a high premium on commensality. One 61 year old retired state government officer spoke whimsically of his life prior to diabetes where he could have food at parties to his heart's content. He succinctly described his resolution of the excess-restraint dilemma while also portraying the pressures related to food and social occasions in India:

These marriages - these lunches are very tempting. Everyone says "Take, Take". There are two sweet courses or so. There are often times when - you know they say "The best way of overcoming temptation is to succumb to it". There have been occasions when I have succumbed to it. Then what I do at night is starve. Sweetmeats are my own special weakness.

A number of patients yearned for their childhood days of unrestrained access to joint-family kitchens where, in their memories at least, there was an unlimited supply of delicious and usually sweet food. Others spoke longingly of their desire to eat deep-fried savouries sold on street stalls - forbidden to them not only on account of their diabetes but on account of general health concerns and on grounds of purity and pollution concerns with respect to caste (Marriott, 1968).

LONG-TERM ADJUSTMENT

Relationship between causal reasoning and long-term adjustment

Turnquist et al. (1988) note that adjustment to illness is a complex process which may demand changes in many spheres of life. As stated earlier, insulin involved diabetes requires life-long monitoring of diet, carefully timed injections etc. In order to investigate adjustment patients were asked whether the treatment disturbed or interfered with their life, whether having diabetes stopped them doing anything that they wanted to do, and whether their life would have been different in any important way if they had not had diabetes.

Patients varied considerably in their reactions to the diabetic regime. One young Englishman commented:

You are kind of tied because you can't ... you have to be at home every morning, you can't just say I'm off for three days. You can't really go off on your own, certainly not on a holiday even if you wanted to, because it is very tricky ... something might happen, things can happen that you can't control, a hypo. So it does limit you .. It does limit your career... Diabetics are not allowed in the police or the army - so there is a stop there. And I think I did have some aspirations to the army. (28 year old, male, assistant computer programmer)

Such a transcript can be compared with the reply of another Englishman who said:

No, I'm a fighter. I look round at some of the other people who haven't got it, and they don't do as much exercise as I do. Any sport I play it, because I don't like being beaten by it... I don't really think about it, except in the morning when I give myself the first injection then I forget about it till the next one. Its just a way of life now ... if you look after yourself you are no different to anyone else. (29 year old, male, toolmaker)

Seventy four per cent of the English patients reported some kind of adjustment problems and their predominant concerns were with lost opportunities they had experienced as individuals in their career and sporting aspirations. Sixty nine per cent of the Indian patients reported adjustment problems but their emphasis was on failed obligations in the area of social and family roles. One elderly Indian woman living in a joint-family commented:

> I feel I am unable to do my duty towards my children. If one can't do even that duty what good is that person for? ... I have to take my 5 year old grand-daughter to school. I do it. But now I'm not confident about the other grandchildren and whether I'll be able to look after them or not.

Even when Indian patients did talk of career difficulties associated with diabetes they rarely blamed diabetes for lack of career advancement but instead tended to talk of technical difficulties associated with injections and diet when their jobs forced them to travel outside Bombay. The emphasis on the workplace for the English patient, and on the family for the Indian patient in answers to the adjustment questions, echoes the cultural differences already discussed in connection with the notion of stress as a causal agent.

The original hypothesis had been that, for the English sample, having a causal theory would be predictive of better adjustment and this was supported. There was a tendency for the poorly adjusted a) to be disproportionately represented amongst those who could not nominate a cause for their own diabetes, b) to state that nothing had happened in their lives to bring the diabetes on, and c) to comment that their diabetes could not have been prevented. For example, amongst those who thought they could not have prevented their diabetes, 79% reported adjustment problems, whereas amongst those who thought they could have prevented their diabetes only 55% reported adjustment problems. The data therefore support other research in Western cultures which suggests that having a causal theory is related to better adjustment and coping and, conversely, that having no causal theory is related to poorer adjustment (Turnquist et al. 1988). However, as already pointed out, self-blame as such was very rare in the English sample. The Indian data present a different pattern of results. Overall levels of adjustment were the same as in England but do not relate to causal theory. Answers to the question about the cause of their diabetes and to subsequent questions about whether anything happened to bring on the diabetes and whether the diabetes could have been prevented were not related to measures of adjustment. Having a causal theory about one's own diabetes was predictive of neither good nor bad adjustment and in this way it can be seen that the relationship between attributional style and behaviour which is characteristic of Western society does not seem to be, in this study, characteristic of Indian society. Self-blame in the Indian sample was also not related to adjustment.

It has been suggested that one of the benefits of having a causal theory is that it may confirm the patient in the ideology that the world is a controllable place in which future bad outcomes can be avoided.

However, as Turnquist et al. (1988) have pointed out empirical support for this, or any other mechanism, is not strong. Since diabetic patients do face the prospect of medical complications associated with their condition, it is possible to question patients directly about the degree of control they expect to have over the future of the illness and relate this to their causal reasoning. Forty nine per cent of the English patients were worried by the thought of diabetic complications and there was a slight tendency for these patients not to have an answer to the initial question on the cause of their diabetes. However, there was no association between patients having a causal theory for their own diabetes and their outlook on future control since all but one of the patients thought that they could do something to avoid these complications. Their outlook can in part be related to the very optimistic atmosphere of the clinic they attended and the data suggest that the relationship between causal theorising and adjustment is not mediated by patients' beliefs about the control they expect to have over their illness.

Of the 40 Indian patients who knew about diabetic complications, 40% were worried about them but worry bore no relation to the causal reasoning offered earlier. Only four patients thought that nothing could be done about avoiding complications and these patients were not distinctive in terms of having or not having a causal theory. In both cultures patients talked of the importance of a restricted diet and taking exercise. However, English patients placed great importance on having regular blood tests while Indian patients talked more generally of "following the doctor's advice" and also talked of the use of aruyvedic medicine and remedies such as karela (bitter gourd). I noted that during their medical consultations, Indian patients referred quite frequently to aruyvedic preparations which the doctors tended to "tolerate" while stressing that the patient must also continue with insulin. Indian patients talked in their interviews about their use of "alternative medicine" and the consultant in one of the clinics, chancing to overhear, would sometimes enter into jocular interchange with the patient about the efficacy or otherwise of karela.

Dietary management

The material on adjustment discussed so far concerns the patients' replies to questions about whether diabetes and its management interferes with their longterm goals. The patients were also asked more specific questions about whether they were currently having difficulties in managing the treatment regime. Fifteen per cent of the English sample reported difficulties in managing their diet on a daily basis and usually talked about "timing" difficulties, for example "at what point do you inject when you are going out to eat - how late will dinner be?" However, 56% of the Indian patients reported difficulties in managing their diet which spread far beyond the timing of injections. A variety of social occasions ranging from visiting family and friends to attending marriage parties were reported as impossible to manage due to the type of food consumed on such occasions and the pressure on guests to partake of the food. When asked about the diet one male patient said:

> *It's damn difficult. When we go out with friends I have to order something different. Everyone looks at me thinking he is different. We can't go to anybody's house for the lunch and so on. We can't accept any invitations.*

A 50 year old police officer spoke of his regret at not being able to enjoy sweet food along with his friends and family. Several patients reported that the pressure to eat at social occasions was so great that they did not go to the lunch part of marriage parties and one lawyer commented on how he could not make visits at Diwali on account of all the food and drink he was offered.

The difficulty which Indian patients face with following the diabetic diet can be related to the very special role of food in Hindu culture and the importance of the specific social roles and rules which constitute social occasions. As Appadurai (1981) has noted, food is the focus of much taxonomic and moral thought and "in contemporary South Asian society, even a casual visitor can only be impressed by the importance of food in daily life and daily discourse" (p. 495). For Hindus the offering of food to a deity is a crucial component of the act of worship (Ferro-Luzzi, 1977). Khare (1976) estimates that there are at least 105 fasts and festivals in the Hindu calendar, with 20 being major observances. Many festivals are celebrated with the eating of deep-fried savouries and particular sweetmeats, none of which should be part of a diabetic's diet. In Maharashtra pedhas and barfi must be consumed at Diwali, sweet chappatis at Holi, modak (sweet rice and coconut balls) at Ganpati. Indeed the happy fat elephant God Ganpati (Ganesh) is the most popular household deity in the Bombay region. Krishna, another favourite deity, is associated with butter, on account of his time as a cowherd. Further, at the festival of Sankrant the ritual exchange of sesame sugar ladoos is an intrinsic part of the occasion wherein people offer a ladoo saying "Til gul ghya, gode bola" - "Take this sweet sesame and speak sweetly to me" (for the year).

In India it is considered a great insult to the host if the guest does not eat the food that is offered. Khare (1976) writes that the pleasure of eating is only complete when associated with "the domestic warmth of one's kind and affines". In addition to festivals, there are many other family gatherings and weddings. It would be inauspicious if at least one sweet dish (e.g. jelabi, sheera) was not offered at a wedding feast. A 24 year old telephone operator told of the social pressures entailed in these occasions:

> *We have to eat. Because weddings when you go and you don't eat. Its not good. Like its for respect. And for weddings they will specially give the card to you. And they'll say come for food. Come for their food ... So in the weddings, especially in India, we find all puris and that, which will get more oil and ghee, and vegetables also they will put full of oil. That's a problem.*

Fifty six per cent of Indian patients reported difficulties with their diet while attending weddings commenting that people pressed them to eat saying that "One day won't make a difference". Only two of the English patients mentioned that occasions such as Christmas presented any difficulty and tended to stress that relatives erred on the side of pressing caution rather than indulgence.

Indians might be expected to be particularly receptive to dietary advice given the historic emphasis in Aruyvedic and folk medicine on diet as treatment, the contemporary stress which cosmopolitan medicine in India places on diet (Goody, 1982), and the importance placed by Indian patients on receiving dietary advice (Nichter, 1980). However, other research in Bombay (Sivakumar et al. 1986) and on predominantly Hindu Gujerati communities in Britain (Peterson et al. 1986; Samanta et al. 1987) has also pointed to the severe difficulties that Asian diabetics have in regulating their diets. Being well-fed is a sign of affluence in Asian society and several patients in the present sample commented on this. However, the interview material clearly revealed that most patients knew that they ought to monitor their diets more carefully and wanted to do so. Their difficulties can only be understood in terms of the complex role of food in Hindu culture.

CONCLUSION

Medical science offers the familial diabetic patient a probabilistic account of the cause of their disease and we see from the scant use of heredity in lay causal explanation that patients are not satisfied with heredity as an explanation of their condition. Wolpert (1992) suggests that scientific and lay reasoning have quite different origins noting that while an idea such as heredity is common in lay explanation, the scientific explanation of family resemblance could not have been achieved by common-sense. The aspect of medical reasoning which the familial patients in this study found hard to grasp is not the term "heredity" as such but the probabilistic nature of the explanation involved. Their dilemma is reminiscent of Malinowski's (1948) "primitive man" who resorts to magic when chance and circumstance are not fully understood, and " ... clings to it, whenever he has to recognise the impotence of his knowledge and of his rational technique" (p. 15).

In order to fully answer the "why me" question to their satisfaction, familial and non-familial diabetic patients in India and England sought to explain the cause of their illness in terms of a variety of factors including diet, stress and shock. The extensive use of diet in both cultures is entirely compatible with the "machine model" of the body (Osherson and AmaraSingham, 1981) within cosmopolitan medicine and the humoural physicalistic model of the body within aruyvedic medicine (Leslie, 1976). The English patients' use of shock as a systemic pathological factor rather than as a psychological stressor further locates their explanations in a strictly physical universe. The Indian patients' use of stress, particularly given the emphasis which they place on problems arising from family obligations, gives an interesting insight into the sometimes precarious relationship between the individual self and the familial self in Hindu society.

For English patients the data suggest a connection between having a causal theory of one's own diabetes and adjustment to the condition. Throughout the interview the English patients focused on the trajectory of their past and future lives and were concerned with what they could achieve for themselves in career terms, and how they as individuals could manage the condition. For the Hindu patients having a causal theory of their diabetes promoted neither good nor bad adjustment. Karma was not offered as a specific cause but did feature when the patients were directly questioned about it. It might be tempting to describe the Hindu patients in terms of indifference with respect to cause and, given their expressed difficulties in managing the regime, as passive with respect to treatment. But the transcripts suggest not so much a passive approach to diet as an active, if sometimes troubled, approach to the fulfilment of social obligation. One Hindu middle-aged woman recounted that the only reason that she adhered to the diabetic diet was to stay alive to care for husband and family.

Much current health education focuses on the problems patients have in translating their goals into actions and recent models in social psychology have stressed the importance of the normative factors which influence the pathway between attitude and behaviour (Ajzen, 1988). The data of the present study reveal how very complex and powerful those normative presures can be. Family and friends may in a general sense desire the patient to act in a healthy manner but will also have conflicting desires for the patient to be a good guest. Diabetic patients in India recount these pressures to be greater than do diabetic patients in England. This research is of some relevance to the manner in which doctors and dieticians advise Indian patients, particularly in inter-cultural settings, where English staff may regard non-compliant patients as weak-willed and overlook the social context of individuals' health care decisions. In prescribing treatment regimes for Indian patients, medical exhortations may be more successful if couched in terms of social obligations rather than in terms, more familiar to Westerners, of individual obligation.

The giving and receiving of food is of tremendous significance in Hindu society. Appadurai (1981) has commented that profound conceptions of self are involved in transactions involving food. In India, on occasions like marriage parties, individuals are not merely representing themselves but their extended families and this alters the options individuals have regarding their own behaviour in these settings. Some patients reported explicitly sending "delegates" to take their place so that they could avoid being put in the position of eating unsuitable food. In order to understand why these pressures are so powerful the construction of the self in Hindu society must be appreciated. While it is the case that Dumont's (1970) polarised description of the autonomous Westerner and the rule-governed Hindu is over-simplistic, Markus and Kitayama (1991) have usefully suggested that for many non-Western cultures "it is the 'other' or the 'self-in-relation-to-other' that is focal in individual experience" (p. 225). The material of these interviews supports research which has suggested that in India individuals construe themselves and others as much in terms of social roles as of individual attributes. Shweder and Bourne (1982) have demonstrated how Hindus describe their friends in social relational rather than personality terms, and Miller (1984) presents data which show that adult Hindus place greater emphasis than Americans on contextual factors in their everyday social explanations. Kon (1984) notes that the self has a negative rather than a positive value in a number of Asian societies and Sinha (1985, cited in Triandis, 1989) suggests that conformity to others in public settings is highly valued in collectivist cultures whereas to be distinct and different is highly valued in individualistic cultures. Roland (1988) has extensively described how individuals in India are very aware of reciprocal obligations and responsibilities and of "the social etiquette of hierarchical relationships" (p. 233). It can be argued that one of the reasons that Hindu diabetic patients find it so difficult to resist eating certain foods on social occasions is that they find it hard to isolate their needs as diabetic patients from their social obligations and to give priority, in Roland's (1988) terms, to their individual self rather than their familial self. One Hindu male diabetic patient in the study encapsulated this view of self when he reported how he was unable to refuse to eat at a wedding not simply because he didn't want to be rude but because he "didn't want to appear as a separate person."

ACKNOWLEDGMENTS

I would like to thank all the patients in Bombay and Brighton who so freely gave their views and time. Dr J. C. Patel (The Bombay Hospital), Dr S. S. Ajgaonkar, (The All-India Institute of Diabetes/S. L. Raheja Hospital) and Dr V. D. Laghate (Jagjivanram Hospital) and the late Dr Joanna Sheldon (The Royal Sussex Hospital) for giving me encouragement and access to their patients. Sunita Joshi, Chattora Ranade, Ann Allen, Freda Gardner and Sophie Green provided excellent research assistance. The Nuffield Foundation is also to be thanked for a supporting grant.

REFERENCES

Affleck, G., Pfeiffer, C., Tennen, H. and Fifield, J. (1987), Attributional processes in rheumatoid arthritis. *Arthritis and Rheumatism*, **30**, 927–931.

Ajzen, I. (1988), *Attitudes, Personality and Behavior*. Milton Keynes: Open University Press.

Appadurai, A. (1981), Gastro-politics in Hindu South Asia, *American Ethnologist* **8**, 494–511.

Beals, A. R. (1976), Strategies of resort to curers in South India. In *Asian Medical Systems: A Comparative Study*, edited by C. Leslie, pp. 184–200. Berkeley and Los Angeles: University of California Press.

Bloom Cerkoney, K. A. and Hart, L. K. (1980), The relationship between the health belief model and compliance of persons with diabetes mellitus. *Diabetes Care* **3** (5) 594–598.

British Diabetic Association (1980), *The Diabetic's Handbook,* London: British Diabetic Association.

Bennett, P. H. (1983), Diabetes in developing countries and unusual populations. In *Diabetes in Epidemiological Perspective,* edited by J. I. Mann, K. Pyorala, and A. Teuscher, pp. 43–57. Edinburgh: Churchill Livingstone.

Bollag, U. (1983), Practicable measures for the detection and care of diabetes mellitus in developing countries. In *Diabetes in Epidemiological Perspective,* edited by J.I. Mann, K. Pyorala, and A. Teuscher, pp. 345–355. Edinburgh: Churchill Livingstone.

Bowes, P. (1977), *The Hindu Religious Tradition,* London: Routledge & Kegan Paul.

Bradley, C. and Marteau, T. (1986), Towards an integration of psychological and medical perspectives of diabetes management. In *Diabetes Annual,* edited by K. G. M. M. Alberti, and L. P. Krall, vol.2, pp. 169–183. Amsterdam: Elsevier Science Publishers.

Bulman, R. J. and Wortman, C. B. (1977), Attribution of blame and coping in the "real world": Severe accident victims react to their lot, *Journal of Personality and Social Psychology,* **35**, 351–363.

Carstairs, G. M. (1957), *The Twice-Born: A Study of a Community of High-caste Hindus,* London: Hogarth Press.

Carstairs, G. M. and Kapur, R. L. (1976), *The Great Universe of Kota:Stress, Change and Mental Disorder in an Indian Village,* London: Hogarth Press.

Cartwright, A. (1967), *Patients and Their Doctors,* London: Routledge & Kegan Paul.

Dumont, L. (1970), *Homo Hierarchicus* London: Weidenfeld & Nicolson.

Dunn, F. L. (1976), Traditional Asian medicine and cosmopolitcan medicine asadaptive systems. In *Asian Medical Systems: A Comparative Study,* edited by C. Leslie, pp. 133–158. Berkeley and Los Angeles: University of California Press.

Eisenberg, L. (1977), Disease and illness: Distinctions between professional and popular ideas of sickness, *Culture, Medicine and Psychiatry,* **1**, 9–23.

Ferro-Luzzi, G. E. (1977), Ritual as language: The case of South Indian food offerings, *Current Anthropology,* **18(3)** 507–514.

Furnham, A. (1982), Explanations for unemployment in Britain, *European Journal of Social Psychology,* **12**, 335–352.

Godbole, A. S. (1976), *Full Life with Diabetes,* Bombay: Popular Prakashan.

Goody, J. (1982), *Cooking, Cuisine and Class: A Study in Comparative Sociology,* Cambridge: Cambridge University Press.

Greenberg, L. W., Jewett, L. S., Gluck, R. S., Champion, L. A. A., Leiken, S. F., Altieri, M. F. et al. (1984), Giving information for a life-threatening diagnosis: Parents' and oncologists' perceptions, *American Journal of Diabetes Care,* **138**, 649–653.

Guzder, J. and Krishna, M. (1991), Sita-Shakti: Cultural paradigms for Indian women, *Transcultural Psychiatric Research Review,* **28**, 257–301.

Hamman, R. F. (1983), Diabetes in affluent societies. In *Diabetes in Epidemiological Perspective,* edited by J. I. Mann, K. Pyorala, and A. Teuscher, pp. 7–42. Edinburgh: Churchill Livingstone.

Harré, R. (1981), Expressive aspects of descriptions of others. In *The Psychology of Ordinary Explanations of Social Behaviour,* edited by C. Antaki, pp. 139–156. London: Academic Press.

Harré, R. and Secord, P. (1972), *The Explanation of Social Behaviour,* Oxford: Blackwell.

Harris, R., Linn, M. W. and Pollack, L. (1984), Relationship between health beliefs and psychological variables in diabetic patients, *British Journal of Medical Psychology,* **57**, 253–259.

Heelas, P. (1981), 'Introduction: Indigenous Psychologies'. In *Indigenous Psychologies: The Anthropology of the Self,* edited by P. Heelas and A. Lock, pp. 3–18. London: Academic Press.

Heider, F. (1958), *The Psychology of Interpersonal Relations,* New York: Wiley.

Helman, C. G. (1978), "Feed a cold, starve a fever" - Folk models of infection in an English suburban community, and their relation to medical treatment, *Culture, Medicine and Psychiatry,* **2**, 107–137.

Helman, C. G. (1990), *Culture, Health and Illness,* Sevenoaks: Wright.

Herzlich, C. (1973), *Health and Illness: A Social Psychological Perspective* London: Academic Press.

Hewstone, M. (1988), *Causal Attribution: From Cognitive Processes to Collective Beliefs* Oxford: Blackwell.

Hopper, S. (1981), Diabetes as a stigmatized condition: The case of low-income clinic patients in the United States, *Social Science and Medicine,* **153**, 11–19.

Horton, R. (1970), African traditional thought and western science. In *Rationality,* edited by B. R. Wilson, pp. 131–171. Oxford: Blackwell.

Jaggi, O. P. (1973), *Indian System of Medicine,* Atma Ram and Sons.

Jain, S. and Patel, J. C. (1984), Economic status, castes and locality of diabetes atttending O. P. D. of All India Institute of Diabetes, *Journal of the Diabetic Association of India,* **XXIV** (1), 9–11.

Jolly, J. (1977), *Indian Medicine,* Manishiram Manoharlal Publishers.

Kakar, S. (1982), *Shamans, Mystics and Doctors: A Psychological Inquiry into India and Its Healing Tradition,* Delhi: Oxford University Press.

Khare, R. S. (1976), *The Hindu Hearth and Home* New Delhi: Vikas.

Kelley, H. H. (1971), Attribution in social interaction. In *Attribution: Perceiving the Causes of Behavior,* edited by E. E. Jones, D. E. Kanouse, H. H. Kelley, R. E. Nisbett, S. Valins, and B. Weiner, pp. 1–26. Morristown, NJ: General Learning Press.

Kon, I. S. (1984), The self as a historical-cultural and ethnopsychological phenomenon. In *Directions in Soviet Social Psychology,* edited by L. H. Strickland, pp. 29–46. Springer Series in Social Psychology, New York: Springer-Verlag.

Lalljee, M. (1981), Attribution theory and the analysis of explanations. In *The Psychology of Ordinary Explanations of Social Behaviour,* edited by C. Antaki, pp. 119–138. London: Academic Press.

Leff, J. (1988), *Psychiatry Around the Globe* London: Gaskell/The Royal College of Psychiatrists.

Leslie, C. (1976), Introduction. In *Asian Medical Systems: A Comparative Study,* edited by C. Leslie, pp. 1–12. Berkeley and Los Angeles: University of California Press.

Lewis, G. (1975), *Knowledge of Illness in a Sepik Society,* London: Athlone Press.

Littlewood, R. and Lipsedge, M. (1982), *Aliens and Alienists: Ethnic Minorities and Psychiatry,* Harmondsworth: Penguin.

Madan, T. N. (1969), Who chooses modern medicine and why? *Economic and Political Weekly,* **4(37)**, 1475–1484.

Malinowski, B. (1948), *Magic, Science and Religion and other essays*, Selected and edited by R. Redfield,. Glencoe, Illinois: The Free Press.

Marriott, M. (1968), Caste ranking and food transactions. In *Structure and Change in Indian Society,* edited by M. Singer and B. S. Cohn, pp. 133–171. Chicago: Aldine Publishing Company.

Mann, J. I. (1984), "Dietary fibre and diabetes" *Dietary Fibre in the Management of Diabetes* Proceedings of the British Diabetic Association Symposium held in London on I June 1984. Oxford: Medical Education Services Ltd.

Markus, H. R. and Kitayama, S. (1991), Culture and the self: Implications for cognition, emotion, and motivation, *Psychological Review,* **98(2)**, 224–253.

Mead, G. H. (1934), *Mind, Self and Society,* Chicago: University of Chicago Press.

Mehta, R. (1976), From purdah to modernity. In Indian Women, edited by B. R. Nanda, pp. 113–128. New Delhi: Vikas.

Miller, J. G. (1984), Culture and the development of everyday social explanation, *Journal of Personality and Social Psychology,* **46(5)**, 961–978.

Miller, J. G., Bersoff, D. M. and Harwood, R. L. (1990), Perceptions of social responsibilities in India and in the United States: Moral imperatives or personal decisions? *Journal of Personality and Social Psychology,* **58(1)**, 33–47.

Mull, J. D. and Mull, D. S. (1988), Mothers' concepts of childhood diarrhea in rural Pakistan: What ORT program planners should know, *Social Science and Medicine,* **27(1)**, 53–67.

Nichter, M. (1980), The layperson's perceptions of medicine as perspective into the utilization of multiple therapy systems in the Indian context, *Social Science and Medicine,* **14B(4)**, 225–233.

Oakley, W. G., Pyke, D. A. and Taylor, K. W. (1978), *Diabetes and its Management,* Oxford: Blackwell Scientific Publications.

Osherson, S. and AmaraSingham, L. (1981), The machine metaphor in medicine. In *Social Contexts of Health, Illness and Patient Care,* edited by E. Mishler, L. R. AmaraSinghman, S. T. Hauser, R. Liem, S. D. Osherson and N. E. Waxler, pp. 218–249. Cambridge: Cambridge University Press.

Patel, J. C. and Talwalkar, N. G. (1966), *Diabetes in the Tropics* Bombay: Diabetic Association of India.

Peterson, D. B., Dattani, J. T., Baylis, J. M. and Jepson, E. M. (1986), Dietary practices of Asian diabetics, *British Medical Journal,* **292**, 170–171.

Pill, R. and Stott, N. C. H. (1982), Concepts of illness causation and responsibility: some preliminary data from a sample of working class mothers, Social Science & Medicine, **16**, 43–52.

Posner, T. (1977), Magical elements in orthodox medicine: Diabetes as a medical thought system. In *Health Care and Health Knowledge,* edited by R. Dingwall, C. Heath, M. Reid, and M. Stacey, pp. 141–158. London: Croom Helm.

Rack, P. (1982), *Race, Culture, and Mental Disorder,* London: Tavistock.

Roland, A. (1988), *In Search of Self in India and Japan: Towards a Cross-Cultural Psychology,* Princeton: Princeton University Press.

Samanta, A., Campbell, J. E., Spalding, D. L., Panja, K. K., Neoggi, S. K. and Burden, A. C. (1987), Dietary habits of Asian diabetics in a general practice clinic, *Human Nutrition: Applied Nutrition,* **41A**, 160–163.

Sanders, K., Mills, J., Martin, F. I. R. and Home, D. J. D. (1975), Emotional attitudes in adult insulin-dependent diabetics, *Journal of Psychosomatic Research,* **19**, 241–246.

Shah, A. (1974), *The Household Dimension of the Family in India* Berkeley and Los Angeles: University of California Press.

Shillitoe, R. W. and Miles, D. W. (1989), Diabetes mellitus. In *Health Psychology: Processes and Applications,* edited by A. K. Browne, pp. 208–233. London: Chapman & Hall.

Shweder, R. A. (1977), Likeness and likelihood in everyday thought: magical thinking and everyday judgments about personality. In *Thinking: Readings in Cognitive*

Science, edited by Wason, P. C. and Johnson-Laird, P. N. pp. 446–467. Cambridge: Cambridge University Press.

Shweder, R. A. and Bourne, E. (1982), Does the concept of the person vary cross-culturally? In *Cultural Conceptions of Mental Health and Therapy,* edited by A. J. Marsella, and G. White, pp. 97–137. Reidel: Dordrecht.

Sivakumar, S. D., Raja, D. V. P. and Kannan, K. (1986), What does an average general hospital diabetic subject think of his illness – a survey, *Journal of the Diabetic Association of India,* **XXVI** (1), 30–34.

Sonksen, P. H. and West, T. E. T. (1978), Carbohydrate metabolism and diabetes mellitus. In *Recent Advances in Endocrinology and Metabolism,* edited by J. H. L. O'Riordan. London: Churchill Livingstone.

Spencer, K. and Cudworth, A. (1983), The aetiology of insulin dependent diabetes mellitus. In *Diabetes in Epidemiological Perspective,* edited by J. I. Mann, K. Pyorala, and A. Teuscher, pp. 99–164. Edinburgh: Churchill Livingstone.

Stainton Rogers, W. (1991), *Explaining Health and Illness: An Exploration of Diversity,* Hemel Hempstead: Harvester Wheatsheaf.

Stimson, G. and Webb, B. (1975), *Going to See the Doctor: The Consultation Process in General Prcatice,* London: Routledge & Kegan Paul.

Strauss, A. L. (1987), *Qualitative Analysis for Social Scientists.* Cambridge: Cambridge University Press.

Taylor, C. (1985), The person. In *The Category of the Person. Anthropology, Philosophy, History,* edited by M. Carrithers, S. Collins, and S. Lukes, pp. 257–281. Cambridge: Cambridge University Press.

Taylor, S. E., Lichtman, R. R. and Wood, J. V. (1984), Attributions, beliefs about control, and adjustment to breast cancer, *Journal of Personality and Social Psychology,* **46**, 489–502.

Tennen, H. and Affleck, G. (1990), Blaming others for threatening events, *Psychological Bulletin,* **108** (2), 209–232.

Tennen, H., Affleck, G., Allen, D. A., McGrade, B. J. and Ratzan, S. (1984), Causal attributions and coping with insulin-dependent diabetes, *Basic and Applied Psychology,* **5**, 131–142.

Tennen, H., Affleck, G. and Gershman, K. (1986), Self-blame among parents of infants with perinatal complications: The role of self-protective motives, *Journal of Personality and Social Psychology,* **50**, 690–696.

Totman, R. (1982), Philosophical foundations of attribution therapies. In *Attributions and Psychological Change: Applications of Attributional Theories to Clinical and Educational Practice,* edited by C. Antaki, and C. Brewin, pp. 45–59. London: Academic Press.

Triandis, H. (1989), The self and social behaviour in differing cultural contexts, *Psychological Review,* **96(3)**, 506–520.

Turnquist, D. C., Harvey, J. H. and Andersen, B. L., (1988), Attributions and adjustment to life-threatening illness, *British Journal of Clinical Psychology,* **27(1)**, 55–65.

Waitzkin, H. and Stoeckle, D. (1976), Information control and the micropolitics of health care: Summary of an on-going research project, *Social Science and Medicine,* **10**, 263–276.

Watkins, J. D., Roberts, D. E., Williams, T. F., Martin, D. A. and Coyle, V. (1967), Observation of medication errors made by diabetic patients in the home, *Diabetes,* **16**, 882–885.

Watkins, J. D., Williams, T. F., Martin, D. A., Hogan, M. D. and Anderson, E. (1967), A study of diabetic patients at home, *American Journal of Public Health,* **57**, 441–451.

Watts, F. N. (1982), Attributional aspects of medicine. In *Attributions and Psychological Change: Applications of Attributional Theories to Clinical and Education Practice,* edited by C. Antaki, and C. Brewin, pp. 135–155. London: Academic Press.

Williams, G. H. (1986), Lay beliefs about the causes of rheumatoid arthritis: Their implications for rehabilitation, *International Rehabilitation Medicine* **8**, 65–68.

Wolpert, L. (1992), *The Unnatural Nature of Science,* London: Faber and Faber.

Wortman, C. B. (1976), Causal attributions and personal control. In *New Directions in Attribution Research,* Volume 1, edited by J. H. Harvey, W. J. Ickes, and R. F. Kidd, pp. 23–52. Hillsdale, NJ: Erlbaum.

Part III — Representations of Human Agency and of the Quality of Life

TEN   **Human Agency and the Quality of Life: A Theoretical Overview**   **191**
Ivana Marková

ELEVEN   **Quality of Life: Hope for the Future or an Echo from the Distant Past?**   **205**
Andrew Jahoda

TWELVE   **Quality of Life and Mental Health: Evaluating the Impact of Long-Term Care**   **225**
Margaret M. Barry and Charles Crosby

THIRTEEN   **Coping and Human Agency**   **249**
Ladislav Valach

CHAPTER TEN

Human Agency and the Quality of Life: A Theoretical Overview

Ivana MARKOVÁ

Department of Psychology, University of Stirling, Stirling, FK9 4LA

INTRODUCTION

Questions such as what constitutes a good quality of life and well-being, for a long time now, have had important places in the philosophical thought of Western civilization. Without much analytical effort one can easily discern two extreme philosophical viewpoints on this subject, with the remainder falling somewhere between the two. The first viewpoint derives well-being, happiness and pleasure entirely from an individual's attitude of mind. For example, the Epicurean philosophers in ancient Greece thought that a wise and self-controlled individual could be happy and feel well irrespective of any adverse situation in which he or she happens to be placed, including, say, physical torture. According to Epicurus, even being burned or tortured within the very bull of Phalaris, the wise man will say: 'How sweet, how indifferent I am to this!' (Cicero, Tusculan Disputations, II, VII, 17). For the Epicureans, therefore, the individual's well-being was independent of environmental or societal factors and it was fully determined by the individual him- or herself. Since Aristotle, philosophers have thought that happiness should be the aim of human life although, as Aristotle himself was aware, for different people happiness could mean quite different things.

The other extreme viewpoint was taken up much later by the utilitarian philosophy which sought the origin of well-being in the extent to which environment and social welfare satisfied the individual's needs. Utilitarianism assessed objects in terms of their utility, that is whether they tended to produce 'benefit, advantage, pleasure, good or happiness and prevented evil or unhappiness' (Bentham, 1970, p.12). Utilitarian philosophy emphasized that individuals are themselves the best judges of their own well-being and they are able to decide for themselves the value of material objects and to choose among them accordingly. Human actions should conform with the principle of utility: they should augment happiness and diminish unhappiness, both in themselves and in the community at large.

The meaning of the notion 'well-being' and the ways well-being can be achieved are thus highly variable, and one wonders whether any common ground can be found between two such disparate positions. Part III of this book will address the question as to which kinds of factors, e.g. individual, cultural or socio-historical, contribute to what is thought to be 'well-being' and how the meaning of this term changes over time.

QUALITY OF LIFE: THE RIGHT OF EVERY CITIZEN

Well-being is no longer merely a subject of philosophical speculation. With the development of the welfare state, terms such as 'a good quality of life', 'life satisfaction', 'happiness' and 'well-being', are all used to express what are now thought to be *fundamental rights of every citizen.* Terms such as 'social welfare', 'an unpolluted environment', 'care for the sick, disabled and elderly', feature significantly in the manifestos of political parties struggling to obtain the popular vote. In turn, dissatisfaction with societal institutions, services, unhealthy food and pollution, are all expressed in terms of an inadequate quality of life and a lack of well-being.

Societal responsibility for the quality of life and well-being has been brought into the focus of an industrialized world, in the last two decades or so, mainly by the increased public questioning of the consequences of technological advancement in various spheres of life. While technological advancement leads to more comfort and well-being, it also causes destruction of the natural environment and, increasingly, creates moral problems. For example, how can one draw a line between the benefits of technology and the exploitation of the natural environment with its attendant hazards to health? Or, given the availability of advanced technology, should a baby with brain-damage be put on a life-support machine when the experts claim that this will only add to her suffering? Such issues have significant implications, for better or for worse, not only for the lives of people today but also for future generations. As a result, more and more existing practices, concepts and moral codes are being highlighted, leading to increased public awareness of existing and potential dangers to humankind and of the problematic issues concerning quality of life and well-being.

Yet while a good quality of life and well-being are claimed to be individual rights, they are not packages given to individuals as gifts by the welfare state. That the individual him- or herself is perceived as being responsible for his or her own health is implied by the very existence of health education. In order to enjoy a good quality of life and well-being, individuals should carry out certain kinds of activities, e.g. take physical exercise, eat healthy food, and avoid other activities, e.g. consuming alcohol or smoking. The Government can issue health warnings. Individuals either heed or ignore these warnings.

However, the question of how mutual responsibilities, for a good quality of life and well-being, should be distributed between the individual and society, does not permit an easy answer. For example, the individual, in order to live in an unpolluted environment, may move his or her home to the country. Yet events like Chernobyl or other kinds of collectively produced pollution can reduce to nothing such individual efforts. Or the individual may buy organically grown vegetables, yet global pollution will, again, make fruitless such efforts to live healthily. Moreover, it is by no means obvious what particular rights individuals have with respect to a good quality of life and well-being, what these rights include and exclude. A part of the problem is that both social sciences and social practices interchangeably operate with diverse concepts of an individual right. The question of diverse concepts of a right is rarely being attended to, indeed, there is little awareness of the problems it poses. Diverse concepts, such as that of *an ego-centrically based individual right* and of *a dialogical concept of right*, presuppose a different distribution of individual and societal responsibilities. Consequently, they imply different moral obligations of an individual and society for well-being and a good quality of life.

INDIVIDUAL RIGHT AS AN EGO-CENTRED CONCEPT

In his book on *Taking Rights Seriously*, Dworkin (1978) maintains that the modern concept of right is based on the Kantian idea of human dignity. The basic assumption of this idea is that all individuals should be recognized and treated as full members of the human community. The recognition of human dignity, on which Kant (1788/1873) placed such a tremendous emphasis, was implied by his conviction that rationality, intentional acting and autonomous thought are supreme capacities of human beings, i.e. they are the End in Itself. Thus it is inconsistent with the idea of human dignity to deprive people, in any way, of such a recognition or treatment. If people have a right with respect to something then it is wrong to interfere with it. While this position says nothing about what particular rights individuals may have, it is important that according to this view, *rights belong solely to individuals*. That rights are usually understood to be 'properties – powers of immunities, liberties or entitlements – of individuals', (Singer, 1993, p. 99) has become commonly accepted as a mainstream perspective in social science and politics. It also follows from this point of view that rights are of an adversarial nature. They are claims of individuals either against the state or against other people with respect to the entitlements that they perceive as being denied to them.

Kantian ethics, based on the idea of human dignity, was a culmination of the perspective of *individualism* that had previously been nurtured in European culture for two or three centuries. Two main sources of the individualist perspective have been identified in the scholarly analyses of individualism.

One source of individualism has been described by historians and sociologists as a spectrum of factors in the socio-economic-cultural sphere that affected ordinary life. Amongst these factors four in particular are worthy of mention. Firstly, newly arising economic pressures resulted in the movement of populations from villages to towns and in the decline of traditional communities. While in medieval society personal identity was tied to roles that were passed on from one generation to the next, new economic conditions freed individuals from these roles. They provided them with new opportunities of choosing their ways of life and of sharing essential civil rights. Secondly, Calvinist theology, focusing on the individual's will and self-determination, encouraged introspection and self-examination of the individual's conduct. Thirdly, the invention of print and the growth of mass literacy inspired reading and promoted reflective activities such as letter writing and keeping diaries. Fourthly, personal privacy became a new value, at least for the higher classes, who now separated activities that were, from activities that were not, intended for public eyes.

Historians (e.g. Stone, 1977; Eisenstein, 1979; 1983) have argued that the growth of individualism in European culture was accompanied by essential changes in interpersonal family relationships. With more freedom granted to people with respect to their choice of marriage partners, their personal relationships grew more affectionate. Marriage became a voluntary contract between husband and wife rather than being arranged by others. Second, changes occurred in child rearing with the child becoming a centre of family activities, leading again to stronger emotional bonds within a family. Referring to these changes in interpersonal relationships, Taylor (1989) points out that, of course, it does not mean to say that before individualism people would not love each other or would not care for their children. Rather, these relationships were now given a prominence they had not had before: they took a central place in human awareness.

The second source of individualism was to be found in Renaissance philosophy, science and art. It was contained in the idea that the individual is a free agent who is responsible for his or her own fate. For example, the Renaissance philosopher Pico della Mirandola claimed that the individual, who is a 'microcosm in the centre of the macrocosm' (Pico della Mirandola (1486), *On the Dignity of Man*), makes and decides his or her own destiny. Individualism became a celebration of free will. For Descartes, free will is 'the noblest thing we can have because it makes us in a certain manner equal to God' (Descartes, 1647/1970, p.228). Since human actions are intentional and goal-directed, the individual is responsible for what he or she does. Thus, free will and choosing his or her way of life commits an individual to moral actions. Taylor (1989, p.185) maintains that, spiritually, there were three sides to this emerging individualism. Two of them stem from the medieval Augustinian radical reflexivity encouraging self-examination and self-control. The third one, a central force of the Reformation, was a personal commitment: it is the power of will that is required for acting with the whole concentration of mind and for acting morally. All of these sides, taken together, formed the basis of a self-centred individualism. Its consequences for the individualist conception of right and for the notion of well-being have been far reaching (Farr, 1991).

Amongst those who have been particularly preoccupied with a close link between freedom, equality and morality was one of the classics of the theory of democracy De Tocqueville (1835/1966). He argued that while Christianity established equality between people in spiritual terms, modern morality must provide people with equality in material terms. Democratic revolutions are morally obligated to ensure people's equality in well-being and in the available public wealth. De Tocqueville's ideas have been incorporated into the notion of morality that has become a basis of the modern welfare state.

THE DIALOGICAL NATURE OF AN INDIVIDUAL RIGHT

We have emphasized that self-centred individualism, claiming that the individual is the microcosm in the middle of the macrocosm, was a quest for freedom, independence and dignity. However, while individualism may appear to be by nature self-centred, this appearance is no more than an illusion. We have to remember that individualism was a historical – cultural revolt against the medieval tradition in which individuality had not been prominent in the ways Renaissance made it to be. As this tradition was breaking down, a celebration of the I had occurred against this background. The I that thinks, acts, makes decisions and is morally responsible, was a most meaningful and effective way of combating the outdated medieval world. At that time of the exhilarated glorification of the individual, it did not appear to be so important that one can become an individual, the self, only through a *dialogical process* of interaction of one self with other selves. Appreciation of the idea of the interdependence between an individual and his or her natural and societal contexts had to wait for a couple of hundred years. It became part of the Romantic movement that, in the eighteenth century penetrated the humanities, arts, literature, politics and social sciences. Thus, the main feature of Hegel's (1807/1977) social dialectic was to show how the self, in the complex journey of self-education, achieves self-consciousness through mutual interaction with other human beings and through the acknowledgement of one person by the other. By seeing oneself through the eyes of others, one becomes aware of one's own and of others' obligations. It was Mead's (1934) notion of the "generalized other" that was an expression of this dialogically based morality. Consequently, one can have rights only to the extent that they are shared and recognized by others. Thus individualism based on freedom, equality and dignity can exist only if everybody mutually recognizes each other's rights. A welfare state can function properly only if rights are dialogically maintained and monitored.

Let us consider, as an illustration of this point, Mead's notion of "public property". In order for this notion to have any meaning it has to be accepted by all members of the community. For the claim "this is mine" to have any sense, everybody must have the same attitude towards it, including the individual in question. From this common attitude the rights and obligations of individuals follow: if someone has property, it is his or her right to control it and nobody else can. It follows from this common attitude that one may covet another's property, and may accept or give gifts but taking another's property is not permitted: that is stealing. Thus, the individual must adopt the other person's perspective and both parties must understand that the situation would be the same if their positions were reversed. According to Mead's point of view, a right does not belong solely to individuals but is dialogically maintained. A right belongs both to the individual and to the other (Marková, 1987).

This point of view has been recently developed by Singer (1993). Singer maintains that what is ordinarily called a right is only what is meant by the individual's entitlement but not the dialogical process involving both the individual and others. She insists that the notion of right as inherently adversarial is a distortion. To assert a right means to call upon others to acknowledge our right.

Mead's analysis of social action is based on the idea that an individual act is part of a dialogical process between the self and others. The individual action is only started by the self but its meaning is jointly co-determined by the agent and by the one who responds to that action. The actions of one individual have consequences for others and can be a threat to others; they can have consequences that go beyond the intentions of the action. Consequently, actions are never perceived as neutral but are always perceived as intentional and interpreted in moral terms.

This issue of agency and its social nature is taken up in Part III by Valach. He argues that health-related strategies, such as *coping*, although they are the activities of an individual, to conceive of them as individualistic is mistaken. The activities of the individual are always situated in several social contexts. Firstly, the individual is born into a particular socio-cultural environment and learns existing patterns of behaviour. Secondly, any new kind of activity that he or she may begin is grounded in inter-personal interaction and therefore, oriented both towards the self and others. As Valach shows, *coping* is a social process in which the individual's activities are partly determined by the socio-cultural conditions in which the individual lives. In addition, coping is an active process and not an automatic adaptation to socio-cultural conditions. It is influenced by, and at the same time influences, the relationship between self and others.

DILEMMAS OF DIALOGICAL INTERDEPENDENCIES: THE CASE OF PRE-NATAL DIAGNOSING

Human actions are always situated in several socio-cultural contexts. These contexts include technological advancements and these can have a remarkable effect on what is considered a good quality of life. Moreover, these advancements may affect the perceived distribution of responsibility for an action. Differences in perspective between the individual and the collective on perceived responsibility often lead to dilemmas. Let us consider the effect, on an individual's decision-making, of one particular kind of technological advancement: the pre-natal diagnosing of genetic disorders.

Since the middle of this century the development of sophisticated medical technology has made it possible, with considerable 'justification', to prevent the birth of physically and mentally unfit fetuses. For some time now, fetuses with various genetic disorders such as Down's syndrome, haemophilia and spina bifida, can be identified using advanced technological procedures which include ultrasound, amniocentesis and chorionic villus sampling. These procedures are being refined all the time, leading to the possibility of diagnosing, at earlier and earlier stages of pregnancy, more disorders, with even greater accuracy. Prospective parents are thus given the possibility of deciding two things. Firstly, whether they wish to undergo such diagnostic procedures. Secondly, if they do and the fetus is found to be affected by a physical or mental disorder, whether they wish to go for abortion. The abortion of affected fetuses is being 'justified' in terms of the poor quality of life of the child and of his or her parents if the child were born.

The availability of modern diagnostic procedures may also determine the quality of life of a person affected by a genetic disorder even a long time before any symptoms of his or her disorder manifest themselves. For example, McKie (1988) discusses the case of a 2-month old baby whose mother had Huntington's chorea. The prospective adoptive parents were interested in having the baby only if she were not going to be affected by Huntington's chorea. Therefore, the adoption agency requested that a probe be carried out on the girl to determine whether or not she had inherited the Huntington's chorea gene. In this particular instance the baby in the end, was not tested on ethical grounds. The geneticist successfully argued that it was unethical to test such a young baby. The individual should decide for him- or herself whether he or she wished to be tested.

The issue of testing goes far beyond the individual's knowing or not knowing about his or her genetic disorder. Once the individual knows about it, there are profound implications for his or her employment, life assurance, health insurance and so on. With these technological advances even some doctors worry that scientific concerns are becoming more important than human ones. There are many persons who may have a good life until middle age before showing any signs of the disease, and who, therefore, can be very successful in their career until then. However, "scientists now determine the quality of life that society should allow, and they programme society carefully and insidiously to accept their guidance on these matters" (McKie, 1988, p.85).

Yet, at the same time, there are families in which the experience of Huntington's chorea has been so devastating that they would wish to prevent the birth of affected individuals (e.g. Thomas, 1982). There remains a deep division amongst the professionals, and amongst the individuals concerned, about the ethics of predictive testing for Huntington's chorea and other incurable hereditary diseases.

This case shows that well-being can be defined differently not only by professionals and clients but the clients, as individuals, may adopt different perspectives on the same issue depending on their experience or moral preferences. Later in Part III, Jahoda raises the issue of different perspectives with respect to the quality of life when discussing problems of people with learning difficulties.

HOW MUCH CHOICE?

When one talks about individual rights as entitlements, usually one or other of the following two cases is meant: firstly, a right to choose a course of action that puts a great deal of emphasis on the individual's agency; secondly, a right may refer to an entitlement of receiving something from society, i.e. welfare benefits or protection guaranteed by law and order. The emphasis on human agency in the present Western culture underlines the close association between the quality of life and the individual's freedom of choice. It is held that the individual should be free to choose his or her own lifestyle and to make free decisions concerning his or her activities. If the person is disabled he or she should have a selection of social services and care facilities from which to choose. What has not been fully explored, though, is *what level of choice* should count as a feature of a good quality of life? Choosing with respect to one's activities implies having responsibilities for one's actions. Either of the two extreme positions with respect to freedom of choice may occur. For example, in the case of pre-natal diagnosing, the individual may perceive him- or herself as having too much choice, too many responsibilities and moral obligations resulting from his or her decisions. Alternatively, he or she may have too little or no choice at all with respect to the activities and facilities available, thus feeling powerless and unable to affect his or her environment. In this case the individual may feel that he or she is treated as a non-agent or a non-person.

Let us take up again the case of pre-natal diagnosing. A number of research findings indicate that the availability of pre-natal diagnosis imposes pressure on women to use these facilities, often against their own wishes. As Green (1990) points out, the purpose of pre-natal diagnosis is usually presented to prospective mothers as a matter of securing the well-being of her unborn baby. In reality, however, it is a screening procedure for genetic defects and if the fetus is diagnosed as being affected, abortion is the only way of avoiding it. Research by Sanden and Bjurulf (1988) indicates that some pregnant women wish to take the diagnostic test but will not consider abortion even if malformation of the fetus is found. Their reason for having an amniocentesis is to find out if the fetus is healthy. Such reasons, however, are not considered to be cost-effective from the scientific and economic points of view. Pre-natal diagnosing is justified to the public in terms of reducing genetic defects and not in terms of the mother having early knowledge about the presence of a defect in the baby.

In the study by Marková et al. (1984) it was found that undergoing pre-natal testing may be interpreted, not as enabling the prospective parents to decide freely whether or not to have an affected child, but as a commitment to abortion. A number of women carriers of haemophilia, a genetic blood clotting disorder, felt that availing themselves of an amniocentesis committed them to abortion should the fetus prove to be affected. The study showed that about 60% of Scottish and Canadian female carriers of haemophilia, many of whom were already mothers of sons with haemophilia, claimed that haemophilia is not a sufficiently severe disorder to justify the termination of a pregnancy. Moreover, none of the patients with haemophilia agreed with the termination of a pregnancy in the case of haemophilia. Understandably, these patients may have realized that had amniocentesis existed years ago they themselves might not have been born (Marková et al., 1984) and, of course, this was a very offensive point of view to many of them.

Green (1990) maintains that at present it is not considered acceptable to allow a newborn handicapped baby to die, yet it is considered highly desirable to terminate a pregnancy if the fetus is affected by a disorder. Women who reject the idea of abortion and who decline pre-natal diagnosis may be viewed as being responsible for the birth of a handicapped child and for the situation resulting from it. Green (1990, p. 37) argues that:

> *from here is but a short step to assuming that any mother of a handicapped child could have avoided her situation had she so chosen.*

Such assumptions can be justified on the grounds that high technology enables us to identify the most serious genetic abnormalities very early in pregnancy and that its benefits, therefore, should be used by the prospective parents concerned.

Women are conscious of such pressures, as has been shown in our own study quoted above and, more recently, in a Swedish study carried out by Sjögren and Uddenberg (1987). This study has shown that about 30% of participants have recognised that the very existence of pre-natal diagnosis can lead to more negative attitudes towards disabled people.

Green (1990) argues that the existence of fetal diagnosis has changed the whole nature of pregnancy itself. It can never be the same even for those mothers who decline to have tests because there will always be the knowledge that they had the opportunity and could have acted:

> *The concept of free choice is a dubious one at the best of times. In the case of pregnant women the social pressures to participate in screening programmes and to terminate an affected pregnancy are considerable (Green, 1990. p.38).*

Perceiving oneself as having too much responsibility also serves as a basis for argument to Watney (1990) who attacks the "practices of freedom" in the UK. Writing about citizenship and the "politics of identity in the age of AIDS", he complains that health education about AIDS contains an implicit accusation that homosexuals have been responsible for the epidemic. Watney maintains that the official campaigns are being run in such a way as to disseminate the government's 'family' and 'traditional moral' values. The discrimination against homosexuals, in Watney's view, is based on "the typically individualistic approach of the work of the Health Education Authority, whose adverts share a common by-line, AIDS: You're as safe as you want to be" (Watney, 1990, p.171).

Having considered some cases in which too much choice is troublesome for the individual concerned, let us turn our attention to the other extreme situation in which the individual perceives him- or herself as having no choice at all or too little choice with respect to his or her life-style and daily activities.

Research into the quality of both the care and the life of people with learning difficulties constantly reveals a lack of freedom to choose, a lack of privacy and poor social relationships. Cattermole et al. (1989) have found these issues to be the least satisfactory aspects of the quality of life of people with learning difficulties before they had moved from long-stay hospitals to hostels in the community. A study into the quality of care and of life of people with moderate to severe learning difficulties (Marková et al., 1992) showed virtually no opportunities of choosing whom they met, in either a hospital or a hostel setting. Much of institutional life was routinised, with routines being very much like rules. Routines, i.e. events and activities that are regularly repeated, totally dominated institutional life. The routine-based hospital regime not only dictated the rhythm of the participants' day but it also made them almost completely dependent on staff. For example, there was only one occasion during the whole of the study when the hospital residents were given a cup of tea or coffee outwith the morning or afternoon tea-breaks. Having been socialized in this way, individuals who were quite capable of asking for a drink did not do so even if they needed one. For instance, a man in one of the wards had stomach problems and was sick on several occasions when being observed by the researchers. The staff were sympathetic and showed concern. However, the man was not offered a drink to remove the unpleasant taste from his mouth after being sick nor did he ask for one but waited for over two hours until he received a drink with his evening meal.

Virtually none of the interpersonal interactions in either the hospital or the hostel were concerned with offering choices or asking people with learning difficulties about their choices. Even the most personal elements of residents' daily routine, such as getting dressed, washed, bathed, shaved and being given drugs were carried out in groups, often using a production line approach. For example, the most frequently used bathing procedure was for one nurse to wash and for another nurse to dry the person concerned. One ward attempted to introduce a more personalised care, with one member of staff taking responsibility for a particular group of residents. However, there was little opportunity for flexibility when the members of staff were working within the organisational constraints of the ward routines. In effect, it meant that one person tended to deal with a group of individuals rather than having the time or continuity of contact to provide more personal care.

In his chapter on the quality of life of people with learning difficulties, Jahoda provides a historical overview of the changes in meaning of 'learning difficulties'. He shows how, since the nineteenth century, professional practices have been influenced by the eugenic movement, by 'morality concerns' with respect to people with learning difficulties, and by attempts to protect society from 'untrainable idiots'. However, Jahoda goes on to show that in spite of considerable changes in both public and professional awareness of learning difficulties, many existing educational and medical models of learning difficulties still enshrine past myths about 'mongols' and the 'mentally retarded'. Like Valach, Jahoda draws attention to the fact that an individual's quality of life is intimately interlinked with an appreciation of the human agency of people with learning difficulties held by their carers and other professionals. He argues that people with learning difficulties must be treated as free agents. They have to decide for themselves what kind of lifestyle they wish to lead. Jahoda cites evidence that people with learning difficulties are well aware of their situation and strongly protest against their lack of choice concerning activities and the identities that others thrust upon them. He argues that psychometric tests, designed for populations other than those to which they directly apply, can provide elegant data but be totally useless at providing information about specific individuals.

In contrast to Jahoda, other researchers claim that quality of life should be assessed both *subjectively* and *objectively*. While the former is based on the experiential evaluation of his or her quality of life by the individual concerned, the latter is assessed in comparative terms. For example, quality of life can be assessed in terms of a comparison between the individual's and others' access to material objects or to social facilities; how much freedom to choose his or her lifestyle the individual concerned has in comparison to others. Quality of life can also be assessed in terms of a comparison between existing and some ideal quality of life for the individuals concerned; and so on. In their chapter, Barry, Crosby and Bogg draw attention to the fact that the meaning of quality of life may be different for various social groups and that researchers are faced with the challenging task of adequately defining it in some measurable terms. They show that the relationship between subjective and objective measures of the quality of life may be quite intricate and one cannot take it for granted that they will corroborate each other.

Concerning the subjective appreciation of the quality of life, individuals do not assess it *in a vacuum* but with respect to some reference point. For example, it is likely that a person living in a hospital for the mentally ill will assess his or her quality of life in comparison to other people with mental illness living in such a hospital. Using such comparative criteria, they may subjectively assess their own living conditions as, say, very good. However, if contrasted, for example, with the living conditions of people outside the hospital, they may judge their conditions as bad.

Objective criteria for assessing the quality of life are usually set by professionals or researchers. They decide, on the basis of their own judgement, what constitutes a good quality of life and what comprises the components of such an assessment. Their assessment criteria are determined by societal values, by the general standard of living and by collective constructions of the meaning of a good quality of life. As Barry, Crosby and Bogg show in their own research, subjective assessments and objective assessments of the quality of life of people with mental illness living in a long-term hospital differed to a considerable degree. They question the validity of the subjective measures of quality of life pointing to a variety of reasons for the lack of match between the figures they had obtained for subjective and objective assessment and they face the challenging task of analyzing these problems.

RESPONSIBILITY AND THE QUALITY OF LIFE

Amongst the multitude of existing approaches to the analysis of responsibility, some focus on the degree of intention, goal-directedness and commitment to the action; others are more preoccupied with personal versus collective responsibility; yet others with the interdependence between the two; and so on. However, despite divergencies, there is a common feature in all of these approaches. Responsibility is an essential characteristic of human agents whose actions are defined *not* in neutral but in moral terms. Responsibility *always* implies a certain kind of moral or ethical concern.

Being responsible means that an action for which responsibility is assumed can be evaluated in terms of good or bad, right or wrong. The question, of course, is: good or bad, right or wrong, for whom? Clearly, individual and societal concerns in regard to well-being and the quality of life may differ considerably. For example, screening for HIV may not be 'good' for the HIV seropositive individual concerned but may be 'good' for others who might be infected by the person carrying the virus. Or, screening for HIV may not be 'good' for the infected individual at the time of screening but may be 'good' for the same individual from the long-term point of view. Such an individual may, as a result of screening, undergo essential changes in his or her lifestyle and make arrangements in case AIDS were to develop.

Another question concerns the relationship between time span and responsibility. Do individuals and societies have responsibility for the quality of life of people today or of those in the future? Considering that quality of life is a social construction dependent on certain socio-cultural conditions, what can one say, today, about the likely criteria governing the quality of life and well-being of future generations? Similarly, on the basis of which criteria can the prospective parent today make decisions about the quality of life of a fetus affected by a genetic disorder? One cannot predict how technology in the future may affect quality of life. Thus, assuming responsibilities for today's actions, individuals and groups are faced with two kinds of uncertainty about the future: uncertainty about the consequences of today's actions and uncertainty about the criteria of quality of life in the future.

The question "who is responsible?", does not usually arise when activities proceed smoothly, habitually and produce expected outcomes. The question is usually raised when, for one reason or other, the action, or its consequences, awaken awareness and reflexive thought. When this happens accounts of agents' involvement and environmental factors are required in order to attribute responsibility and thus satisfactorily to explain the event.

In the last two decades it has become apparent more than ever before that judgements concerning well-being and the quality of life cannot be settled *a priori*, whether by agents of the welfare state, by doctors, lawyers, clergymen or members of any other profession. Today, such judgements are affected by a variety of factors. For example, many decisions about well-being and the quality of life are associated with political and economic considerations, such as how much money local governments are prepared to spend on hostels for people with learning difficulties and mental illness. Self-help groups, the provocative actions of particular individuals, coverage in the mass media of communication all increase reflexive thought about the quality of life and lead to public debates. All these matters lead directly back to the relationship between individual and society, either in regard to priorities or responsibilities or social constructions of well-being and the quality of life.

REFERENCES

Bentham, J. (1970), *An Introduction to the Principles of Morals and Legislation*, ed. J. H. Burns and H. J. A. Hart, London: University of London, The Athlone Press.

Cattermole, M., Jahoda, A. and Marková, I. (1989). Quality of life for people with learning difficulties moving to community homes. *Disability, Handicap and Society*, **5**, 137–152.

Cicero, *Tusculan Disputations*, trs. J. E. King, London: William Heineman, 1927.

Descartes, R., Letter to Christine of Sweden, 20th November 1647. In Kenny, A. (trs. and ed.), *Descartes: Philosophical Letters*, Oxford: Clarendon Press, 1970.

De Tocqueville, A. (1835, 1840), *Democracy in America*, eds. J. P. Mayer and M. Lerner; transl. G. Lawrence, New York: Harper and Row, 1966.

Dworkin, R. (1978), *Taking Rights Seriously*, Cambridge Mass.: Harvard University Press.

Eisenstein, E. L. (1979), *The Printing Press as an Agent of Change*, Cambridge and New York: Cambridge University Press.

Eisenstein, E. L. (1983), *The Printing Revolution in Early Modern Europe*, Cambridge and New York: Cambridge University Press.

Farr, R. M., (1991). Individualism as a collective representation. In V. Aebischer, J. P. Deconchy & E. M. Lipiansky (Eds.), *Idéologies et Représentations Sociales*. (pp. 129–143). Cousset: Delval.

Green, J. (1990), *Calming or Harming?*, London: Galton Institute.

Hegel, G. W. F. (1807), *Phenomenology of Spirit*, trs. A. V. Miller, Oxford: Clarendon Press, 1977.

Kant, I.(1788), *Critique of Practical Reason*, trs. Abbott, T. K., London: Longmans, Green, 1873.

Marková, I., Forbes, C. and Inwood, M. (1984), Consumers' views of genetic counselling in haemophilia, *American Journal of Medical Genetics*, **17**, 741–752.

Marková, I., Jahoda, A., Woodward, D. and Cattermole, M. (1992), Living in hospital and hostel: the pattern of interactions of people with learning difficulties, *Journal of Mental Deficiency Research*, **36**, 115–127.

Marková, I. (1987), *Human Awareness*, London: Hutchinson Education.

McKie, R. (1988), *The Genetic Jigsaw*, Oxford: Oxford University Press.

Mead, G. H. (1934), *Mind, Self and Society*, Chicago: Chicago University Press.

Pico della Mirandola, G. (1486), *On the Dignity of Man*, Hs Wallis C. G., Indianapolis and New York: Bobbs - Merrill, 1965.

Sanden, M. L. and Bjurulf, P. (1988), Pregnant women's attitudes for accepting or declining a serum-alpha-fetoprotein test, *Scandinavian Journal of Social Medicine*, **16**, 265–71.

Singer, B. (1993), The democratic solution to ethnic pluralism, **19**, *Philosophy and Social Criticism* (2) pp. 97–114.

Sjörgen, B. and Uddenberg, N. (1987), Attitudes towards disabled persons and the possible effects of prenatal diagnosis. An interview study among 53 women participating in prenatal diagnosis and 20 of their husbands, *Journal of Psychosomatic Obstetric Gynaecology*, **6**, 187–96.

Stone, L. (1977), *The Family, Sex, and Marriage in England 1500–1800)*, London: Weidenfeld and Nicolson.

Taylor, C. (1989), *Sources of the Self*, Cambridge: Cambridge University Press.

Thomas, S. (1982), *Ethics of a predictive test for Huntington's chorea*, British Medical Journal, **284**, 1383–85.

Watney, S. (1990), Practices of freedom: "Citizenship" and the politics of identity in the age of AIDS. In J. Rutherford (ed.) *Identity: Community, Culture, Difference*. London: Lawrence and Wishart.

CHAPTER ELEVEN

Quality of Life: Hope for the Future or an Echo from the Distant Past?

Andrew JAHODA

Strathmartine Hospital Dundee DD3 0PG

The concept 'quality of life' is used in various contexts, some of which reflect the concerns and contradictions of today's society. The phrase is often used in a negative sense to refer to adverse environmental factors which detract from a reasonable standard of life. These may relate to day-to-day problems like overcrowded roads and poor public transport, or to larger issues such as CO_2 emissions and global warming which pose a threat to the basic health and happiness of millions. Along with a growing awareness of the delicate ecological balance which ensures the continued existence of human kind, there is a yearning for the amenities and standards of life which reflect an affluent consumer society: the 'quality' of the market place.

In the area of learning difficulties 'quality of life' is also an issue, and there are a growing number of measures designed to examine the social and physical environments provided by various services (Raynes, 1988). However, as Ignatieff (1984) explained, the needs of a particular group are not determined solely in relation to the wider society, but have a history of their own.

> We are... the only species whose needs have a history. It is the needs we have created for ourselves and the language of entitlements we have derived from them, which give us any claim to respect and dignity as species and individuals. Needs language, therefore, is a distinctively historical and relative language of the common good. (p. 14)

A logical extension of this argument is that the changing quality of life, which people with learning difficulties have been afforded by society, has mirrored changing perceptions of them as human beings on the part of society. Consequently, this chapter will begin with a brief historical outline. I hope to show how the acknowledgement of the humanity and personhood of people with learning difficulties has radically altered the way in which their needs are defined and how the services are delivered that meet those needs. The importance of individual agency in determining the nature of lifestyles will then be considered, along with ways of eliciting the perspectives of service users. This will be followed by a brief examination of some common conceptions of the quality of life. Finally, the relationship between public policy and the individualistic 'economy of care' will be discussed, and conclusions drawn about likely developments in the future.

THE HISTORICAL BACKGROUND

Scheerenberger (1983), in his wide ranging account of the history of people with learning disabilities in Western societies, pointed out the Judeo-Christian origins of two of the most powerful Western conceptions of disability. The first is based on the emphasis of early Christians on the position of people with learning disabilities as the innocent children of God. The second conception is based on the subsequent doctrine of 'original sin' which contradicted the notion of innocence. Instead, disability could be regarded as a manifestation of a sin or an evil. Luther, one of the architects of the reformation, adopted the latter view, describing a child with multiple disabilities as being possessed by the devil. Luther believed such a child to have had no soul and he argued that it should be killed (Scheerenberger, 1983). These two contrasting beliefs, which provoke an uneasy mixture of pity and fear, provide an important backdrop to the history of services for people with learning disabilities and help us to understand public attitudes concerning these issues. When looking at the historical changes in such services over the last two centuries, people with learning difficulties will be referred to by the terms in use at the time. The changing labels, in their own right, provide a sense of the evolving position of such people in society.

Public Institutions

In the last couple of centuries a number of institutions arose which provided specialist services for people with learning disabilities. The common threads which led to the growth of institutions for such people, who were then referred to as 'idiots and imbeciles', cannot be understood solely by reference to this group. The institutional movement reflected the enormous upheaval caused by the industrial revolution. It is no accident that institutions were also built for the old, the sick, the poor, law breakers and for people who were mentally ill (Foucault, 1977; Ryan and Thomas, 1980; Skull, 1977). The humanitarian endeavours of these early efforts were quite unique in the sense that the first institutions were educational establishments. The pioneering work of Itard and his fellow Frenchman Seguin in the educational sphere gave credence to the possibility of reducing the handicap of people previously considered ineducable and of returning them to society. To these ends, the educationalists pioneered a range of techniques and philosophies of education which, by today's standards, might be considered progressive.

Itard's celebrated attempt to educate Victor, initially believed to be a feral child, was perhaps the first carefully documented effort to educate an 'idiot' (Scheerenberger, 1983). Although his programmes may now be considered regimented, Seguin employed techniques such as modelling and positive reinforcement, which emphasised the importance of sensory stimulation and of language. He was also concerned that students should gain practical social skills and learn to live in the community as good citizens. He advocated that institutions should be small and located close to cities. The rationale for the location was to allow the students to visit events such as exhibitions, theatres and meetings which would inspire them and stimulate their interest in the life of the community (Scheerenberger, 1983). Since the purpose of these establishments was to train people to live in the community, the education was moral as well as useful. It was designed to make people good citizens (Lazerson, 1975).

The concern with morality set the stage for a shift in interest away from the protection of imbeciles and idiots towards the protection of society from such individuals. Despite the fact that the benevolence of many of the early institutions was prompted by Christian principles, others believed that idiots and imbeciles were a throw back to a more primitive state of man and the result of divine retribution for the immorality of their parents (Ryan and Thomas, 1980). Thus in an unscientific form, the concepts of idiocy and of imbecility as forms of moral degeneracy was born. Towards the end of the nineteenth century, simplistic theories of inheritance reinforced these fears. People with Down's syndrome were described as mongols because their features include the epicanthic fold, a characteristic of Asian people. Perhaps this label, a mongol, also reflected Western attitudes towards Asian people.

The alarmist projections of the eugenics movement led to a fear that people with a mild disability, i.e. 'imbeciles' would undermine the fabric of society. They were believed to be the most morally degenerate. A physician in charge of a large institution early this century wrote:

> *The recognition of the moral imbecile, and the absolute necessity of a life long guardianship, protection against temptation and all the horrors of criminal procedure, were strenuously insisted upon...in the name of science, of sociology, as a matter of political economy, of the protection of homes, and all that man holds dear. (Barr, 1904, p.1)*

'Moral imbecile' was a term for a category with several grades:

> *Low grade: ... temperament bestial. (to) High grade:... with a genius for evil. (Barr, 1904, p.1)*

By the turn of the century 'idiots', who had previously been regarded as more pitiable than frightening, also came to be considered a threat to society (Begab, 1975).

The Emergence of the Medical Model

During this period there was a switch in large institutions from an educational to a medical model and a concern with aetiology and treatment became predominant. The metaphor of idiocy and imbecility as a sickness in society was taken literally. Being thus treated as a medical problem, it was considered to fall within the remit of the medical sciences (Barr, 1904). However, despite the occasional use of some rather dubious brain surgery, the predominant concern was with the perceived threat of growing numbers of idiots and imbeciles, who were considered to have abnormal sex drives. Consequently, sterilisation was openly advocated and practised, even though this practice was never legalised. 'Asexualisation' was even suggested to improve the behaviour of imbeciles and rid them of their 'moral degeneracy' (Barr, 1904).

The early twentieth century also saw the development of intelligence tests, originally devised by Binet to separate those requiring special schooling from those who were to enter mainstream education. Unlike the innovative early nineteenth century educational developments for those described as 'idiots', there was apparently little that was 'special' about education for children with mild problems. The primary aim was to provide a form of vocational training for less able children to prevent other children from being held back by being educated in the same classroom (Lazerson, 1975; Ryan and Thomas, 1980). This aim can be seen in Binet's (1905) attempt to identify the employment status of a group of former special school pupils. The results of studies with intelligence tests during the first three decades of this century seemed to support the views espoused by the eugenics movement. People from ethnic minorities, the deprived and the poor, all performed badly on IQ tests (Begab, 1975; Lazerson, 1975; Ryan and Thomas, 1980). The prevalent view was that intelligence tests measured a genetically endowed trait of intelligence which could not be improved by education.

At the turn of the century, people described as 'idiots and imbeciles' were sent to institutions apart from the wider community. This was reflected in the dehumanising nature of these institutions, where the personhood and individuality of residents were destroyed in the daily grind of institutional life. In many respects, however, the nature of the institutional life has remained unchanged until today. The following example is taken not from the beginning but from near the end of the present century. It is drawn from an observational study we carried out in a long-stay hospital in the late 1980s.

It describes the shaving routine in a long-stay hospital:

John saw the nurses walking to the toilets and immediately rose to join the group of residents waiting there for a shave. The smell of urine was inescapable. When his turn came, John sat in one of the three chairs lined up facing the washbasins. Although staff talked amongst themselves, no words passed between John and the busy staff member as shaving foam was routinely slapped on his face and the rapid shave began. The shave took one and a half minutes, and once finished, John went over to the basin, washed his face with water, and dried it with a communal towel. The staff member rinsed the razor with hot water, and began shaving the next resident.

So while we may be deeply shocked, today, by conditions that have been found in hospitals for people with learning difficulties in Roumania and Greece we should be aware that, albeit in a milder form, similar problems persist in the darker recesses of our own services for people with learning difficulties.

The kind of simplistic hereditary theories that held at one time have since been largely discounted. Similarly, the view that people with learning difficulties are immoral and pose a threat to society, is no longer accepted. There is less faith in intelligence tests as accurate measures, since cultural and environmental factors can influence performance (Mittler, 1979). However, some stereotypes from the turn of the century still persist. For instance, fears of the promiscuity and sexual deviance of people with learning difficulties can still be found in some quarters today, and probably derive from the alarmist period of the eugenics movement (Elwood, 1981).

Reform

More enlightened views came to the fore during the 1960s and 1970s, coupled with public exposure of institutions in the United States and Britain. Enquiries into long-stay institutions tended to follow in the wake of publicity about horrendous episodes of ill treatment, which had resulted in either injury or death. However, the reports highlighted the more mundane aspects of institutional life which contributed to a culture of systematic abuse. The report of Enquiry into South Ockenden Hospital (HMSO,1974) pointed to many of the indignities in the daily lives of patients, including toilets which were openly visible from corridors, lining up naked to be bathed in batches and living in overcrowded dormitories with no personal privacy. The status of the residents was reflected in the barren and inhumane conditions in which they lived.

A classic study was that of Goffman, whose 'Asylums' (1961) presented a gruesome portrayal of how residents were ground down by routine and depressed by the bleakness of their surroundings. The growing recognition that those with mental handicaps were 'people, not patients' sparked the first moves towards establishing smaller community-based hostels and towards designing measures of what is now referred to as 'quality of life'. These measures, such as the Revised Child Management Scale (King et al., 1971), were concerned with promoting individual instead of group care practices and with ensuring a dignified existence for children living both in large and in small institutions. This involved introducing more choice into the daily lives of residents. Even having one's own clothes was a luxury rarely afforded to those in institutional care, where most clothes and toiletries were common property. However, these efforts at reform were soon overtaken by the changing philosophy of care, which came to stress that people with mental handicaps had the right to live in home-like environments (Jay Committee, HMSO,1979).

Normalisation

The 'normalisation movement', with its aim of reducing, if not actually reversing, the devalued status of people with a learning difficulty in society, has perhaps been the single most influential school of thought over the last decade for policy makers, pressure groups and professionals who work with people with learning difficulties. In essence this movement advocates the acceptance of people with learning difficulties into mainstream society. Originally a Scandinavian concept, it addressed the right of people with learning difficulties to share the human and legal rights of other citizens, as well as to "normal ... housing, education, working and leisure conditions" (Bank-Mikkelsen, 1990, p.56). It was Wolfensberger (1972; 1990a; 1990b) who shifted the emphasis from human rights to a consideration of how people with learning difficulties could overcome their stigmatised status. As he put it: "... then other desirable things would almost automatically follow, at least within the resources of his/her society" (Wolfensberger, 1983, p.234).

According to Wolfensberger, whose views have tended to become an accepted version of 'normalisation' in Britain, the negative role afforded to people with learning difficulties is maintained through conscious and unconscious imagery. Hence, how people are treated, either as a group in services or on an individual basis, will reflect these negative images. At the end of the day if you expect someone to be incompetent, helpless and child-like, you are likely to further handicap the person, by how you treat him or her. The belief thus becomes a kind of self-fulfilling prophesy. Wolfensberger suggests that to prevent this socially engineered handicap one has to raise the awareness of people of the negative images underlying such treatment. Moreover, by using behavioural techniques and positive interventions, it is possible to increase people's social competence and thus to reduce their apparent disability.

Wolfensberger's greatest contribution to improving the quality of life for those with learning difficulties is the importance he attaches to people's shared humanity, and to their right to live in ordinary housing, to use ordinary facilities such as shops and pubs, and to be an integrated member of the local community. Gurus of the normalisation movement in this country, like Tyne (1981), have also stressed Wolfensberger's concern with counteracting public prejudice and with promoting a positive view of people with learning difficulties. However, the theoretical backbone of Wolfensberger's ideas is that the general public ought to accept people with learning difficulties as valued members of the community through their conformity to societal norms.

Perrin and Nirje (1985) have pointed out that the acronym for Wolfensberger and Thomas' (1983) service quality evaluation scheme, 'pass' is the term coined by Goffman (1963) in his work entitled Stigma. In his book, Goffman argued that to escape from their stigmatised identity people need to conceal their stigmata in order to be accepted within the normative framework used by society. Although much embroidered, and presented as an agenda for social change, many of Wolfensberger's basic premises are to be found in Goffman's (1963) writings.

PASSING (Wolfensberger and Thomas, 1983) evaluation is the successor to PASS. It looks in detail at the service practice, the extent to which the service is an integral part of the local community, how much it conforms to social norms and whether or not it promotes a positive image of service users. The latter not only includes the ways in which the service users are presented (e.g. whether or not they wear colour co-ordinated clothing), but it also includes the presentation of staff members. The following extract from the PASSING manual details the 'impact of worker personal appearance':

> *Workers whose personal appearance is not valued (due to obesity, mannerisms, grooming, sloppy dress, etc.) are apt to impair image of clients, in contrast to workers whose appearance is more culturally valued, e.g., who are clean, wear stylish clothes, have neatly styled and trimmed hair/beard, etc. (Wolfensberger and Thomas, 1983, p.221).*

This quotation illustrates the importance attached to image and to the dictates of the 'conservatism corollary', which requires that people with learning disabilities conform to the most conservative social norms in order to achieve acceptance and status. In practice this would rule out people with learning disabilities taking part in activities which others would take for granted. For example, Perrin and Nirje (1985) have pointed to Wolfensberger's objection to people with learning disabilities working with animals, due to the negative connotations of such an association. However, even if evidence was produced to indicate some damaging link, should individual's dignity, choice and sponteneity be made secondary to good appearances? The aspirations of the individual and what passes as keeping up appearances are not always compatible. These and other points have been discussed by Bayley (1991) and by Robinson (1989).

If one acknowledges the influence of Goffman on the work of Wolfensberger, then one must understand Goffman himself as a man of his times, albeit a brilliant scholar. When Goffman wrote about stigma, he reflected the attitudes and beliefs of his own time, that society's norms are static and may not change to accommodate stigmatised individuals. Now many people are aware of the power of minority groups in changing attitudes. The new movement aimed at counteracting stigma is to be found among people with learning disabilities themselves. Self-advocacy has become an increasingly powerful voice, lobbying against prejudice and demanding an increasing role inside services and organisations for people with learning disabilities (Williams and Shoultz, 1982; Kennedy, 1990).

Charting these historical developments should have demonstrated the link between how people with learning disabilities are perceived and the nature of the support and services considered appropriate for them. Perhaps one aspect of the self which has received less attention is that of self as agent, and the part which people with learning disabilities can play in determining their own lifestyles.

TABLE 11.1 – Variables related to adaptation in research studies on deinstitutionalisation (Source: Cattermole, M., Jahoda, A. and Marková, I. (1990))

Type of study	Examples	Criteria used to assess adaptation
Studies using Adaptive Behaviour Scale (ABS)	Vitello et al. (1983) Eyman et al. (1979)	Independent functioning, domestic activity, self-direction, responsibility, socialisation
Studies using Progress Assessment Chart (PAC)	Locker et al. (1984)	Self-help, communication, socialisation
Other studies	Schalock & Harper (1978)	Personal maintenance, clothing care and use, socially appropriate behaviour, money management, apartment cleanliness, meal preparation
	Willer & Intagliata (1981)	Self-care, behavioural control, community-living skills, use of community resources, social support
	Challis & Shepherd (1983)	Sexual behaviour, behaviour, leisure activities, catering activity

INDIVIDUALITY AND AGENCY

The role of individual agency is often ignored when residents from long-stay hospitals are being resettled in the community. Table 11.1 provides a summary of some criteria used to assess adaptation of long-stay hospital residents moving to community residences.

The most commonly used tool has been the Adaptive Behaviour Scale, although other studies have used quite similar criteria to assess adaptation, most of them being concerned with the development of self-help skills and appropriate behaviours. This list represents achievements the significance of which is largely unknown for people with learning difficulties moving into community residences. In order to find out more about this, we carried out a study (Cattermole et al., 1990) examining the views of people with learning difficulties before and after they moved from the parental home or a hospital to live more independently in the community.

Table 11.2 summarises the issues about which participants expressed dissatisfaction both before and after their move from either hospital or home to the community. The table shows that the learning of self-help skills came low down on the list of issues about which participants were concerned. For them social life was of greatest importance. Other issues, such as freedom and choice, were of particular concern to the hospital residents before they moved out. One woman said:

> *You want your own freedom, don't you. It's a free country, I ken, but you're no free with the nurses taking you everywhere you go and asking where you've been...They have more freedom outside the hospital...The people outside...can go anywhere they like. They don't have people telling them where to go or when to come in, when to go to bed.*

TABLE 11.2 – Factors relating to quality of life (Source: Cattermole, M., Jahoda, A. and Marková, I. (1990))

Aspects of their circumstances about which participants expressed dissatisfaction	Number of participants expressing negative statements		
	Home group (N=7)	Hospital group (N=8)	Total
(i) Before move (living at home/in hospital)			
Social life and friendships	6	6	12
Relationships with carers [1]	6	6	12
Freedom and choice	4	7	11
Privacy	3	8	11
Opportunity to use/learn self-help skills	4	6	10
Stigmatization	4	6	10
Amount of spending money	1	5	6
Daytime activities	3	1	4
(ii) After move (living in community residences)			
Stigmatization	6	7	13
Social life and friendships	6	5	11
Daytime activities	6	5	11
Privacy	6	4	10
Amount of spending money	6	4	10
Relationships with carers [2]	5	4	9
Freedom and choice	5	3	8
Opportunity to use/learn self-help skills	3	4	7

[1] Parents (Home group); Ward staff (Hospital group).

[2] Staff in community residences.

It was pointed out earlier that many features of an institutional life in a long-stay hospital have remained virtually unchanged for centuries until today. Similarly, the sentiments of residents living in such institutions and wishing for more freedom, were expressed a long time ago.

It may be surprising to learn that the following letter was written about a hundred years ago by a young American, living in a long-stay hospital, who proposed to form a "running away club". The letter was reported in a book written by the physician in charge of a large institution at the beginning of this century:

Here is one thing that I want to be successful in a short time from now:- I contemplate a running-away club to different parts of the United States and also to the Philipines (where his father lived). I want all the boys who are in favor of starting this club today, to stand up and I will put down the names, and do not be afraid to stand up...Here are the reasons:- For more liberty, more independence, more sight-seeing of this wide world, more walks... (Barr, 1904, p.335).

The physician introduced the letter by describing it as having been written "by a high-grade boy aged 15, who, most erratic, has a very vivid imagination". While no one in the study we carried out matched this boy's considerable literary skills, there is a clear overlap in sentiment. They express their own social position relative to the wider social world of which they are a part. What makes the awareness-of-self-in-relation-to-others critical for their perception of the quality of life, is that it is within this relative framework that they will judge the value of their lives and develop their aspirations for the future.

TAKING PEOPLE SERIOUSLY

After looking at the importance of agency in determining the nature and quality of people's lives, it is worth reflecting on why consumers' perceptions of services should be taken into account. The wishes and aspirations of service users do not necessarily coincide with the aims and objectives of either carers or services, nor should we expect them to. Indeed, there may also be misapprehensions about people's interpretations of events. For example, a hospital training flat may be seen by the residents as a trial period to test if they are capable of living in a community setting. Hence, a move back to the wards might be viewed by the staff as a 'valuable learning experience' and by the person concerned as a devastating personal failure. Flynn's (1989) exploration of the lives of people with learning disabilities living in their own homes in the Manchester area highlighted another example of misunderstood intentions. The social work staff regarded their primary aim as fostering their clients' self-sufficiency, with the ultimate goal of withdrawing from their lives. In contrast to this, the clients had come to regard the social workers as an important and reliable source of social support and friendship. Therefore to ensure a 'quality' service, which meets the needs of people with learning disabilities, it is vital to obtain insight into the meaning of people's life experiences.

The problem facing those carrying out an evaluation of a service, or support system, is how best to obtain the views of people with learning disabilities. There are drawbacks to using a formally worded and highly structured format of interview which makes no allowance for communication difficulties. The onus is on the interviewer to make it possible for the participants to express their own opinions and feelings and a variety of strategies may have to be utilised. Re-phrasing or even approaching a question from a different tack may be necessary to facilitate comprehension. In order to maintain the flow of the interview, to make sense of the participants' responses and to explore areas of interest, the interviewer must understand the wider context of the participant's life. For example, such knowledge would be vital if interviewing people living in a long-stay hospital within an institutional culture. In this setting the very language used to address people with learning difficulties has its specific terminology, e.g. 'high-grade', 'low-grade', 'fit case', 'boys and girls', 'outsiders', 'out on pass', 'the box room', 'the needle', 'being booked', 'getting high'. The measure used to evaluate quality of life should be sensitive to the unique experience of the particular people whose views one wishes to examine. There is little point in using a broad measure of quality of life with excellent psychometric qualities, standardised for the general population, if it is only partially relevant to the lives of those participating in the study.

One reason commonly given for ignoring the views of people with learning difficulties is their compliance, i.e. the tendency to agree with whatever is suggested to them. The interview, however, is a social situation and does not take place in vacuo but in the wider framework of people's lives (Farr, 1982). Most staff, professionals and non-handicapped people are likely to be in a position of power over people with learning difficulties. Consequently, people with learning difficulties cannot be expected to make outspoken and critical comments. If they are to have the confidence to express their views openly, the interviewer must create the conditions for an interview. He or she must convince them that he or she is not part of the establishment, coming to obtain their views which may be used in evidence against them. Nor must the researcher appear as a tester, i.e. a someone with all the right answers.

Edgerton (1967), in his classic work "The Cloak Of Competence", introduced the participant observational approach from anthropology to studying the lives of people with learning difficulties. The original study was concerned with the experience of people with learning disabilities who had been discharged from a long-stay hospital in California. The sensitive and thorough approach used by Edgerton and his followers has generated a great wealth of insight. The thoroughness and detail of the observations brings with it a humanity which allows the researchers to establish the core issues in the lives of those being studied. In a more recent book, following up a number of elderly members of the original cohort, Edgerton described the method adopted by his research team:

> *Their research spanned long periods, relied on unobtrusive observation and conversation, not tests or interviews...research of this kind requires close rapport, and rapport requires reciprocity and intimacy. As anyone who has engaged in participant observation knows, complete objectivity is chimeral. We care about the people we study and to a degree we become involved in their lives...However, when we prepare reports...we make every effort to achieve objectivity, and with the help of our colleagues who sometimes challenge our interpretations, we believe that our descriptions are as accurate as care and understanding can make them...Without the context and detail that more extended portraits can provide, the texture and meaning of these lives with their moments of triumph and torment, like their routines and tedium, are lost. (Edgerton 1991, p.ix)*

The detailed reports provided also allow the reader to make his or her own interpretations of the data. Although this method is especially well adapted to studying the lives of people with more severe learning disabilities who have communication problems, Goode (1979) has also used it to examine the experience of the congenitally deaf and blind. In such cases a close rapport with the participants facilitates the observer's understanding of the communicative intent of their actions.

CONCEPTIONS OF QUALITY OF LIFE

The differences in perspectives between carers, professionals and people with learning disabilities themselves, highlight the fact that quality of life is a relative social construct. It is therefore not possible to attempt a definitive or even an objective account of it. However, it is worth relating some current themes in the debate about quality of life as it relates to those with learning disabilities.

A number of features such as dignity, privacy, choice, or individual versus group care are generally agreed to be essential features of 'quality' services. These features are mutually interdependent. For example, the privacy of one's own bedroom may not only allow greater choice in terms of offering a retreat with the prospect of obtaining peace and quiet, but also a place where one can listen to music. The dignity of being on a supported employment scheme, on the other hand, may be accompanied by responsibilities which conflict with personal wishes regarding dress and time keeping.

In order to consider various quality indicators, measures such as Index of the Physical Environment (Pratt et al., 1980) and the Revised Residence Management Practices Scale (Raynes et al., 1979) have been developed. They include items such as whether there are sufficient bathrooms to enable people with learning difficulties to have a bath individually, rather than in batches or according to a rota, and whether people have their own clothes and personal possessions. These straightforward measures seem designed more to correct past wrongs than to strive for excellence (Bradley and Bersani, 1990).

Less tangible quality issues receive less scrutiny. For example, the nature of relationships with carers, or with professionals working with people with learning disabilities are rarely discussed. This is surprising given that such relationships are a vital determinant of the lives which people with learning difficulties lead. In addition, staff members and professionals often attach great importance to the viewpoints or philosophies on which they base their relationships with people with learning difficulties. The lack of debate about the nature of relationships may in part be due to the dogmatic expression of theories underlying widely held viewpoints, such as normalisation. Such dogma can prevent questions being raised about inherent difficulties (Robinson, 1989). For example, the internal contradictions between normalcy and individual agency implicit in Wolfensberger's interpretation of normalisation, pose a dilemma for the carer. Should people be enabled to express their individuality by wearing comfortable old clothes for pottering about in the garden or should they wear something smarter for the sake of the neighbours?

For some time now 'independence' has been one of the core themes in services for people with learning disabilities. The aim of developing the individual to the maximum of his or her potential, or a focus on training, has provided a goal for carers and professionals. Efforts to achieve these aims have been considered a benchmark of quality. The ultimate aim of such training is that the person should acquire sufficient self-help skills to require a minimum of staff support. Consequently, the underlying concept of independence appears to refer to domestic self-sufficency and competence to 'survive' in the community (Cattermole et al., 1987). Apart from ignoring, or assigning only a secondary role to the socio-emotional needs of people with learning disabilities who often lack social support and friendship (Jahoda et al., 1990), there have been other more subtle consequences for service users. In particular, people with learning difficulties are placed in the position of learners and the staff in the position of teachers and arbitrators of appropriate skills and behaviour. While staff need to help people learn new skills and to provide guidance, to be constantly in the role of teacher and moral superior can create social boundaries. How can the staff member appreciate their tenants' feelings of boredom and frustration, when they are making desperate efforts to teach them to budget their meagre income? The last thing the staff member may be willing to countenance is any activity which may result in additional money being spent. Indeed, it has been suggested that extreme staff efforts to promote independence may reflect attitudes which are as judgmental and authoritarian as staff who are overprotective and smothering (Brechin and Swain, 1988).

Another extreme attitude towards independence was found by Cattermole et al. (1990), when looking at the lives of people with mild learning disabilities moving from home and hospital to the community. The authors found that a number of staff believed it was not their role to tell tenants what to do, since they thought that tenants should be left to make their own way and learn from their own mistakes. Therefore staff held back from direct intervention in the lives of the tenants, except when help was requested or when a crisis arose. It is through interdependence that most people gain the necessary social and practical support they need to live independently. Some of the most important tasks which support staff can fulfil are the following: being a companion for shopping trips; sharing a meal; helping to find employment or day-time activity; and to accompany the tenant to a new social event.

The training model may leave people with learning difficulties in the position of life-long learners. This may in fact be regarded as a laudable aim in life. Amongst people with more severe learning disabilities this approach has achieved some success. The almost complete absence of activity and interaction in the lives of people with more severe learning disabilities living in traditional services has come to be regarded as a key shortcoming in their quality of life (Felce et al., 1985; 1986). Hence, to improve their quality of life, Felce et al. have successfully implement a training model based entirely on behavioural methods. There may be compelling arguments for the use of behavioural interventions in overcoming particular difficulties (Cullen, 1990). Nevertheless, there is also a danger that behavioural approaches do not sufficiently appreciate people as against schedules of reinforcement. Human relationships are based on intersubjectivity, and for them to last, there has to be a mutual interest in their maintenance. Perhaps the main idea which emerges from Gentle Teaching (Cheseldine, 1991), an approach developed for working with people who display the most difficult behaviours, is that learning to value the person is as important in maintaining the motivation and interest of staff members as it is for those with whom they are working.

For those who do, in the end, achieve independence, yet lack socio-emotional support, the question inevitably poses itself: 'Free for what?'. Edgerton et al. (1984) carried out a long-term follow-up of fifteen people with learning difficulties discharged from a Californian hospital. These now elderly people were reported to be relatively satisfied with their lives. However, a more detailed description of six of these people's lives (Edgerton, 1991) uncovered a bleaker picture, with episodes of exploitation and of isolation. Indeed, these individuals made clear their wish to balance a sense of autonomy with supportive relationships which would give security in their old age and give meaning to their lives. Flynn (1989) uncovered a similar set of attitudes prevailing among people living in their own homes in the Manchester area. They demonstrated a similar resilience and pride in having their own homes, and would not countenance a move back to hostel type accommodation, even when facing victimisation. What many of Flynn's interviewees desperately desired was greater social support.

One way to avoid conflicting views about a person's future is to obtain a clear understanding of his or her strengths and needs. Traditional assessment procedures for adults with learning disabilities, based on normative data, have largely been superseded by more individualistic approaches such as Life Planning Manual (Chaimberlain, 1985). These client-centred methods demand that 'plans' should be drawn-up with the co-operation of the individual with a learning disability. However, Cattermole (1989) has demonstrated the difficulty which professionals experience in developing such a cooperative relationship and that they can be totally unaware of their own domineering and directive attitude. Ward (1986) was so concerned with the behaviour of professionals in Individual Programme Planning meetings (a similar approach to Life Plans) that she attempted to train professionals in how to behave in such meetings. Hence, while purporting to be client centred, the position of the person with learning disabilities in Individual Programme Planning or the Life Planning Programme remains unclear.

The complex paper work and assessments entailed in a system such as Life Plans, inevitably remains under the control of staff or carers. Moreover, there is usually no mechanism for dealing with the conflicting views and aspirations which are expressed by people with learning difficulties, staff and carers. This situation often leads to marginalisation of the person with learning difficulties. Brechin and Swain (1986) have tried to redress this balance by developing an approach which places as much emphasis on the process of defining co-operative goals and objectives as on achieving them. The process places the person with learning disabilities in a pivotal role, and forces all the participants to carefully assess and reconcile the different views and ideas which are presented, in order to reach a more truly shared agenda for action.

PUBLIC AND PRIVATE DIMENSIONS OF CARE

Inspired by the Griffiths Report, H.M.S.O (1988), government policy in Britain is indeed moving towards the assessment of individual needs, and through the case management approach to develop a package of care suited to the individual. The role of the case manager in assessing the individual and in purchasing services on his or her behalf brings us back to the 'quality of life' of the market place.

The other fashionable term in the new 'mixed economy of care' is 'quality assurance'. While efforts to ensure a high standard of service is imperative, Bradley (1990) has pointed to a number of potential flaws in the centralised standardisation of services. For example, a system aimed at evaluating a range of services is likely to be calibrated at the 'lowest common denominator'. In addition, the more ordinary or flexible the service, the more difficult it might be to measure it precisely. Following this line of thought, an examining body attempting to ensure choice and a reasonable standard of food may demand that a service produce a set menu for the week ahead. This may penalise a flexible service, where people in a staffed house are helped to purchase and to cook their own food on an individual basis. Finally, Cullen (1990) warned of lessons to be learned from the American system, where the public funding of services in particular states is tied to recording detailed information about the work being carried out with individuals. If a complex and ongoing monitoring system is implemented, there is a danger that an extra tier of bureaucracy will be put into place, demanding numerous hours of staff time filling in measures and scales. This could easily become a paper exercise, necessitating long office hours and detracting from the real job of working with people.

On the other hand, the new competitive element introduced into services makes a system of independent monitoring, despite all its pitfalls, of vital importance. In traditional services the hierarchical medical and social services models may have made it difficult, if not impossible, for service users, their families and professionals working within the system, to make the powers that be listen to their criticisms (Ryan and Thomas, 1980). With the diversification of services, and with government policy aimed at creating more client-centred approaches, one might have imagined a greater openness. However, in the new commercial climate, where hospitals, voluntary sector organisations and private facilities routinely employ people to enhance their public image, services may be just as unlikely to brook any criticism. The new competitive market means that a poor press could result in fewer people using a service and a consequent loss of funding. Instead, it is likely that many managers of human services will wish, or be forced, to do just the opposite. For example, there are now very large and old long-stay hospitals for people with learning disabilities that describe themselves as 'centres of excellence'. The dilemma for staff will be between the demands of loyalty to the organisation and their public duty to defend the rights and enhance the lives of people with learning disabilities. Psychologists, along with other professionals working in services, do not require objective measures of the quality of life to realise the grim reality of living in a highly institutionalised hostel or hospital ward. However, with the exception of a brave few, people are only likely to speak out where management proves responsive towards users and staff.

The monitoring of services and support provided on an individual basis in terms of housing and employment should be carried out on a local basis. If the monitoring is localised, it can be tailored to the particular service, thereby avoiding the pitfalls of setting the standard to the lowest common denominator and encouraging more ordinary or more flexible services. Any evaluation should also take account of the views of staff, carers, service users and people advocating on behalf of people with learning disabilities. Finally, the monitoring should be carried out in a sensitive fashion with the cooperation of those concerned, and avoid blundering into people's houses in the fashion described by Kennedy (1990), who had first hand experience of his house being inspected.

While the seductive language of the market place may provide the illusion of consumer rights, we should not lose sight of the fact that people with learning difficulties usually depend on the benefits system for their income. Consequently, they are living on the poverty line. For example, people living in a registered care home receive a personal income of £12.20 a week for all necessities such as clothing and toiletries, and luxuries such as going out or saving for holidays. If other people on limited benefits find it impossible to budget on such incomes, how can people with learning disabilities be expected to do this? Moreover, at a human level, relationships and friendships cannot be bought, nor demanded by any Citizen's Charter.

The fact remains that people with learning difficulties continue to suffer stigmatisation in society at large. Wolfensberger (1983) argued that stigmata could become valued, using the example of the bound feet of Chinese women. However, the bound feet of Chinese women were not stigmata but status symbols. These women's feet were positively regarded because they were symbols of the women's socio-economic status. Stigmata have a particular social history within any culture. People are stigmatised because they fail to meet, contradict, or break what, at any given time, are societal norms. The acceptance of people with learning disabilities and the enhancement of their quality of life depends on the further evolution of societal attitudes.

CONCLUSION

What future does the concept of 'quality of life' have in the area of learning disabilities? There are some who would argue that the new technology of hand held computers will greatly contribute to the monitoring and development of services. Stanley and Roy (1988), are part of another movement which claims that 'social validation', or comparing the lives of people with learning disabilities with the average person in the street, will add a new objectivity to evaluating 'quality of life'. However, it is not the technologies which in recent years have dramatically changed the position of people with learning disabilities in society, but how they are perceived as persons. Little attempts were made to provide activity or to compare their lives with the average person in the street until people with learning disabilities were considered worthy of activity and of leading more ordinary lives.

The future will be built on past and present attempts to promote the collective and individual position of people with learning disabilities in society. A more polemical approach may be required to change services and challenge societal discrimination and prejudice. In contrast, it is sensitivity, balance and imagination which may make it possible for individuals to become an accepted part of their street, neighbourhood, village, town or workplace. Perhaps the aspect of personhood which deserves greater attention is people's sense of their own agency, and the role they should play in determining the nature of their own lifestyle. The following words come from a man who took part in a study examining the self-concepts of people with learning disabilities (Jahoda 1988). His inspiring statement shows the dignity which so many people are able to maintain in the face of terrific odds:

> *...because I never got on at school or anything like that. They found out that I was too slow. The thing was, slow then was frowned upon, but it's not really (sic) because I may have been slow but I got there. What's the matter about rushing about on to reach the same target as the rest and then make mistakes? Rushing can cause mistakes and disasters...slow people get there eventually, what's the mad rush?*

REFERENCES

Bank-Mikkelsen, N. E. (1990), Denmark. In I. Flynn and R. J. Nitsch (eds.), *Normalisation, Social Integration and Community Services*, Baltimore: University Park Press.

Barr, M. W. (1904), *Mental Defectives: Their History, Treatment and Training*, Philadelphia: Blakinston's Son and Co.

Bayley, M. (1991), Normalisation as 'social role valorisation': an adequate philosophy? In S. Baldwin & J. Hattersley (eds.), *Mental Handicap: Social Science Perspectives*, London: Routledge.

Begab, M. J. (1975), The mentally retarded and society: Trends and Issues. In M. J. Begab and S. A. Richardson (eds.), *The Mentally Retarded and Society: A Social Science Perspective*, Baltimore: University Park Press.

Binet, A. S. T. (1905), Enquête sur le mode d'existence des sujets sortis d'une école d'arrièreés, *L'Annee Psychologie*, XI, 137–145.

Bradley, V. J. (1990), Conceptual issues in quality assurance. In V. J. Bradley and H. A. Bersani (eds.), *Quality Assurance for Individuals with Developmental Disabilities*, Baltimore: Brookes.

Bradley, V. J. and Bersani, H. A. (1990), The future of quality assurance: It's everybody's business. In V. J Bradley and H. A. Bersani (eds.), *Quality Assurance for Individuals with Developmental Disabilities*, Baltimore: Brookes.

Brechin, A. and Swain, J. (1986), *Changing Relationships: Shared Action Planning with People with a Mental Handicap*, London: Harper & Row.

Brechin, A. and Swain, J. (1988), Professional/client relationships, creating a 'working alliance' with people with learning difficulties. *Disability, Handicap and Society*, **3**, 213–216.

Cattermole, M. (1989), *Social skills training for people with a mental handicap*, Unpublished M. Sc thesis, University of Stirling.

Cattermole, M., Jahoda, A. and Marková, I. (1987), *Training for Independent Living in Mental Handicap Hospitals and Adult Training Centres*, Unpublished Final Report to Scottish Home and Health Department: University of Stirling.

Cattermole, M., Jahoda, A. and Marková, I. (1990), Quality of life for people with learning difficulties moving to community homes. *Disability, Handicap and Society*, **5**, 137–152.

Chaimberlain, P. (1985), *Life Planning Manual*, British Association for Behavioural Psychotheraphy, Rossendale, Lancs, England.

Cheseldine, S. E. (1991), Gentle teaching for challenging behaviour. In J. Watson (ed.), *Innovatory Practice and Severe Learning Difficulties*, Edinburgh: Moray House Publications.

Challis, D. and Shepherd, R. (1983), An assessment of the potential for community living of mentally handicapped patients in hospital. *British Journal of Social Work*, **13**, pp.501–520.

Cullen, C. (1990), The relation between ideology and clinical interventions for people with mental retardation. *Current Opinion in Psychiatry*, **3**, 777–780.

Edgerton, R. B. (1967), *The Cloak of Competence*, Berkeley: University of California Press.

Edgerton, R. B. (1991), Preface. In R. B. Edgerton and M. A. Gaston (eds.) *I've Seen It All! : Lives of Older Persons with Mental Retardation in the Community*. London: Brookes.

Edgerton, R. B., Bollinger, M. and Herr, B. (1984), The Cloak of Competence After Two Decades. *American Journal of Mental Deficiency*, **88**, 345–351.

Elwood, S. (1981), Sex and the mentally handicaped, *Bulletin of the British Psychological Society*, **34**, 169–171.

Eyman, R. K., Demaine, G. C. and Lei, T-J (1979), Relationship between community environments and resident changes in adaptive behaviour: a path model, *American Journal of Mental Deficiency*, **83**, pp. 330–338.

Felce, D., Thomas, M., de Kock, U. and Saxby, H. (1985), An ecological comparison of small community based houses and traditional institutions. *Behaviour Research and Therapy*, **24**, 141–143.

Felce, D., de Kock, U. and Repp, A. C. (1986), An eco-behavioural analysis of small community-based houses and traditional large hospitals for severely and profoundly mentally handicapped adults, *Applied Research in Mental Retardation*, **7**, 393–408.

Flynn, M. C. (1989), *Independent Living For Adults With Mental Handicap*, London: Cassell.

Farr, R. M. (1982), Interviewing: the social psychology of the interview. In F. Fransella (ed.), *Psychology for Occupational Therapists*, Exeter: The British Psychological Society and McMillan.

Foucault, M. (1977), *Discipline and Punish; the Birth of the Prison*, London: Penguin Books.

Goffman, E. (1961), *Asylums*, Harmondsworth; Penguin.

Goffman, E. (1963), *Stigma: Notes on the Management of a Spoiled Identity*, Englewood Cliffs: Prentice-Hall.

Goode, D. (1979), The world of the congenitally deaf-blind. In H. Schwartz & J. Jacobs (eds.), *Qualitative Sociology: A Method to the Madness*, Free Press.

Greengross, W. (1976), *Entitled to Love: The Sexual and Emotional Needs of the Handicaped*, London: Malaby Press.

H. M. S. O. (1974), *Report of the Committee of Inquiry into South Ockendon Hospital*, London: H. M. S. O.

H. M. S. O. (1988), *Community Care: Agenda For Action. A Report To The Secretary Of State For Social Services By Sir Roy Griffiths*, London: H. M. S. O.

Ignatieff, M. (1984), *The Needs of Strangers*, London: Hogarth.

Jahoda, A. Cattermole, M. and Marková, I. (1990), Moving out: an opportunity for friendship and broadening social horizons? *Journal of Mental Deficiency Research*, **34**, pp. 127–139.

Jahoda, A. (1988), *Experience of stigma and the self-concept of people with a mild mental handicap*, Unpubished PhD thesis, University of Stirling.

Jahoda, A., Marková, I. and Cattermole, C. (1988), Stigma and the self-concept of people with a mild mental handicap, *Journal of Mental Deficiency Research*, **32**, pp 103–115.

Jay Committee (1979), *Report of The Committee of Enquiry into Mental Handicap Nursing and Care*, Cmnd 7468 I and II. London: H. M. S. O.

Kennedy, M. J. (1990), What quality assurance means to me: Expectation of consumers. In V. J. Bradley and H. V. Bersani (eds.) *Quality Assurance for Individuals With Developmental Disabilities*, Baltimore: Brookes.

King, R. D., Raynes, N. V. and Tizard, J. (1971), The Revised Child Management Scale, In King, R. D., Raynes, N. V., and Tizard, J. (1971). *Patterns of Residential Care*, London: Routledge & Kegan Paul.

Lazerson, M. (1975), Educational institutions and mental subnormality: Notes on writing a history. In M. J. Begab and S. A. Richardson (eds.), *The Mentally Retarded and Society: A Social Science Perspective*, Baltimore: University Park Press.

Locker, D., Roa, B. and Veddel, J. M. (1984), Evaluating community care for the mentally handicapped adult: comparison of hostel, home and hospital care, *Journal of Mental Deficiency Research*, **28**, pp. 189–198.

Mittler, P. (1979), *People Not Patients*, London: Methuen.

O'Brien, J. (1990), Developing high quality services for people with developmental disabities. In V. S. Bradley and H. A. Bersani (eds.), *Quality Assurance for Individuals With Developmental Disabilities*, Baltimore: Brookes.

Perrin, B. and Nirje B. (1985), Setting the record straight: a critique of some frequent misconceptions of the normalisation principle. *Australian and New Zealand Journal of Developmental Disabilities*, **11**, 69–74.

Pratt, M. W. Luszcz, M. A. and Brown, M. E. (1980), Measuring dimensions of the quality of care in small community residences, *American Journal of Mental Deficiency*, **85**, 188–194.

Raynes, N. V. (1988), *Annotated Directory of Measures of Environmental Quality*, Manchester: Department of Social Policy.

Raynes, N. V., Pratt, M. and Roses, S. (1979), *Organisational Structure of the Care of the Mentally Retarded*. London: Croom Helm.

Robinson, T. (1989), Normalisation: the whole answer? In A. Brechin and J. Swain (eds.), *Making Connections*, London: Hodder & Stoughton.

Ryan, J. and Thomas, F. (1980), *The Politics of Mental Handicap*, Harmondsworth: Penguin Books.

Schalock, R. L. and Harper, R. S. (1978), Placement from community-based mental retardation programmes: how well do clients do? *American Journal of Mental Deficiency*, **83**, pp. 240–247.

Scheerenberger, R. C. (1983), *A History of Mental Retardation*. London: Brookes.

Skull, A. T. (1977), *Decarceration*, New Jersey: Prentice-Hall.

Stanley, B. and Roy, Y. (1988), Evaluating the quality of life of people with mental handicaps: a social validation study, *Mental Handicap Research*, **1:2**, 197–210.

Tyne, A. (1981), The impact of the normalisation principle on service for the mentally handicapped in the United Kingdom. In J. Lishman (ed.), *Research Highlights Number Two: Normalisation*, Aberdeen: Aberdeen People's Press.

Vitello, S. J. Atthowe, J. M. and Cadwell, J. (1983), Determinants of community placement of institutionalised mentally retarded persons, *American Jounral of Mental Deficiency*, **87**, pp. 539–545.

Ward, L. (1986), Alternatives to C. M. H. T.'s : Developing a community support service in South Bristol. In G. Grant, S. Humphreys and M. McGrath (eds.), *Community Mental Handicap Teams: Theory and Practice*, Kidderminster: British Institute of Mental Handicap.

Willer, B. and Intagliata, J. (1981), Social-environmental factors as predictors of adjustment of deinstitutionalised mentally retarded adults, *American Journal of Mental Deficiency*, **86**, pp. 252–259.

Williams, P. and Shoultz, B. (1982), *We Can Speak For Ourselves*, London: Souvenir Press.

Wolfensberger, W. (1972), *Normalisation: The Principle of Normalisation in Human Services*, Toronto: National Institute on Mental Retardation.

Wolfensberger, W. (1983), Social role valorization: a proposed new term for the principle of normalisation, *Mental Retardation*. **21**, 234–239.

Wolfensberger, W. (1990a), A brief overview of the principle of normalisation. In I. Flynn and R. J. Nitsch (eds), *Normalisation, Social Integration and Community Services*, Baltimore: University Park Press.

Wolfensberger, W. (1990b), The definition of normalisation. In I. Flynn and R. J. Nitsch (eds.), *Normalisation, Social Integration and Community Services*, Baltimore: University Park Press.

Wolfensberger, W. and Glenn, L. (1978), *Programme analysis of service systems (PASS): A method for the quantitative evaluation of human services (3rd ed.)*, Toronto: National Institute on Mental Retardation.

Wolfensberger, W. and Thomas, S. (1983), *Program Analysis of Service Systems' Implementation of Normalisation Goals* 2nd Edition, Toronto: National Insititute on Mental Retardation.

CHAPTER TWELVE

Quality of Life and Mental Health: Evaluating the Impact of Long-Term Care

Margaret M BARRY[1] and Charles CROSBY[2]

[1]*Department of Psychology, Trinity College, Dublin 2, Ireland.* [2]*Health Services Research Unit, Department of Psychology, University College of North Wales, Bangor, Gwynedd, LL57 2DG*

INTRODUCTION

Quality of life has emerged in recent years as an important construct in relation to both the conceptualisation and the evaluation of mental health care. Improved quality of life has become an explicit priority of the community alternatives to hospital-based care, it is one of the most frequently cited justifications for deinstitutionalisation (Anthony, 1980; Bachrach, 1980; Shadish et al. 1985), and it is increasingly identified as a critical outcome variable for evaluating community support services for chronic psychiatric clients. A concept such as quality of life accentuates a holistic approach to mental health care, embracing the physical, social, cognitive, emotional and material aspects of well-being. At a practical level, in the area of service evaluation, quality of life issues focus attention on how the service is influencing the lives of its clients, looking beyond illness-related outcomes to consider the broader impact of the service on a number of life areas. As such, quality of life directs awareness towards an examination of needs and standards of care. Therefore as an evaluative measure it holds much promise, potentially providing a useful evaluative framework against which to assess the outcomes of care.

The use of quality of life as a criterion for evaluating the impact of mental health care highlights the importance of accurately defining and measuring the determinants of quality of life for service users. In applying the concept of quality of life as an outcome measure, attention needs to be given to the validity of the measures, elucidating the factors that influence judgements of subjective well-being, and monitoring the sensitivity of the measures in evaluating change. As pointed out by George and Bearon (1980), "if quality of life is to be an organising rubric for research, planning and practice, the distribution, predictors and correlations and implications of life quality need to be carefully delineated" (p. 202). In order to identify the particular service components which are critical to ensuring a good quality of life for clients it is necessary first to address the general question of what constitutes and determines good quality of life for different client populations. These considerations are of particular importance in relation to people with chronic mental health problems who are service-dependent, as the objective of maximising their quality of life is seen as an important service goal. If we are to establish empirically whether or not community mental health services are adequately meeting their objective of improving the quality of life of service users, we need to define accurately the determinants of life quality for individual clients and to develop valid and reliable measures of assessing their quality of life.

In this chapter we focus on the quality of life of a group of long-stay psychiatric patients being resettled from hospital into a range of community residential facilities. As this group have experienced many years of hospital care and are heavily service-dependent, the objective of enhancing their quality of life in the community placements is seen as a critical service goal. The process of moving the group from hospital to community settings provides an ideal opportunity for monitoring and evaluating how their perceptions of the quality of their lives change as a function of the change in care settings and style of care delivery. Evaluation of the resettlement process also permits an examination of how care in the community settings compares with hospital care in terms of its impact on the quality of life of this group of long-stay patients.

While there is a growing body of discussion and work concerning the quality of life of chronic psychiatric clients living in the community, there are few longitudinal studies which trace the impact on individual clients of being moved from an institutional setting to living in the community. Jones, Robinson and Golightley (1986) point out that while the closure of psychiatric hospitals has given rise to a considerable literature on policy, detailed tracer studies of the effects on patients and the conditions under which they live after discharge are rare. There is a paucity of studies detailing the patterns of patients' lives and the factors that contribute to overall good quality of life following discharge from hospital. This chapter addresses the methodological issues involved in assessing the quality of life of a group of long-stay patients and examines how their experience of institutional care affects their perceptions of life quality both in the hospital setting and later in the community placements. The chapter draws on findings from an on-going longitudinal study being carried out at the Health Services Research Unit, University College of North Wales (Crosby and Barry, 1994) and reports on the quality of life of a group of long-stay patients in the hospital setting and initially at six months following their discharge to the community. In an international context the study by Zani and her colleagues in Bologna (Chapter 8) and by Jodelet (1991) in rural France are important. In France and in Italy the process of deinstitutionalisation started much earlier than it did in the United Kingdom.

CONCEPTUALISING AND MEASURING THE QUALITY OF LIFE OF A PSYCHIATRIC POPULATION

A generally accepted definition of quality of life is that it refers to "the sense of well-being and satisfaction experienced by people under their current life conditions" (Lehman, 1983b, p.143). Zautra and Goodhart (1979) emphasise the importance of defining the quality of life experience, "both as subjectively evaluated and objectively determined by an assessment of external conditions" (p.1). The methods used for assessing quality of life have taken their lead from a number of national surveys on quality of life in the USA. The approach adopted by researchers such as Andrews and Withey (1976) and Campbell, Converse and Rodgers (1976), was to consider general or global measures of well-being together with life satisfaction measures and objective indicators of external life circumstances in a number of life areas. Though the specific domains used to describe quality of life have varied, they have tended to include life areas such as living situation, health, work, finance, social and family relations, leisure, safety, etc. A number of satisfaction measures, rating scales and semantic differential scales have been designed for this purpose.

This approach to assessing quality of life has been adapted by researchers in relation to chronic psychiatric patients. A number of quality of life schedules have been developed specifically for use with a chronic psychiatric population, e.g. the Oregon Quality of Life Questionnaire (Bigelow et al., 1982) and the Satisfaction with Life Domains Scale (Baker and Intagliata, 1982). However, *Lehman's quality of life interview* is probably the most widely used scale in this area and its psychometric properties have been most extensively examined. Lehman (1983a) developed a general quality of life model based on national survey data. According to this model, quality of life is ultimately "a subjective matter, reflected in a sense of global well-being" (Lehman 1983a, p. 369). The model views the experience of general well-being as a product of three types of variables: personal characteristics such as age, sex, etc., objective quality of life in various life domains, and subjective quality of life in the same life domains. From this model Lehman developed a scale for assessing the quality of life of chronic psychiatric clients resident in the community. The scale, which consists of a structured interview format, collects objective and subjective data covering nine life domains in addition to measures of general well-being.

Much of the quality of life research that has been carried out with psychiatric populations has largely focused on community studies, evaluating the impact of community care on the quality of life of chronic clients who are currently living in the community. Such studies point to the many social problems affecting the quality of life of chronic clients. Both Lehman et al (1982) Lehman (1983a,b) and Baker and Intagliata (1982) report that life areas such as finance, unemployment, personal safety and health are consistent sources of dissatisfaction for discharged clients. However, Lehman et al (1982) report that while psychiatric clients were less satisfied than the general public with most life areas, over half the clients surveyed reported being "mostly satisfied" in most life areas. Studies of clients discharged from hospital also report that they generally express high levels of satisfaction with being out of hospital (Petch, 1990).

Studies comparing chronic clients in different care settings have found that clients in hospital care report a lower quality of life than those living in the community (Lehman et al., 1986; Simpson et al., 1989). Lack of comfort and personal safety in the hospital setting were found to detract from patients' quality of life. It should be noted, however, that such studies are of comparisons between groups of clients in hospital, hostels and community settings and, as such, the findings are limited by the fact that the groups sampled are usually not randomly allocated to the different care facilities. Placement within certain types of facilities tends to correspond with the severity of psychopathology, and this may in turn affect the quality of the living environment, thereby confounding the validity of the findings. Also of importance is the fact that comparisons between groups do not allow for the influence of individual differences in perception of life quality in different settings.

Longitudinal studies by Okin, Dolnick and Pearsall (1983) and Gibbons and Butler (1987) followed up groups of patients as they were discharged from hospital, evaluating the effect of the move from hospital on their perceived quality of life. On the whole, clients reported significant positive changes in their quality of life. These studies draw attention to the often neglected aspect of the institutionalisation debate, i.e. the problematic living conditions of psychiatric hospitals and the need for a more balanced attention to the problems faced by hospitalised patients as well as by those living in the community. There is a need for longitudinal studies which trace the same clients as they move from the hospital into community settings, allowing a more direct comparison of quality of life under different care regimes. Such prospective longitudinal studies provide a clearer picture of the influence of different forms of care delivery on clients' quality of life, and therefore can inform the debate as to whether community-based care does succeed in enhancing the quality of life of chronic clients over and above that offered by traditional hospital care.

Determinants of Quality of Life for a Long-stay Psychiatric Population

Lehman's model of quality of life, which is based on normative data from a survey of the general population, was applied originally in relation to chronic clients living in the community. The application of this model to a hospitalised long-stay population needs to be considered. Lehman's model is founded on a conceptual base which integrates access to resources and opportunities, fulfilment of social roles in multiple life domains, and expressed satisfaction with life in various domains. Access to resources for long-stay patients may be constrained by virtue of their current level of functioning or living situation, and the resources that are available may be limited or not under their own direct control. The availability of various life opportunities to a long-stay population may also be severely limited, e.g. limited employment, training and leisure opportunities, and a restricted network of social relationships.

With regard to the fulfilment of social roles in multiple life domains, the long-term psychiatric patient may be seen as the occupant of an ascribed and all encompassing social role, that of psychiatric patient or being "mentally ill" (Goffman, 1961). The average long-stay patient rarely has an occupational or domestic role apart from this, e.g. the majority are unemployed, unmarried, etc. This is particularly relevant for patients in receipt of hospital or residential care, as the usual segmentation of life into domestic, occupational and recreational sections rarely occurs and the person is placed in one continuous context, that of resident of a psychiatric hospital or care facility. Looking, therefore, at the dimensions that are commonly used to define quality of life, one has to question if these dimensions are especially central in the assessment of the quality of life of long-term psychiatric patients. The relative importance of life domains such as work, financial, recreational, social, and family relations for a group of people who have lost or never had occupational status, income, good health and are virtually socially isolated need to be examined rather than assumed. Baker and Intagliata (1982) raise the question of whether we know enough about how individuals view their lives, particularly those dealing with a major mental health problem, to be able to select appropriate dimensions for measuring life quality.

Life Satisfaction

The concept of life satisfaction also needs to be examined in this context. Andrews and McKennell (1980) suggest that social indicators of perceived well-being reflect two basic types of influence: affect and cognition. Life satisfaction may be taken as referring to a cognitive assessment of one's overall conditions of existence and progress toward desired goals (Andrews and Withey, 1976). Andrews and McKennell (1980) point out that the concept of satisfaction involves some notion of comparison, either explicit or implicit, between a level of achievement and a set of needs or aspirations. Expressed satisfaction may therefore be perceived as being particularly dependent upon social comparison. In this respect one has to query the standards of comparisons used by people who have spent a large proportion of their life in a psychiatric institution. The richness and variety of their lives will undoubtedly have been curtailed by years of hospitalisation. Satisfaction also involves an affective component regarding the fulfilment of needs, desires, expectations and hopes of the individual. Campbell et al. (1976) refer to the 'limited horizons and low aspirations' of chronic psychiatric patients, and how expectations have been progressively lowered to fit the realities of the situation. It is plausible to suspect that 30–40 years in a psychiatric hospital would lead to a change in the way reality is perceived, changing the relationship between living conditions and their evaluation. However, this important fact is rarely discussed in the quality of life literature. The majority of the research studies in this area has been concerned with the quality of life experiences of chronic psychiatric clients currently living in the community. The previous life experiences and expectations of these clients are rarely taken into account in the assessment of their current quality of life. In relation to long-stay patients, the fact that many have spent a substantial proportion of their adult life in a psychiatric institution would appear to be one of the most significant influences to be considered in assessing their quality of life. The experience of institutional care is likely to influence how long-stay patients will come to judge the quality of their lives in the new community settings and it is therefore important to take this factor into consideration.

THE NORTH WALES STUDY ON QUALITY OF LIFE

A study of 62 long-stay residents of a large psychiatric hospital in North Wales was carried out in order to examine their perceptions of their quality of life. The quality of life study forms part of a larger project concerning the evaluation of the resettlement of long-stay patients. Details of the study are described in full elsewhere (Lowe et al., 1988; Crosby et al., 1990). Briefly, the study is concerned with monitoring and evaluating the impact of the resettlement process on the lives of the individual patients as they are discharged from hospital. Patients' quality of life together with levels of psychiatric and behavioural functioning are assessed on the hospital ward prior to discharge, and follow-up assessments are carried out following their discharge from hospital, thus allowing a comparison between the hospital and community settings. At present the study is working to three baseline measures prior to discharge and three repeat measures post-discharge, at six weeks, six months and one year. The following discussion draws on findings from the first research cohort, and reports on the quality of life experienced by patients on the hospital wards prior to discharge and at six months following their move to the community. (The term 'patients' will be used to describe the study's sample while in the hospital setting while the term 'clients' will be used once they have been discharged from hospital.)

The quality of life schedule was administered to 62 long-stay psychiatric in-patients selected for resettlement from hospital. The majority of the hospital sample (83%) had a clinical diagnosis of schizophrenia, ranged in age from 27 to 87 years (mean = 56 years), had spent lengthy periods in hospital (mean total years in hospital = 25.6 years) and demonstrated low levels of social and behavioural functioning. The design of the quality of life study is in accordance with the overall design of the evaluation project, i.e. a repeated measures longitudinal design, permitting the collection of data from the same individuals at a number of points prior to, and following, their discharge from hospital.

Lehman et al's Quality of Life Interview (1982) was adapted and modified for use in the study. As Lehman's scale was devised initially for use with chronic clients resident in the community, its use with a sample of long-stay hospital residents, many of whom were quite elderly and dependent, raised a number of questions concerning its appropriateness. Following pilot trials, the questions and their response formats were modified in order to ensure comprehensibility and ease of administration for the hospital sample. A number of open-ended questions were also included in the schedule in order to explore individual perceptions of significant life events and experiences, attitude to discharge and reactions to discharge from hospital. Further details of the adaptation of the schedule and its psychometric properties can be found in Barry, Crosby and Bogg (1993). The redesigned schedule, which contains 96 items in all, retains the same basic structure as Lehman's scale covering subjective and objective indices for nine life areas, together with an index of general life satisfaction.

For the purposes of data analysis, objective and subjective composite scores were computed for each life domain. Composite indices were compiled by summing the scores of the individual items in each life area, thereby permitting sub-scores to be calculated for both the objective and subjective indices in each life domain. Internal consistency reliabilities (Cronbach's alpha) were computed for each of the objective and subjective life domain scores based upon the initial baseline interview (Barry et al., 1993). The reliability coefficients were generally high, with only the scale of objective living ($r = 0.55$) having a reliability coefficient of less than 0.60; however, it is noted that Lehman (1988) also reports reliability estimates of less than 0.50 for sub-scales of objective living such as autonomy, privacy and influence. The coefficient reliabilities for the remainder of the scales ranged from 0.63 to 0.95.

Perceived Quality of Life in the Hospital Setting

Details of the quality of life in the hospital settings are reported in Barry et al. (1992, 1993) but the main findings will be summarised here. The initial baseline assessment of quality of life on the hospital wards showed that patients' quality of life as measured by the objective indicators appeared to be severely restricted. There were low levels of privacy and independence on the hospital wards, with dormitory sleeping arrangements and inadequate facilities for self-catering. Many of the patients were socially isolated with few social contacts within or outside the hospital. Although some of the patients reported having friends, further questioning revealed that they rarely met or had contact with such friends. There were low levels of social interaction on the wards. The most frequent source of daily interaction was with staff, with 39% of patients reporting not interacting socially with other in-patients on the ward. Social interactions outside the hospital were infrequent, as was contact by phone and writing. Apart from family there were few sources of social support outside the hospital. The frequency of family contact tended to vary between patients, e.g. 26% had not received any visits in the last year, while 39% received weekly or twice monthly visits, with the remainder receiving visits on a more infrequent basis, one to three times a year. Few of the patients engaged in active leisure activities, and none was in employment at the time of interview. However, 36% of the group carried out work in the hospital for which they received a small payment. The majority of the patients (71%) received less than £20 per week and for some this was a source of dissatisfaction as they felt they 'didn't get enough money to spend' and 'could do with more money' to buy cigarettes, coffees, etc. when they visited the local town.

Yet, despite the objective living conditions, self-reported levels of satisfaction were high in most life areas, with the highest levels of satisfaction being expressed in relation to social relations (73%) and living situation (72%). Sources of dissatisfaction concerned finances and frequency of family contact, with residents expressing a desire for more money and greater contact with family members. However, even in these life areas, the majority appeared to be satisfied with their current situation (Figure 12.1). Generally, patients were reluctant to report sources of dissatisfaction or to point to areas of their lives that they considered unsatisfactory in some way. This was especially evident when patients were questioned directly concerning what they disliked most about life in the hospital. Few of the patients pointed to sources of dissatisfaction; comments such as 'I don't dislike anything about it' and 'I like everything here' were common with 79% of responses coded as either don't know (24%) or nothing specified (55%).

Levels of expressed satisfaction with life in general were also high (61%) but were often accompanied by comments which suggested that patients had resigned themselves to their present situation and had lowered their expectations accordingly: "life is nearly over, things could have been better", "I'm in hospital and that's about it", "I wish I was outside (the hospital) but I feel I'm making a good job of the situation". The overall impression from the hospital results is of a group of patients who rate low on quality of life as objectively measured, yet evaluate their subjective life quality in a positive manner.

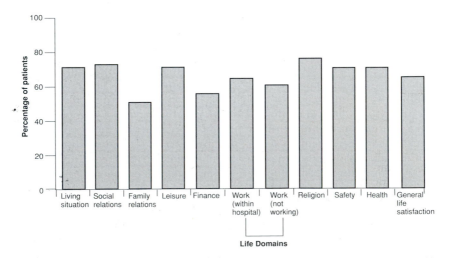

Figure 12.1 – Hospital baseline levels of satisfaction: domain-specific and general life satisfaction. (N = 62)

Examination of the qualitative data concerning important life areas and aspirations suggests that while life areas such as family, social relations and leisure emerged as being of importance to patients, aspects of the more immediate living environment may be more salient determinants of life quality for this hospitalised group. For example, in response to questions concerning sources of enjoyment or unhappiness, residents tended to refer to events in the immediate environment, e.g. complaints about the other residents or general complaints concerning hospital life were the most common sources of displeasure, while cigarettes, teas and coffees were cited as the most popular sources of enjoyment. A striking 51% of the hospital group were either unable or unwilling to specify what was the most important thing in their lives. However, for those who did respond, replies generally referred to family, work, leisure and relationships. The expressed aspirations of patients were quite low and many seemed resigned to life in hospital, with the older residents who had been hospitalised for lengthy periods expressing less favourable attitudes toward discharge. However, the data do support the contention that life areas such as social relations, family and leisure are of importance to this group of in-patients, thereby validating the inclusion of these life areas in the quality of life schedule.

Reports of general life satisfaction were found to be most strongly correlated with the domain specific subjective indices, but were not strongly correlated with either the domain specific objective indicators or demographic variables such as age or length of stay in hospital. These results are consistent with previous findings (Andrews and Withey, 1976; Campbell et al., 1976; Lehman et al. 1982; Lehman 1983a, b; Baker and Intagliata, 1982). However, general life satisfaction was found to be influenced by level of psychiatric functioning, with a negative correlation emerging between reports of general life satisfaction and psychiatric symptoms such as depression ($r = -0.29$, $p = 0.02$) and thought disorder ($r = -0.53$, $p = 0.001$) as measured on the Brief Psychiatric Rating Scale (Overall and Gorham, 1962). Those patients with higher ratings of depression and thought disorder were more likely to report lower levels of life satisfaction. These findings, which are reported in detail in Barry, Crosby and Bogg (1993), may be compared with those reported by Lehman (1983b). Using the Rand Health Insurance Study Mental Health Battery as an index of psychopathology, Lehman reported significant negative correlations between general life satisfaction and symptoms of depression and anxiety but not in relation to thought disorder. However, Lehman (ibid.) did suggest that the use of different measures of psychopathology might give rise to different relationships with the quality of life measures. The findings from the present study using the Brief Psychiatric Rating Scale are therefore of interest in this context.

The study also examined the effects of dependency on perceptions of life quality. The variable of functional dependency was considered important in view of the lengthy periods that the residents had spent in hospital. A significant positive correlation was found between overall level of dependency as measured by the total general behaviour score on the Rehab scale (Hall and Baker, 1983) and general life satisfaction ($r = 0.23$, p = 0.05). The more dependent residents were found to report higher levels of life satisfaction than residents who were rated as more able and independent. A related finding concerned the relationship between attitude to discharge and general life satisfaction. Those residents who expressed higher levels of life satisfaction were also more likely to express a desire to remain in hospital (r = 0.38, p < 0.01) and were less positive concerning their discharge from hospital (r = -0.23, p < 0.05). As pointed out by Wing and Brown (1970), an unfavourable attitude toward discharge is one of the central features of institutionalisation. These findings, therefore, raise the question of the extent to which the high levels of satisfaction are a product of the effects of institutionalisation, reflecting patients' adaptation and resignation to a dependent and restricted life style.

Implications of Findings

The difficulty in reconciling the high rates of satisfaction expressed by the majority of hospital patients with the quality of life as measured by the objective indices in hospital raises a number of questions concerning the validity of the self-report measures and how the quality of life data should best be interpreted. The frequently reported lack of correlation between the objective and subjective indices of the quality of life is usually interpreted as testimony to the fact that the two sets of indices are measuring different aspects of the quality of life (Andrews and Withey, 1976; Campbell et al., 1976; Lehman, 1988). However, one could argue that, given the lack of correlation between the two sets of measures, it is not possible to clarify the nature of the relationship between the objective conditions in different life areas and their subjective perception and evaluation. Do states of well-being have a clear-cut objective counterpart? Is satisfaction with social relations necessarily determined by the frequency of social contact? As Glatzer (1991) points out, it is the combination of the objective and subjective components of welfare that defines quality of life.

The complex question of how subjective well-being is related to the objective components of quality of life remains unanswered at this stage. The fact that individuals may experience feelings of satisfaction and deprivation at the same time has also been reported by other researchers (e.g. Andrews and Withey, 1976; Campbell et al., 1976; Bradburn, 1969; Glatzer, 1991). Glatzer (1991) suggests that the positive and negative aspects of well-being may be independent of each other and that both well-being and ill-being may have many components. In the area of job satisfaction, for example, Herzberg et al. (1957) point to the fact that while job satisfaction depends on a certain set of conditions, job dissatisfaction may be related to an entirely different set of conditions. In relation to general life satisfaction there is a need to identify which factors lead to satisfaction and which factors lead to dissatisfaction and to examine the process by which these are determined. The relationship between objective conditions and their subjective evaluations also requires further examination in order to delineate the mediating mechanisms by which the different components of the quality of life are appraised.

The lack of correlation between the quality of life indices also begs the question as to how much weight should be given to each set of indicators for the purpose of service evaluation studies. The subjective measures are generally regarded as the more sensitive indicators of life quality. However, Strack et al. (1990) caution that reports of subjective well-being, used as subjective indicators, may be a function of temporary influences at the time of judgement. Wilde and Svanberg (1990) point to the fact that subjective quality of life ratings have been reported to be vulnerable to a number of sources of distortion, including acquiescent response set (Ware, 1978) and social desirability (Carstenson and Cone, 1983). The problem of positive response bias is frequently encountered in relation to satisfaction measures in this area, with levels of reported satisfaction ranging from 60-100%. Should these high levels of expressed satisfaction be accepted at face value as an expression of satisfaction with the current quality of life? Baker and Intagliata (1982) in discussing this issue concluded that "there appears to be no way to completely determine whether the high levels of positive feelings represent a sincere evaluation of aspects of the clients' lives and reflect the clients' actual perceptions of the environment or are due to grateful testimonials or other biasing factors. The answer probably lies somewhere in between" (p. 78).

The demand characteristics of the interview situation need to be taken into account, as validity may be threatened by the 'yea-saying' effect. Hospital patients may be unwilling to express dissatisfaction or be seen to complain, as acceptance of one's lot may be an inevitable part of the process of adapting to and surviving institutional life. Goffman (1961) uses the concept of 'mortification' to describe this process of adapting to life in a psychiatric hospital. Coping with a major mental health problem over an extended period, together with the process of adapting to a dependent lifestyle in hospital, may lower levels of expectation and aspirations, thereby leading patients to be less critical of their situation. The expectation gap between what someone has and what someone expects may therefore be quite narrow, resulting in relatively high levels of life satisfaction.

It is also important to consider the standards against which the judgements of satisfaction are being made. According to Schwarz and Strack's (1990) judgement model, social comparison standards play a major role in the evaluation of subjective well-being and reports of satisfaction are based on the relevant information which is accessible at the time of judgement. The social comparison standards operating in the hospital context are therefore of relevance. When people are institutionalised their freedom in choosing others as a comparison group may be greatly restricted and hospital patients may simply compare themselves with other patients in the hospital. Comparison with a hospital-based reference group may therefore result in relatively high levels of satisfaction with a standard of living that, outside the hospital context, would be considered unsatisfactory. All of these factors should be considered when attempting to interpret the satisfaction data and their role in informing the evaluation process.

These points have quite serious implications concerning the validity of the quality of life measures and how the data should best be interpreted. The subjective measures do, however, appear to be sensitive to the effects of psychopathology and dependency and, despite the clustering of positive responses, they do succeed in highlighting areas where most dissatisfaction exists. It was also found that the information obtained from patients concerning the objective indices of quality of life concurred with the information derived from staff, which gives some confidence in the validity of reportage by patients. A prospective follow-up of the same patients, as planned in the present study, monitoring the changes in the reported levels of satisfaction over time and with changing living conditions, may help address some of the methodological concerns raised earlier in this paper relating to the validity of the subjective measures and their sensitivity to changes in external circumstances.

Temporal Stability of Quality of Life Indices

The stability of the quality of life measures over time was also examined. The design of the study permits the collection of data from the same individuals at regular intervals. Establishing the stability of the measures was of interest for the following reasons:

(1) to examine the extent to which the subjective measures of quality of life were subject to temporary influences, (Strack et al., 1990);
(2) to determine the extent to which reported quality of life fluctuates independently of significant changes in external circumstances such as a move to a different care setting; and
(3) to establish a stable baseline against which to assess changes in reported quality of life following the move to the community, thereby strengthening the study's design.

The same individuals were interviewed at three-monthly intervals prior to their discharge from hospital. In all, over this six month period, the first set of interviews were carried out with the original group of 62 patients at the initial baseline assessment, the second set with 44 of these patients at first repeat baseline assessment and the third set of interviews with 40 patients at second repeat assessment. The dwindling numbers were due to the gradual discharge of residents from hospital as places in the community became available. The means and standard deviations for the composite scores for each life domain across the three baseline assessment points are presented in Table 12.1. In order to assess the amount of change over time, analysis of variance with repeated measures (MANOVA) was carried out on each of the life domain scores for both the objective and subjective quality of life indices. There were no significant changes in the majority of the scales over the three assessment points. The only subjective scale to show significant change over the six month period was the scale concerning the satisfaction with leisure. The observed fluctuation of decreasing and increasing levels of satisfaction may be linked to the actual frequency of leisure activities at the time of interview. With regard

Table 12.1 – Repeated measures analyses (MANOVA) of life domain composite indices at baseline, 1st repeat and 2nd repeat hospital assessments

	Baseline		1st repeat		2nd repeat		MANOVA
	Mean	(SD)	Mean	(SD)	Mean	(SD)	F-Ratio
Subjective indices							
Living situation	13.55	(2.20)	13.42	(2.51)	13.27	(2.52)	0.19
Social relations	8.40	(1.61)	8.34	(1.63)	8.49	(1.01)	0.12
Family relations	5.13	(1.23)	5.00	(1.56)	4.88	(1.12)	0.32
Leisure	5.56	(0.99)	4.82	(1.08)	5.15	(1.35)	3.60*
Finances	2.44	(0.96)	2.50	(0.93)	2.41	(1.02)	0.10
Religion	2.74	(0.75)	2.47	(1.80)	2.53	(1.05)	0.96
Health	13.76	(1.72)	12.60	(3.18)	13.00	(2.94)	1.36
Personal safety	5.35	(1.18)	5.35	(1.48)	5.35	(1.30)	0.00
Objective indices							
Living situation†	–	–	7.33	(1.65)	6.29	(1.93)	6.88*
Frequency of social contacts	17.06	(5.03)	17.12	(4.21)	17.67	(4.26)	0.40
Frequency of family contact	6.00	(2.35)	6.31	(2.74)	5.92	(2.77)	0.50
Leisure activities	19.34	(2.57)	19.19	(2.19)	19.50	(2.59)	0.26
Weekly spending money	12.91	(9.22)	13.12	(9.84)	14.66	(9.05)	0.85
Frequency of religious involvement	2.46	(1.47)	2.14	(1.61)	2.23	(1.38)	0.74
Physical illness in past year	3.72	(0.68)	3.84	(0.52)	3.78	(0.61)	0.44
Victim of robbery/attack	1.32	(0.48)	1.65	(0.49)	1.71	(0.58)	6.58**
Global quality of life	2.66	(0.83)	2.53	(0.88)	2.50	(0.92)	0.32

Notes: Due to the small number of residents engaged in work, the work scale was not included in the analysis.

† The living objective scale used at baseline differs slightly from that used at 1st and 2nd repeats, therefore comparison across all three points was not carried out.

*p = 0.05, ** p = 0.01

to the objective indices, the variation in the objective living index may be explained by the observable deterioration in living conditions on the hospital wards over the period of the assessments, two of the wards being combined in the run up to hospital closure. The change in the safety measures may represent the occurrence of recent thefts or aggressive outbursts on the wards as these were patients' main sources of concern regarding personal safety.

Overall, the results of the repeated measures analyses across the three assessment points showed that both the subjective and objective quality of life indices were stable over time, thereby allowing greater confidence to be placed in the validity of the study's findings. The results, therefore, provide a stable picture of patients' quality of life in hospital against which to compare the impact of community placement.

An additional factor to be considered in interpreting the stability of the subjective data is the observed influence of levels of dependency and psychopathology on the general life satisfaction measures. The pattern of relationships between the subjective quality of life indices and level of dependency and psychiatric functioning requires closer examination. To what extent are fluctuations in the reported levels of subjective well-being related to the level of depressive or psychotic symptoms and how do changes in the level of dependency affect general well-being? A detailed investigation of the interrelationship between these measures over time is required if the critical determinants of psychological well-being for chronic psychiatric clients is to be elucidated further. It is envisaged that the relationship between these different outcome variables in the present study will form an important part of the overall evaluation project.

THE IMPACT OF COMMUNITY PLACEMENT ON QUALITY OF LIFE

The original group of long-stay residents were followed up as they were discharged from hospital. The follow-up study attempted to determine the impact of resettlement on the quality of life of the discharged clients and to examine the sensitivity of the quality of life indices to changes in the care setting and living situation. As pointed out by Baker and Intagliata (1982), an important consideration in the use of quality of life as an outcome measure is the development of measures that are sensitive to the changes being evaluated. The post-discharge follow-up examined the sensitivity of the subjective and objective quality of life indices in discriminating life areas affected by changes in the care setting. The study sought to address the question of how the move to the community affects the quality of life of clients and this paper reports on the findings at six months after their discharge from hospital.

From the original group of 62 long-stay residents, 30 of the 34 discharged were followed up in the community. The remainder of the sample stayed in hospital awaiting community placements. No significant differences were found between the characteristics of 'leavers' and 'stayers' at baseline in terms of demographic and clinical characteristics, attitude to discharge, overall level of dependency or in the level of active psychiatric symptomatology.

The community placements included a health authority housing scheme, a group home run by a voluntary agency, private care homes and a small number of independent living settings. The care environments contrasted sharply with those of the hospital wards. In particular, the newly established residential schemes (i.e. the housing scheme and the group home) offered a better quality physical environment in more domestic style settings, affording more opportunity for privacy, independence, personalisation and greater access to community facilities. The care regimes were also found to be far less restrictive for residents, with a more client-orientated style of care management being implemented. The impact of these changes on clients' quality of life are reported in Barry and Crosby (1993).

At six months post-discharge clients made very favourable comments about their life in the new community settings. 93% described their lives as being either much better (80%) or somewhat better (13%) than in hospital, despite an initial unwillingness on the part of many of them to leave the hospital. Levels of expressed satisfaction in the different life areas were generally higher compared to hospital (Figure 12.2), ranging from 60–93%, with the highest levels of satisfaction being expressed in relation to living situation (93%) and social relations (90%). Clients expressed satisfaction with their personal safety in the community homes (90%), with their relationships with the care staff (90%) and the other residents in the scheme (87%), and with the treatment received (73%). The life areas that elicited the highest levels of dissatisfaction were lack of employment (25%), finance (20%) and family contact (27% dissatisfied). The levels of family contact had not changed appreciably following the move to the community. The majority of the clients would have liked more contact with their family. Likewise, clients still expressed a desire for more money, receiving on average £26.67 per week. The dissatisfaction with not having a job was voiced mainly by the younger clients, many of whom had been attending the industrial therapy unit in the hospital. Occupational or training services had not been replaced following the move from hospital

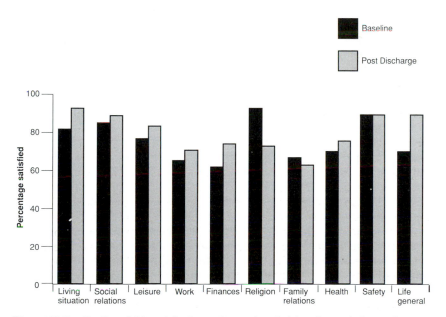

Figure 12.2 – Quality of life satisfaction ratings at hospital baseline and six months post-discharge in the community. (N = 30)

and this was obviously missed by the younger clients. With regard to life in general, clients expressed higher rates of satisfaction with their life overall in the community (87%) compared to that expressed when in hospital (71%).

A number of questions sought to determine in what ways clients perceived their quality of life to have changed. When questioned about which areas of their lives were most affected by the move to the community, the majority of the responses referred to the greater freedom and independence afforded by the community settings; "they were too strict in hospital, your life wasn't your own, there's real freedom here", "got the privacy, don't have to sleep in a dormitory, can cook my own food, can watch TV and radio, can go shopping, I get the money and more contact with staff". Many of the clients also described the change as being more global; "I'm much happier here....my life has changed and I feel as if its a new life".

In order to assess the statistical significance of the changes in quality of life, repeated measures analyses of variance were carried out on the objective and subjective composite indices for each life domain, comparing the hospital baseline findings for the 30 discharged clients with their quality of life at six months post-discharge. The results are presented in Table 12.2. The study revealed that the movement to the community resulted in improvements in objective standards of living for the resettled group, i.e. more comfortable living conditions, higher levels of interactive contact within the facility, and greater freedom and independence. These changes were reflected in clients' comments concerning their quality of life. The majority appeared to be adapting well to their life in the community, which is worthy of comment given the relatively lengthy periods this group had spent in hospital as against the relatively short time they had spent living in the community. As expected, the most significant change to emerge at this early stage was in relation to the immediate living situation, and satisfaction with living situation showing a statistically significant improvement. Clients also reported higher levels of interaction among residents and staff in the community residences and increased participation in leisure activities. Significant improvements in general well-being were also reported. However, significant changes were not found in all life areas, e.g. family contact and finance remained common sources of dissatisfaction. This finding is consistent with that reported by previous studies, and as pointed out by Petch (1990) and Okin et al. (1983), changes in longer-term patterns of behaviour will take longer than six months to be attained.

A follow-up of the quality of life of the patients remaining in hospital was also carried out. While the repeated measures design in the present study essentially meant that the discharged group acted as their own control, it was also of interest to determine how the patients who remained in hospital awaiting discharge progressed or deteriorated over the same time period. Statistical analysis revealed no significant improvements in reported life satisfaction for the hospital group. The only improvement to emerge in objective life quality was in relation to finance, with an increase

Table 12.2 – Life domain composite indices at baseline and six months post-discharge for hospital 'leavers' (N = 30) resettled in the community

Life domain	Hospital baseline		Community		MANOVA
	Mean	(SD)	Mean	(SD)	F-Ratio
Subjective indices					
Living situation	13.14	(2.58)	14.43	(0.92)	6.20*
Social relations	8.40	(1.44)	8.92	(0.28)	2.99
Family relations	4.84	(1.39)	4.95	(1.72)	0.06
Leisure	5.21	(1.13)	5.64	(0.91)	2.63
Finances	2.29	(0.98)	2.54	(0.84)	2.03
Religion	2.89	(0.43)	2.65	(0.80)	2.37
Health	13.48	(1.69)	13.56	(2.06)	0.07
Personal safety	5.46	(1.07)	5.57	(0.92)	0.17
Objective indices					
Living situation	7.80	(1.48)	8.90	(0.99)	3.77
Frequency of social contacts	17.67	(5.31)	21.29	(4.67)	18.62***
Within the facility	8.62	(3.62)	11.31	(3.03)	14.74***
Outside the facility	4.89	(2.69)	6.12	(2.63)	10.41**
Frequency of family contact	5.46	(2.62)	5.71	(2.48)	0.71
Leisure activities	19.52	(2.69)	20.48	(2.31)	4.68*
Physical illness in past year	3.75	(0.65)	3.86	(0.45)	1.00
Frequency of religious practice	2.41	(1.50)	1.91	(1.27)	2.01
Victim of robbery/attack	1.43	(0.50)	1.75	(0.65)	3.53
Global quality of life	2.36	(0.99)	2.82	(0.55)	6.53*

Notes: Due to the small number engaged in employment, the work scale was not included in the analysis.
*p = 0.05, **p = 0.01, ***p = 0.001

in reported weekly spending money. However, the objective indices of living situation showed a significant deterioration since the baseline findings (F = 30.10, p < 0.001). The assessment of the hospital living environment at baseline pointed to the poor quality of the physical environment which afforded little in the way of personal privacy or opportunity for expression of individual identity (Crosby et al., 1990). Patients still in hospital awaiting discharge reported a further deterioration in their living conditions. The institutional environment of the hospital appeared to offer less in the way of comfort, independence and freedom for its residents in comparison with the community settings and this may be particularly the case in the period prior to hospital closure.

Generally, the findings suggest that the quality of life measures can discriminate life areas which have been affected by a change in external circumstances. The findings from the repeated measures carried out at baseline, which showed a stable level of quality of life, allow greater confidence to be placed in the findings of the community study. What emerges quite clearly from clients' comments concerning the differences between hospital life and life in the community, is the greater independence and freedom afforded by the community setting. Although lack of freedom *per se* did not emerge in residents' accounts of life in the hospital, it would appear that once they were discharged from hospital, independence and being able to do things for themselves was an important consideration for this group of chronically ill clients. Burckhardt, Woods, Schultz and Ziebarth (1989), in a study of the quality of life of people with chronic physical illnesses, also found that the theme of independence emerged as a salient feature of life quality. Although implied in some of the life domain scales, the addition of items specifically tapping independence and freedom might increase the content validity of quality of life scales for chronic psychiatric clients.

Clients' comments about their experience of resettlement provide valuable insight into their perceptions of the specific changes in their lives and is a useful addition to the more quantitative information derived from the life domain indices. It will be interesting to observe whether the standards of comparison employed by the community residents in their judgements of life quality will change as a result of increasing levels of independence and greater exposure to the standards of living in the local community. Analysis of the one year follow-up data which is currently being published helps to cast some light on this question of the pattern of change over time (see Barry and Crosby, 1994).

The findings from this phase of the study suggest that movement to the community has led to an improvement in quality of life for the clients in this study. The improvements in living and social conditions, the increased levels of satisfaction with living situation and life in general, together with clients' comments concerning greater freedom and independence, point to the contrasts between hospital and community living. These results confirm reports from previous studies of positive changes in clients' quality of life following discharge from hospital to appropriately designed community facilities (Okin et al., 1983; Gibbons and Butler, 1987; Petch, 1990). The observed improvements in quality of life were also reflected in the other evaluation measures used in the study, such as the quality of care provided and improvements in clients' levels of behavioural and social functioning (a more detailed account of these outcomes may be found in Crosby et al., 1993). Although the findings from the present study are tentative, owing to the small sample and the relatively short period of time spent by clients in the community, the study does demonstrate that the quality of life of quite dependent, chronic psychiatric clients can be enhanced in the community through the provision of appropriate community residential schemes. It will be necessary to await later results to ascertain if initial outcome patterns are maintained over a longer period of time. Generalisation of these findings to other community care schemes is, of course, dependent on the quality of care provided.

Small scale, carefully designed studies, such as the present one, help to provide useful empirical information on the utility of quality of life indices in evaluating the impact of service changes on individual clients. The measures appear to be able to discriminate the areas of life most affected by the move from hospital and such information is of considerable value to service providers and planners concerned with the consequences of resettlement for client groups with specific needs. As pointed out by Jones et al. (1986), the provision of rapid feedback is particularly valuable in view of the major policy shift being implemented. More detailed studies are needed in order to determine which groups of clients benefit most from which type of care setting and to determine which variables are most critical for ensuring a high quality of life for clients requiring long-term care.

CONCLUSIONS

The gathering of data on how individuals perceive their lives is obviously a central part of assessing quality of life. It would appear, however, that self-assessments of quality of life do have certain limitations that need to be taken into account in interpreting the data. The appraisal process involved in making self-assessed judgements of quality of life requires further investigation. Research in this area needs to elucidate the types of social and cognitive judgements that are made and how these are influenced by external life circumstances, social comparison standards, subjective perceptual processes and internal referents such as values and attitudes, personal aspirations, and perceived control. The discrepancy between the objective and subjective indices that has been reported in the literature to date needs to be explored more fully in order to determine the possible psychological and social mediators of perceived quality of life and to delineate more clearly the sources of life satisfaction and dissatisfaction.

The findings to date also suggest the importance of relating the information derived from the quality of life interview to other outcome measures, such as levels of psychiatric and behavioural functioning, and characteristics of the residential setting. Variables such as staff attitudes and management practices may also exercise an important influence on the quality of life of service recipients, particularly those in residential care. Such an approach permits the development of a more comprehensive model of quality of life, which would enable one to look at the critical determinants of quality of life and how these interact in producing positive or negative effects on the client's life.

An overview of the existing studies suggests the need for developing and refining current methods of assessing quality of life. A case may be made for the use of more exploratory methods of data gathering, so that we can arrive at a better understanding of the relevant dimensions of quality of life for different populations. Used in conjunction with structured interview schedules, qualitative approaches may offer the possibility of exploring the more individualistic determinants of quality of life. The qualitative data in the present study were found to be a useful addition to the information derived from the quantitative scales, highlighting the importance of independence as a significant dimension of quality of life for chronic psychiatric clients. McGee et al. (1991) comment that current methods of measuring quality of life run the risk of imposing an external value system on individuals. Schedules based on a standard list of aspects of life deemed to be important to life quality may not include aspects of importance to the individual. McGee et al. (ibid.) describe the development of a new method of assessing quality of life (SEIQoL), which elicits an individualized judgement of quality of life based on the relative importance of particular life areas for each individual. The application of such novel approaches to assessing the quality of life of psychiatric clients may reveal interesting new perspectives in this area of work.

The information derived from the quality of life schedule, as well as providing useful outcome data, also provides a rich array of information on clients' perceptions of their lives and what areas they perceive as important. This information is of considerable value to service practitioners directly involved in the planning and implementation of services programmes for this group. The findings to date suggest a number of life areas on which intervention and rehabilitation strategies may focus. Attention is drawn to the problematic living conditions in large psychiatric hospitals which may have a deleterious effect on the quality of life of residents. The objective quality of life indices suggest that resettlement programmes should direct attention to the social needs of chronic clients, focusing on life areas such as maintaining and encouraging any existing family contact, since this emerged as an area of considerable importance and relevance to clients' life quality. The data on clients' social relations also highlight the need to assess carefully clients' abilities to relate socially and develop friendships during the preparation and planning of community placements. The prospect of social isolation following discharge, as a result of clients' restricted social contacts during years of hospitalisation, presents an area of concern. Expressed dissatisfaction regarding finance highlights the importance of assessing and monitoring clients' abilities in budgeting their limited funds. The need for structured recreational and educational/vocational activities for clients following discharge is also suggested from the quality of life data, particularly in relation to the younger clients. In addition, the findings from the subjective indices of life quality point to the necessity of addressing clients' attitudes and expectations. It would appear that the experience of lengthy periods of institutional care may have robbed individuals of their expectations, aspirations, and desire for achievement. Although the ability of clients to make choices and decisions concerning their own lives may be severely curtailed by past experiences and basic dependency needs, the importance of facilitating the development of these abilities cannot be ignored.

In summary, quality of life emerges as an important and meaningful construct in the provision and evaluation of mental health care. The increasing emphasis on quality of life issues in the mental health literature signals a shift to a more holistic model of care. Elucidating the meaning and measurement of a multidimensional construct such as quality of life may be an important step in the development of a more empirical model of positive mental health.

ACKNOWLEDGEMENTS

The work reported in this paper forms part of a longitudinal study commissioned by the Welsh Office, The Department of Health, Clwyd and Gwynedd Health Authorities, and Clwyd and Gwynedd Social Services Departments. The cooperation and assistance of the residents and staff of the North Wales Hospital and the community residential schemes in Clwyd is gratefully acknowledged. The views expressed in this paper represent those of the authors and do not necessarily reflect those of the sponsors.

REFERENCES

Andrews, R. F. and Withey, S. B. (1976), *Social Indicators of Well-being: Americans' Perceptions of Life Quality*. New York: Plenum Press.

Andrews, F. M. and McKennell, A. C. (1980), Measures of self-reported well-being: Their affective, cognitive and other components. *Social Indicators Research*, **8**, 127–155.

Anthony, W. A. (1980), *The Principles of Psychiatric Rehabilitation*. Baltimore: University Park Press.

Bachrach, L. L. (1980), Is the least restrictive environment always the best? Sociological and semantic implications. *Hospital and Community Psychiatry*, **31**, 97–103.

Baker, F. and Intagliata, J. (1982), Quality of life in the evaluation of community support systems. *Evaluation and Program Planning*, **5**, 69–79.

Barry, M. M., Crosby, C. and Mitchell, D. A. (1992), Quality of life issues in the evaluation of mental health services. In D. R. Trent (Ed.) *Promotion of Mental Health*, Vol. 1. (pp. 153–163). Aldershot: Avebury.

Barry, M. M., Crosby, C. and Bogg, J. (1993), Methodological issues in evaluating the quality of life of long-stay psychiatric patients. *Journal of Mental Health*, **2**, 43–56.

Barry, M. M. and Crosby, C. (1993), Community mental health care: Promoting a better quality of life for long-term clients. In D. R. Trent and C. Reed (Eds.) *Promotion of Mental Health*, Vol. 2. (pp. 113–130) Avebury.

Barry, M. M. and Crosby, C. (1994), Assessing the impact of community placement on quality of life. In Crosby, C. and Barry, M. M. (Eds.) *Evaluation of community resettlement from the North Wales Psychiatric Hospital*. Avebury Community Care Series.

Bigelow, D. A., Brodsky, G., Stewart, L. and Olson, M. (1982), The concept and measurement of quality of life as a dependent variable in evaluation of mental health services. In G. J. Tash and W. R. Tash (Eds.) *Innovative Approaches to Mental Health Evaluation* (pp. 345–366). New York: Academic Press.

Burckhardt, C. S., Woods, S. L., Schultz, A. A. and Ziebarth, D. M. (1989), Quality of life of adults with chronic illness: A psychometric study. *Research in Nursing and Health*, **12**, 347–354.

Bradburn, N. M. (1969), *The Structure of Psychological Well-being*. Chicago: Aldine.

Campbell, A., Converse, P. E., and Rodgers, W. L. (1976), *The Quality of American Life*. New York: Russell Sage Foundation.

Carstenson, L. L. and Cone, J. D. (1983), Social desirability and the measurement of psychological well-being in elderly persons. *Journal of Gerontology*, 38, 713–715.

Crosby, C., Barry, M. M., Mitchell, D. A., Grant, P., Horrocks, F. A. and Litterjohns, C. J. (1990), *Evaluation of the Clwyd mental health community service: An interim report*. Health Services Research Unit, Department of Psychology, University College of North Wales: Unpublished Report.

Crosby, C., Barry, M. M., Carter, M. F. and Lowe, C. F. (1993), Psychiatric rehabilitation and community care: Resettlement from the North Wales Hospital. *Health and Social Care*, 1, 335–363.

Crosby, C. and Barry, M. M. (Eds.) (1994), *Evaluation of Community Resettlement from the North Wales Psychiatric Hospital*. Avebury Community Care Series.

George, L. K. and Bearon, L. B. (1980), *Quality of Life in Older Persons: Meaning and Measurement*. London: Human Sciences Press.

Gibbons, J. S. and Butler, J. P. (1987), Quality of life for 'new' long-stay psychiatric in-patients: The effects of moving to a hostel. *British Journal of Psychiatry*, 157, 347–354.

Glatzer, W. (1991), Quality of life in advanced industrialised countries: the case of West Germany. In F. Strack, M. Argyle and N. Schwarz (Eds.) *Subjective Well-Being* (pp. 261–279). Oxford: Pergamon.

Goffman, E. (1961), *Asylums: Essays on the Social Situation of Mental Patients and Other Inmates*. Chicago: Aldine.

Herzberg, F., Mausner, B., Pederson, R. and Capwell, D. (1957), *Job Attitudes: Review of Research and Opinion*. Pittsburgh: Pittsburgh Psychological Services.

Jodelet, D. (1991), *Madness and Social Representations*. London: Harvester.

Jones, K., Robinson, M. and Golightley, M. (1986), Long-term psychiatric patients in the community. *British Journal of Psychiatry*, 149, 537–540.

Hall, J. N. and Baker, R. (1983), *REHAB*. Aberdeen: Vine Publishing Company.

Lehman, A. F. (1983a), The well-being of chronic mental patients: Assessing their quality of life. *Archives of General Psychiatry*, 40, 369–373.

Lehman, A. F. (1983b), The effects of psychiatric symptoms on quality of life assessments among the chronically mentally ill. *Evaluation and Program Planning*, 6, 143–151.

Lehman, A. F. (1988), A quality of life interview for the chronically mentally ill. *Evaluation and Program Planning*, 11, 51–62.

Lehman, A. F., Ward, N. C. and Linn, L. S. (1982), Chronic mental patients: The quality of life issue. *American Journal of Psychiatry*, 139, 1271–1276.

Lehman, A. F., Possidente, S. and Hawker, F. (1986), The quality of life of chronic patients in a state hospital and in community residences. *Hospital and Community Psychiatry*, 37, 901–907.

Lowe, C. F., Grant, G., Morrell, J. B., Alladin, W. G. and Ellis, N. A. (1988), *Evaluation of the mental health community service in Clwyd: A research proposal*. Department of Psychology, University College of North Wales.

McGee, H. M., O'Boyle, C. A., Hickey, A., O'Malley, K. and Joyce, C.R.B. (1991), Assessing the quality of life of the individual: The SEIQoL with a healthy and a gastroenterology unit population. *Psychological Medicine*, 21, 749–759.

Okin, R. L., Dolnick, J. A. and Pearsall, D. T. (1983), Patients' perspectives on community alternatives to hospitalisation: A follow-up study. *American Journal of Psychiatry*, 140, 1460–1464.

Overall, J. and Gorham, D. (1962), The Brief Psychiatric Rating Scale. *Psychological Reports*, 10, 799–812.

Petch, A. (1990), '*Heaven Compared to a Hospital Ward*': *An evaluation of eleven supported accommodation projects for those with mental health problems*. Social Work Research Centre, Stirling University.

Schwarz, N. and Strack, F. (1990), Evaluating one's life: A judgement model of subjective well-being. In F. Strack, M. Argyle and N. Schwarz (Eds.) *Subjective Well-Being* (pp. 27–47). Oxford: Pergammon.

Shadish, W. R., Orwin, R. G., Silber, B. G. and Bootzin, R. R. (1985), The subjective well-being of mental patients in nursing homes. *Evaluation and Program Planning*, **8**, 239–250.

Simpson, C. J., Hyde, C. E. and Farragher, E. B. (1989), The chronically mentally ill in community facilities: A study of quality of life. *British Journal of Psychiatry*, **154**, 77–82.

Strack, F., Schwarz, N., Chassein, B., Kern, D. and Wagner, D. (1990), Salience of comparison standards and the activation of social norms: Consequences for judgements of happiness and their communication. *British Journal of Social Psychology*, **29**, 303–314.

Ware, J. (1978), Effects of acquiescent response set on patient satisfaction ratings. *Medical Care*, **16**, 327–336.

Wing, J. K. and Brown, G. W. (1970), *Institutionalisation and Schizophrenia: A comparative study of three mental hospitals 1960–1980*. London: Cambridge University Press.

Wilde, E. D. and Svanberg, P. O. (1990), Never mind the width - measure the quality. *Clinical Psychology Forum*, 2–5.

Zautra, A. and Goodhart, D. (1979), Quality of Life Indicators: A review of the literature. *Community Mental Health Review*, **4**, 1–10.

CHAPTER THIRTEEN

Coping and Human Agency

Ladislav VALACH

Psychiatrische Universitätspoliklinik Bern, Murtenstrasse 21, 3010 Bern, Switzerland

INTRODUCTION

Health and illness are central issues in many societies and cultures. The majority of their citizens consider health to be of the highest value. A large proportion of each country's gross national product is spent on its health services. Consequently, ways of dealing with health and illness are socially well represented. However, the frame of reference for dealing with health and illness has changed substantially during the last 30 years: from a conception of professionalized repair by a specialist to whom patients delegated all responsibility and control, to the stance of an active and self-responsible person who cares for health and copes with problems and illnesses.

Previous research has shown that one of the most frequently used conceptions in making sense of everyday life is a naive theory of goal directed action (von Cranach and Valach, 1983; Valach et al., 1988b). This naive theory is anchored in related social representations (Farr and Moscovici, 1984) of action. These in turn have an effect on the execution of actions (Thommen et al., 1988, 1992). Actions or intentional processes also play a role when directed towards health problems and in particular in theories of coping. Coping as a psychological and psychosocial process has been studied for a quarter of a century in various institutional settings and is now also studied in medical practice as a part of the social representation of this professional group (Heim and Willy, 1986).

Lazarus and Folkman (1984) consider coping as 'a constantly changing cognitive and behavioral effort to manage specific external and/or internal demands that are appraised as taxing or exceeding the resources of the person.' (p. 141). This definition, process- rather than trait-oriented, implies a distinction between coping and automatized adaptive behaviour and it does not identify coping with a successful outcome.

Lazarus also discusses the social dimension of coping in the relation of individual and society. Firstly, he views society as a way of serving people's basic survival-related adaptational needs. Secondly, he views it as shaping persons and groups; social rules and institutions regulate relationships and shape emotions and behaviour. Thirdly, Lazarus describes the influence of people and groups on the social system, in order to highlight the idea of bidirectionality. He argues that stress is created by mismatches between individual and social identities. A social system not only poses demands upon the individual but also provides resources for the individual. If demands upon the individual create conflicts, are ambiguous, or lead to overload, they can result in stress. In addition, social change can lead to stress by making new demands on people. However, the social system also facilitates social relationships which are necessary for the individual. Leventhal et al. (1984) offer an account of coping as a system of self-regulation processing using the concept of an individual as a self-regulating system which is actively trying to reach specific goals. The elements of this model are regulation, phases of processing, and a distinction between objective and emotional processing. The regulation system is conceived as a feedback system. It contains a number of serially ordered parts. In the input phase the stimulus field is interpreted and goals are set. In the response or coping phase the coping answers are planned, selected and executed. The monitoring phase comprises attending to the consequences of action in regard to the set goals. An important part of the model is the distinction between the processing of the environmental characteristics and the processing of the emotional reaction, the informational and emotional systems being processed simultaneously. These two systems create a conscious experience of illness.

Although the conceptualization of coping originally developed from a cognitively oriented model of emotion (Lazarus, 1966), it is often treated in empirical studies as if it were a process of rational and economical decision making which is mostly individual (Krohne, 1978). Although Lazarus's conception of coping implies that social-environmental processes are necessary characteristics of coping, in most work on coping this important issue is largely forgotten. This omission of the study of social processes is not simply due to neglect. It is a direct consequence of interpreting coping as an individual level phenomenon. This misconception stems from a false dichotomy between the individual and society and from treating them as separate entities when it comes to the study of human processes. We shall argue in this chapter that coping is a social phenomenon and that it should be considered in terms of the action of self-active systems.

THE SOCIAL NATURE OF COPING

Psychological thinking on health and illness has long been dominated by models in which human consciousness and awareness play only a secondary role. An example of this model is the influential work of Alexander (1952), who made a breakthrough in psychosomatic reasoning. Much of the later research on coping is based on information processing models in which individuals follow a rationalistic logic and are steered by personality predispositions (Fleischman, 1984). In opposition to this view, it is suggested in this chapter that coping (a) is social in origin, (b) is a social process and (c) has social consequences.

Coping is Social in Origin

The theory of social developmental processes also applies to coping, originating in the social representations of particular social strata. Ways of dealing with health problems are acquired and developed in the course of social interaction. The appropriate conceptions of human social (inter)action have been outlined by Baldwin, Mead and Vygotsky (Baldwin, 1910; Mead, 1913; Vygotsky 1978; Wertsch, 1985; see also Marková, 1990). Research in developmental health psychology illustrates how coping is learned and constructed together with the development of schemata concerning illnesses. Eiser (1990), for example, who has studied children's conceptions of illness, argues that these conceptions already contain differentiated scripts. It has also been shown that even very small children develop strategies for coping with stress in interactions with others (Gianino and Tronick, 1988).

Moreover, differences in coping found in various social groups and subcultures indicate the extent of the social embeddedness of coping modalities. This can be illustrated by examples of classical social categories such as social strata and gender (Pearlin and Schooler, 1978). In searching for empirical work on the social origins of coping in work on the social representation of social groups, it became obvious that such research is less common than might be expected. Beutel (1988) remarks that the influence of sociodemographic variables, such as gender, age, social strata and education, on coping has not been satisfactorily clarified.

Social strata and coping

There are some studies indicating that people from lower social strata lack the resources needed for coping (Marmot and Theorell, 1988) and, therefore, cope less well than people from higher social strata (Carmel et al., 1990; Breznitz-Svidovsky, 1982; McLeod and Kessler, 1990). It was found by Westbrook (1979) that patients from lower social strata use more avoidance and more fatalistic modes of coping. Rim (1990) reports that in coping in difficult situations, blue-collar workers were higher on "minimizing", "suppression" and "blame". White-collar workers were higher on "replacement", "substitution", "mapping" and "reversal".

In a follow-up study of patients operated on for disc herniation 9–19 years earlier (Valach et al., 1988a; Dvorak et al., 1988), white-collar patients differed from blue-collar patients in several coping modalities, indicating the influence of social strata on coping. The white-collar patients, who were without pain at the time of the study, reported having coped with their pain by OPTIMISM, DIVERTING their THOUGHTS and RELEASING their ANGER; while the blue-collar patients mentioned coping by ACCEPTING and by looking for and receiving ATTENTION AND CARE. The white-collar patients, who at the time of the study were experiencing pain, used the following strategies of coping more than blue-collar patients: RELIGIOUSNESS, RELEASE OF ANGER, THOUGHT AS DIVERSION, ATTENTION AND CARE; but less often used: ACTIVITY AS DIVERSION, ACCEPTANCE and SOCIAL WITHDRAWAL. The various modes of coping are listed in Appendix I of this chapter.

One can assume that there are preferred modalities of coping which are anchored in different social strata, thus showing the social origin of some of the coping modalities (Westbrook, 1979; d'Houtaud and Field, 1984). Strata-related social representations of coping also play a role in: (1) the use of coping modalities in ongoing action, (2) long term processes such as illness careers, (3) the narrative of coping and (4) the joint reconstruction of coping processes.

The influence of social strata on coping can be conceptualized in several ways. Although we would not like to exclude from consideration any models of strata influence (whether of strata as a structural feature or as a discursive community), the one we would like to emphasize most is related to a stratum-specific system of knowledge and attitude conceptualized as a social representation (Farr and Moscovici, 1984).

Gender identities and coping

There are several findings on coping as being gender specific (Billings and Moos, 1981; Kleinke et al., 1982) but there are others which find no relationships between gender and coping (Keefe et al., 1991; Hamilton and Fagot, 1988). Littlewood et al. (1991) analyzed how parents cope with the death of their child. They found that women used comforting cognitions less than men. Vingerhoets and Van Heck (1990) report that males preferred problem-focused coping strategies, planned and rational actions, positive thinking, personal growth and humor, day dreaming and fantasies. Females preferred emotion-focused coping solutions, self-blame in the expression of their emotions and wishful thinking. They also sought social support. Schwab (1990) found that dealing with the same source of distress, mothers, compared to fathers, cried more, read more, wrote more on loss and grief, helped others more and stayed alone more. In coping with work stress Parkers (1990) reported that men used more suppression strategies than women. Bird and Harris (1990) showed that early adolescent females used social support more often and ventilation less often than males. Female undergraduates are reported to use more emotion-oriented and avoidance-oriented coping behaviours than males (Endler and Parker, 1990) and the unemployed females relied more on symptom-focused activities such as seeking social support, while unemployed men relied more on problem-focused activities such as job searching.

There is further empirical work on gender specific coping but only a few reports are concerned specifically with health problems. Our study on low back pain patients shows (Dvorak, Valach and Heim, 1988) several differences in coping between men and women. Operated men, presently without pain, used ACTIVITY AS DIVERSION, ACCEPTANCE and OPTIMISM. Operated women without pain used more THOUGHT AS DIVERSION, ALTRUISM, EMOTIONAL RELEASE, MAINTAINING COMPOSURE and COMPENSATION. ATTENTION AND CARE, which is the most social form of coping, was the only coping mode which was used very often by men and women alike. Retired men used more ACTIVITY AS DIVERSION, whilst retired women used more THOUGHT AS DIVERSION, RUMINATION, ALTRUISM, EMOTIONAL RELEASE, TACKLING, PRESERVING COMPOSURE and PASSIVE COOPERATION. ATTENTION AND CARE, together with ACCEPTANCE, were used by both groups equally often.

There seems to be enough evidence pointing to some gender differences in coping with various problems. However, the circumstances in which these differences occur can vary. Comparable events can pose different problems for women than they do for men. In addition, these problems can have a different significance for the two genders who can interpret them differently. Men and women have different ways of mobilizing resources and may, therefore, use different coping strategies. Further, there are a number of phases in every coping model during which these differences can be constructed. Finally, men and women can belong to different coping groups or define themselves and be defined by others as fulfilling different functions. For instance, as the family task of men is often seen by themselves and by others to be that of "providing" and of women that of "supporting", their coping is also oriented towards these functions and towards both conserving and improving the resources at their disposal to fulfil these functions. Therefore, in the case of unemployment, the men will seek new employment while the women will seek emotional balance by receiving support from others, as reported by Endler and Parker (1990). Nevertheless, these differences are part of a gender-specific social representation, further indicating the social origin of some coping processes.

Conventions, culture and coping

The basic assumption of a socially grounded theory of action can be formulated as a convention theorem: members of a social community share social representations related to certain issues, in this particular case to social steering and the control of action (von Cranach and Valach, 1983). Coping modalities can be either conventions or individual processes. We propose that the distribution of coping modalities might indicate a polarization between these two kinds of process.

In the reported follow-up study on the outcome of operations for lumbar disc herniation (Dvorak et al., 1988; Valach et al., 1988a), we found that some sub-groups of the operated patients considered certain coping modalities as their way of coping prior to the operation. For example, the preferred modes of coping prior to the operation by complaint-free patients were mostly ACTIVITY AS DIVERSION, THOUGHTS AS DIVERSION, ACCEPTANCE and ATTENTION AND CARE. These modalities could be said to be based on conventions. In a longitudinal study on coping by women operated on for breast cancer, the following coping modalities were found: ATTENTION AND CARE, ACCEPTANCE, PROBLEM ANALYSIS, PASSIVE COOPERATION, SELF VALIDATION, PRESERVING COMPOSURE, OPTIMISM, TACKLING, THOUGHTS AS DIVERSION, RELATIVIZING, EMOTIONAL RELEASE (Heim et al., 1987, 1988). These modalities, again, were based on conventions.

Seiffge-Krenke and Shulman (1990) have compared the coping of adolescents in Germany and in Israel. They report differences in coping between the two samples. Germans show more approach-avoidance coping and react to situational demands, while Israelis show less variability in coping behaviour across situations and lay greater stress on cognitive factors. Comparing the coping of women operated on for breast cancer in Berne and in Prague we found that the Czech women displayed much longer PASSIVE COOPERATION and DIVERSION (in thoughts or action) in the course of their illness and less PROBLEM ANALYSIS than Swiss women, both after surgery and months and years later (Valach et al., 1992b; 1992c).

Changes in the history of coping with health problems indicate the social character of coping. Shared knowledge and social representation of healing play an important role in the process of coping. The dichotomy between the expenditure and the conservation of energy on the one hand and growing resources and training on the other, influenced the handling of myocardial infarction and is now being used in thinking about and dealing with low back pain (Waddell, 1987). Resting, as a healing remedy, is being restricted, and exercise and training, which previously were believed to be damaging to the patient, are now being emphasized. However, the relationship between available knowledge of both the healing and coping is often trivialized by health planners and others who, in their ambition to prevent illness, overlook the social origin of both knowledge and action. Information which is not integrated into the social action of the agents (the action of the person as well as the action of the groups in which the person is participating) may influence their views but will seldom influence action itself. Changing the character of coping in relation to changing knowledge, it is important to respect its social and cultural nature. The socially embedded and rooted nature of coping is not a byproduct of individual knowledge.

The majority of coping models are wholly individualistic conceptions involving such processes as perception, attention, selection of information, memory, execution and evaluation. The evidence considered in this chapter will enable us to place the concept of coping within the context of human reasoning. Moreover, it will have therapeutic implications for clinicians in their effort to clarify for their clients the social nature of the embeddeddness of coping.

Coping as a Social Process

That coping is a social process is evident from four examples which also illustrate different conceptualization of the coping process:

(a) In several studies we found the coping modality of seeking and receiving ATTENTION AND CARE to be one of the most important. It was used frequently by operated on Low Back Pain-patients (LBP). It was the second most common coping mode reported by these patients whether they had or had not pain at the time of the interview (Valach et al., 1988a). It was also the most frequently cited mode of coping immediately after the operation in women who had been operated on for breast cancer (Heim et al., 1987). Illness problem-related coping is connected with socially oriented coping and cannot be seen as the rational problem-solving of an individual alone. This point has been recognized in numerous studies analyzing social support and its role in health and illness (Bloom, 1982; Funch and Mettlin, 1982; Ell et al., 1989). However, social support is often defined as a structural property and not as the action of individuals and groups dealing with problems (Cohen and Syme, 1985).

(b) Coping is related to the social situation of patients. LBP-patients, patients operated on for breast cancer, patients with multiple sclerosis or patients after myocardial infarction must not only cope with pain, discomfort, disability and the fear of death and dying but also with problems accompanying these complaints in different spheres of their life such as work, family, career, education of children, friendship, etc. It is recognized in the literature on coping that illness is not equally stressful for everyone (Fallowfield et al., 1987). In studying the specific goals of coping it has been found that social problems are often more salient than physical problems and pain (Meyerowitz, Heinrich and Schag, 1983).

(c) Coping is often the joint achievement of a group such as a family or a couple. The relevance of ATTENTION AND CARE and the descriptions above show that coping is first of all an interactive phenomenon. When talking to couples where the wives suffered from multiple sclerosis, the "we" forms of coping were often used (Kilchenmann, 1989; see also Scott and Badura, 1988). We observed how the families of patients restructured their lives in coping with the new tasks posed by the partner's illness (Valach et al., 1992a).

(d) Coping is a supra-individual process. Communities and whole societies deal collectively with the problems of health and illness. Some of these collective solutions are already institutionalized. Others are in the process of forming. The manner in which people face new threats such as AIDS best exemplifies the development of a process of societal coping (Marková and Wilkie, 1987). This societal level has often been neglected in social psychology (Harré, 1984).

Social Consequences of Coping

Coping is orientated towards future states and processes. With the increasing attention now given to psychosocial factors as relevant criteria of the successful outcome of medical treatment, the quality of life has become a relevant issue (Spilker, 1990). In this new situation the function of coping must now be evaluated in regard to physical and psychological well-being and to the social life of patients (Wortman and Dunkel-Schetter, 1979). It has been reported that the coping strategy of 'seeking information' is related to good social adaptation in women after mastectomy (Zemore and Shepel, 1987). 'Open communication' was found to be related to a good social adaptation in breast cancer patients (Orr, 1986). However, when emotions rather than facts were in the centre of a patient's attention, other kinds of coping were more adaptive, such as "avoid speaking about threat" or "refuse accepting further implications".

In our studies we found a relation between various forms of coping and several areas of social life or degrees of social adaptation. Those patients with pain after low back surgery who maintained that they were OPTIMISTIC, ACCEPTED their complaints, tried to MAINTAIN their COMPOSURE, were able to RELEASE their ANGER and engaged in ATTENTION AND CARE, were judged as better adapted socially than patients who RUMINATED or tended to cope with their problems by SOCIAL WITHDRAWAL. It could be suggested the forms of coping which involve social engagement are connected with better social standing at work, in one's relationship to a partner, in the family and with friends. Disenganging forms of coping which involved social isolation led to lower satisfaction with these life areas (Valach et al., 1990). We observed in a longitudinal study of women with operated breast cancer (Heim et al., 1987; Valach et al., 1992c) that those women who, immediately after surgery, used ACTIVITY AS DIVERSION, ALTRUISM, MAINTAINING COMPOSURE, PROBLEM ANALYSIS, GIVING MEANING, SELF VALIDATION, TACKLING, ATTENTION AND CARE or RELATIVIZING, showed, one year after the operation, a better social adaptation in work, in their marital relationships, and in their relations to children and friends than women who used THOUGHTS AS DIVERSION, REBELLING, EMOTIONAL RELEASE, COMPENSATION or RELEASE OF ANGER.

According to both of these studies, patients who attempt to PRESERVE their COMPOSURE and to seek and to receive ATTENTION AND CARE from others, show better immediate as well as longer term social adaptation in both illness groups. These results can be seen only as correlates of coping. It is possible that these women already differed in their social adaptation prior to their operations. More research is needed to prove conclusively that the origins of good social adaptation are to be found in particular kinds of coping. Nevertheless, the results of our research – a correlational study and a prospective study – can be interpreted as arising from a functional relation between coping and social adaptation. However, the social consequences of coping are not restricted to a change in the patient's social situation. People's attempts to deal with health problems create new social situations and initiate new social processes. Some societal structures and institutions depend on a particular way of coping with health and with illness problems.

COPING AS AN ACTIVITY OF SELF ACTIVE SYSTEMS

In suggesting that coping is of a social nature, in describing it as a social process, and finally, in drawing attention to its social consequences, it can be argued that coping is the action of self-active systems (von Cranach et al., 1982; von Cranach et al., 1986; Kalbermatten and Valach, 1985; Valach et al., 1988b; Valach, 1990a). Conceiving of coping as a special case of intentional social action allows us to integrate existing knowledge on systemic external and internal processes and to distinguish between various agents and different time-related systemic orders.

Action theory refers to an actor's consciously goal-directed, planned and intended behaviour which is cognitively and socially steered and controlled (von Cranach and Valach, 1983). It is both motivated and accompanied by emotions. It is also multidimensionally organized in its sequence, hierarchy and parallelity. The notion of sequence refers to the temporal order of an action, the notion of hierarchy to the order of relative subordination and superordination in levels of action, and the notion of parallelity refers to the simultaneous organization of different programmes of action at the various levels of action. Goal directed action occurs in specific settings, for example in the execution of a task or in task structure, socially representing knowledge of "how things are done" and "how an encounter is organized". Actions are consciously represented. Conscious cognition is the highest level of self-monitoring in human knowledge-processing, followed by emotion and by pain. Cognitions are represented through language. These features can also account for group activity. The processing of information by groups and the execution of group activity proceed on two levels (von Cranach et al., 1986). At the individual level they follow the rules of individual action. At the group level, information is processed through action-related communication and group action is executed through the cooperation of group members. The conceptualization of action applies not only to group actions but also to such longer term processes as a career (Valach, 1990a).

The specific methods of action analysis in our studies were designed in accordance with the theory of goal directed action. These include a systematic observation for an analysis of manifest behaviour, naive observation and attribution for collecting data on social meaning, the self-confrontation interview for providing data on linguistic encoding of cognitions (Kalbermatten and Valach, 1985). The consequences of using an action theoretical approach to analyse coping processes are numerous, amongst which the most important are the following:

(a)   The individual cognitive-emotional problem-solving model which lies behind the conceptualization of coping must be revised in order to incorporate both group phenomena and complex non-linear processes.
(b)   The basically social character of coping becomes evident. This is an issue which we are attempting to deal with in the present chapter.
(c)   In anchoring the semantics of coping to particular psychological and social psychological concepts which themselves are connected with particular research methods requires a methodological revision or reinterpretation of existing data on coping.

THE SOCIAL NATURE OF MONITORING ACTIONS AND OF RECONSTRUCTING ACCOUNTS

In discussing the social nature of coping several methodological issues must be raised.

Data on Coping are of Social Origin

Data on coping stem mostly from a social encounter between an interviewer and an interviewee. The coping processes are jointly reconstructed by a patient and his or her doctor engaged in biographical narration within a particular institutional setting. Mutually exchanged knowledge and the goals of both participants are all more involved in the structure and the course of the joint activity than recall and memory. This issue will now be examined with regard to gender.

Gender specific reconstructions of illness careers

We have shown in a study with 250 patients (Noack and Valach, 1985; Valach and Noack 1985) that women and men, in the waiting room of a doctor's practice, reconstructed their illness careers in quite different ways, although both groups were considered by the doctor as acutely or chronically ill in about the same proportions.

While men attributed their illnesses to situational causes, women talked more about dispositions. Speaking about their reasons for visiting the doctor, more women used "because of" language and more men used "in order to" language to describe their motives (Schütz, 1932). More women reported several strategies of coping, while more men mentioned only one strategy for dealing with their complaints. These are some of the differences which we interpret as representing two different systems of conceiving and executing interactions with a doctor on the reconstruction of an illness career. Men tried to take the steering and control of this action into their own hands (using goal-directed, teleological reasoning); described their illness as having come upon them (situational attribution of cause); offered a closed argumentative system (linear reasoning) with a single chain of actions and events (influence of illness on their life, coping strategy); stated the relevance of the problem; and did not hesitate to make an evaluative inference. They also saw their illness as existing over only a relatively short time span. They reported not using any self treatment after an appointment with the doctor. They clearly described their illness and divided responsibilities between themselves and their doctor. Their conception of patient–doctor interaction was a serial order of individual actions: patient–doctor–patient.

Women, on the other hand, attempted to act jointly with their doctor. They brought the illness into the interaction as "part of themselves" ("because of" motive, dispositional attribution, recurrence of symptoms); offered an open description of their problem (fewer inferences, a functional description instead of stating the relevance); gave more general than evaluative thoughts presenting a number of events instead of a logical chain (several changes in their everyday life after the illness, several coping strategies); and continued their own treatment even after an appointment with a doctor. They seemed to report as if acting toward a shared goal with their doctor. They presented raw information, leaving the integration, the inferences and the evaluation to the doctor.

Any monitoring of coping processes involves categorizing, which relies on social meaning. However, it is the joint and interactive attempts at reconstructing a career or identifying strategies, as in an interview on coping, that imply that the processes of coping are social reconstructions. If data on coping are gathered in a socially relevant and naturalistic way, as in an interview, they are invariably a joint production of the interviewer and the interviewee (Chapter 7). A doctor's interview may not be realistic in terms of past attempts at coping but it is realistic in relating not only to the desired and relevant contents which the patient wishes to communicate but also to the institutionalized setting in which it occurs. Coping narratives are a natural part of the story of an illness career. In the course of an interview the doctor identifies the coping modalities which the patient attributed to him- or herself. One can conclude on the basis of the different reconstructions of illness careers by men and women that monitored coping in an interaction can be seen as a function of this interaction.

Data on Coping are Mostly Data on Social Representations or Conventions

There is a methodological implication of the assumption that coping is social in origin. Data on coping collected in a reconstructive autobiographical interview are not only related to the coping of the individual but represent shared beliefs about coping between the individual and a provider of health care.

It was already pointed out that in our longitudinal study with women operated on for breast cancer, a number of coping modalities were based on conventions. Only a few of them, in the course of the study, proved to be idiosyncratic coping modalities and these were used by only a few women. Also the interviews on coping with patients operated on for low back pain revealed social conventions and social representations concerning good methods of coping, particularly in those patients who were without pain at the time of the interview.

The Social Consequences of the Joint Reconstruction of Coping

The final argument is concerned with the social character of the consequences of holding a coping interview in an ecologically valid institutional setting. Joint attributions about coping by both patient and doctor are of primary relevance quite independently of the quality of the recall. As this task forms part of the institutionalized encounter between doctor and patient, one can hypothesize that it will influence the patient's whole career as a patient, the doctor–patient relationship, and how the doctor will conduct the further course of the patient's treatment. Studies on factors influencing the decision to advise a course of psychotherapy allow us to test this hypothesis (Blaser, 1978). Since the patient's account of coping is a joint product of his or her interview with the doctor, it necessarily has consequences both within and beyond this career, e.g. in the clinician's decisions concerning the course of psychotherapy.

Reconstructing coping as an interaction between a patient and a doctor influences the pool of knowledge in medicine. This truly social process will have further consequences, thus gradually changing medical practice. Perhaps this is the process we are witnessing now. As patients are considered more and more worthy as human beings their stories are regarded as more credible and therefore add to the stock of common knowledge.

CONCLUSION

We have argued that coping processes, although often interpreted in a clinical setting as individual in character, are of a social nature and can best be studied as the actions of self active systems. Since the research procedures on coping can also be seen as social actions, we have concluded that the data of most studies are first and foremost of a social nature. However, coping is an intentional process. It implies the notion of responsibility. As individual processes cannot be understood without some insight into their social nature, so group processes cannot be studied apart from their realization in particular situated actions of particular individuals.

The consequences of the issues discussed in this chapter can be summarized as follows.

(a)   Coping should be seen as a form of social action due to its properties and its social nature as well as its embeddedness in social representations.

(b)   Methods of analysing coping as action and the interpretation of the data collected need to be revised and redesigned in order to capture ongoing actions in the everyday life of patients, including their interactions with health care professionals.

(c)   In any analysis of coping (in the everyday life of patients as well as in their interactions with a doctor) both individual and joint levels of action should be considered.

(d)   It is important that a coping interview be carrried out in ecologically valid environments (Valach, 1990b).

REFERENCES

Alexander, F.(1952), *Psychosomatic Medicine: Its Principles and Applications.* London: Allen and Unwin.

Baldwin, J.M. (1910), *Thought and Things*, Vol. II. London: Swan Sonnenschien.

Beutel, M. (1988), *Bewaeltigungsprozesse bei chronischen Erkrankungen.* Edition Medizin, VCH, Weinheim.

Billings, A. G. and Moos, R. H. (1981), The role of individual coping responses and social resources in attenuating the stress of life events. *Journal of Behavioral Medicine*, **4**, 139–157.

Bird, G. W. and Harris, R. L. (1990), A comparison of role strain and coping strategies by gender and family structure among early adolescents. *Journal of Early Adolescence*, **10**, 141–158.

Blaser, A. (1978), *Indikationsprozesse in der Psychotherapie.* Bern: Huber.

Bloom, J. R. (1982), Social support, accommodation to stress and adjustment to breast cancer. *Social Science and Medicine*, **16**, 1329–38.

Breznitz-Svidovsky, T. (1982), Israeli women on the home front: Coping mechanisms during wartime. Series in Clinical and Community Psychology. *Stress and Anxiety*, **8**, 117–122.

Carmel, S., Barnoon, S. and Zalcman, T. (1990), Social class differences in coping with a physicians' strike in Israel. *Journal of Community Health*, **15**, 45–57.

Cohen, S. and Syme, S. L. (1985), Issues in the study and application of social support. In: S. Cohen, S. L. Syme (eds.) *Social Support and Health.* New York: Academic Press, 3–22.

Cranach, M. von, Kalbermatten, U., Indermuehle, K. and Gubler, B. (1982), *Goal-directed Action.* London: Academic Press.

Cranach, M. von, Ochsenbein, G. and Valach, L. (1986), The group as a self active system: outline of a theory of a group action. *European Journal of Social Psychology*, **16**, 193–229.

Cranach, M. von and Valach, L. (1983), Social dimension of goal-directed action. In: H. Tajfel (ed.) *The Social Dimension of Social Psychology.* Cambridge: Cambridge University Press. 285–299.

Dvorak, J., Valach, L. and Heim, E. (1988), The outcome of operations for lumbar disc herniation. *Spine*, **13**, 1418–1427.

Eiser, C. (1990), Children's knowledge of chronic disease and implications for education. In: L. R. Schmidt, P. Schwenkmetzger, J. Weinman, S. Maes (eds.) *Theoretical and Applied Aspects of Health Psychology.* Switzerland: Harwood Academic Publishers, 215–227.

Ell, K. O., Mantell, J. E. and Hamaritch, M. B. (1989), Social support, sense of control and coping among patients with breast, lung or colorectal cancer. *Journal of Psychosocial Oncology*, **7**, 63–89.

Endler, N. S. and Parker, J. D. (1990), State and trait anxiety, depression and coping style. *Australian Journal of Psychology*, **42**, 207–220.

Fallowfield, L. J., Baum, M. and Maguire, G. P. (1987), Addressing the psychological needs of the conservatively treated breast cancer patient: discussion paper. *Journal of Royal Society of Medicine*, **80**, 696–700.

Farr, R. M. and Moscovici, S. (eds.) (1984), *Social Representations*. Cambridge: Cambridge University Press. Édition de la Maison des Sciences de l'Homme, Paris.

Fleishman, J. A. (1984), Personality characteristics and coping pattern. *Journal of Health and Social Behavior*, **25**, 229–244.

Funch, D. P. and Mettlin, C. (1982), The role of support in relation to recovery from breast surgery. *Social Science and Medicine*, **16**, 91–98.

Gianino, A. and Tronick, E. (1988), The mutual regulation model: The infant's self and interactive regulation and coping and defensive capacities. In: T. M. Field, P. M. McCabe, N. Schneiderman (eds.) (1988), *Stress and Coping Across Development*. Hillsdale N. J: Lawrence Erlbaum. 47–68.

Hamilton, S. and Fagot, B. I. (1988), Chronic stress and coping styles: A comparison of male and female undergraduates. *Journal of Personality and Social Psychology*, **55**, 819–23.

Harré, R. (1984), Some reflections on the concept of "social representation". *Social Research*, **51**, 929–938.

d'Houtaud, A. and Field, M. C. (1984), The image of health: Variations in perception by social class in a French population. *Sociology of Health and Illness*, **6**, 30–60.

Heim, E. and Willy, J. (1986), *Psychosoziale Medizin*. Berlin: Springer-Verlag.

Heim, E., Augustiny, K. F., Blaser, A., Bürki, C., Krohne, D., Rothenbühler, M., Schaffner, L. and Valach, L. (1987), Coping with breast cancer – A longitudinal prospective study. *Psychotherapy and Psychosomatics*, **48**, 44–59.

Heim, E., Augustiny, K. F., Blaser, A., Krohne, D., Rothenbühler, M., Schaffner, L. and Valach, L. (1988), *Erfassung der Krankheitsbeweltigung: Die Berner Bewältigungsformen BEFO*. Bern: Psychiatrische Universittspoliklinik.

Heim, E. and Willy, J. (1986), *Psychosoziale Medizin*. Berlin: Springer-Verlag.

Kalbermatten, U. and Valach, L. (1985), Methods of an interactive approach for the study of social interaction. *Communication and Cognition*, **18**, 281–315.

Keefe, F. J., Caldwell, D. S. Martinez, S. and Nunley, J. (1991), Analyzing pain in rheumatoid arthritis patients: Pain coping strategies in patients who have had knee replacement surgery. *Pain*, **46**, 153–160.

Kilchenmann, A. (1989), *Bewäeltigung bei Paaren mit Multipler Sklerose*. Dissertation, Bern: Department of Psychiatry.

Kleinke, C. L., Staneski, R. A. and Mason, J. K. (1982), Sex differences in coping with depression. *Sex Roles*, **8**, 877–899.

Krohne, H. W. (1978), Individual differences in coping with stress and anxiety. In: C. D. Spielberger, I. G. Sarason (eds.) *Stress and Anxiety Hemisphere*, Washington, 233–260.

Lazarus, R. S. (1966), *Psychological Stress and the Coping Process*. New York: McGraw-Hill.

Lazarus, R. S. and Folkman, S. (1984), *Stress, Appraisal, and Coping*. New York: Springer.

Leventhal, H., Nerenz, D. R. and Steele, D. J. (1984), Illness representations and coping with health threats. In: A. Baum, S. E. Taylor and J. Singer (eds.) *A Handbook of Psychology and Health*. Vol. IV: Social Psychological Aspects of Health, 244–252 Hillsdale N. J: Lawrence Erlbaum.

Littlewood, J. L., Cramer, D., Hoekstra, J. and Humphrey, G. B. (1991), Gender differences in parental coping following their child's death. *British Journal of Guidance and Counselling*, **19**, 139–148.

Marková, I. (1990), The development of self-consciousness: Baldwin, Mead and Vygotsky. In: J. E. Faulconer and R. N. Williams: Reconsidering Psychology. *Perspectives from Continental Philosophy*. Pittsburgh: Duquesne Press, 151–174.

Marková, I. and Wilkie, P. (1987), Representations, concepts and social change: The phenomenon of AIDS. *Journal for the Theory of Social Behaviour*, **17**, 389–407.

Marmot, M. and Theorell, T. (1988), Social class and cardiovascular disease: The contribution of work. *International Journal of Health Services*, **18**, 659–74.

McLeod, J. D. and Kessler, R. C. (1990), Socioeconomic status differences in vulnerability to undesirable life events. *Journal of Health and Social Behavior*, **31**, 162–72.

Mead, G. H. (1913), The social self. *The Journal of Philosophy, Psychology, and Scientific Methods*, **10**, 374–380.

Meyerowitz, B. E., Heinrich, R. L. and Schag, C. C. (1983), A competency-based approach to coping with cancer. In: T. G. Burish, L. A. Bradley (eds.) *Coping with Chronic Disease: Research and applications*. New York: Academic Press. 137–158.

Noack, H. and Valach, L. (1985), Zur Rekonstruktion von Krankheitslaufbahnen in der ambulanten Versorgung. *Sozial- und Preventivmedizin*, **30**, 237–238.

Orr, E. (1986), Open communication as an effective stress management method for breast cancer patients. *Journal of Human Stress*, **12**, 175–185.

Parkers, K. R. (1990), Coping, negative affectivity, and the work environment: Additive and interactive predictors of mental health. *Journal of Applied Psychology*, **75**, 399–409.

Pearlin, L. I. and Schooler, C. (1978), The structure of coping. *Journal of Health and Social Behavior*, **19**, 2–21.

Rim, Y. (1990), Social class differences in coping styles. *Personality and Individual Differences*, **11**, 875–876.

Scott, T. and Badura, B. (1988), Wives of heart attack patients: The stress of caring. In: R. Anderson and M. Bury (eds.) *Living with Chronic Illness*. London: Unwin Hyman.

Schütz, A. (1932), *Der sinnhafte Aufbau der sozialen Welt*. Springer, Wien.

Schwab, R. (1990), Paternal and maternal coping with the death of a child. *Death Studies*, **14**, 407–422.

Seiffge-Krenke, I. and Shulman, S. (1990), Coping style in adolescence: A cross-cultural study. *Journal of Cross-Cultural Psychology*, **21**, 351–377.

Spilker, B. (ed.) (1990), *Quality of Life Assessment in Clinical Trials*. New York: Raven Press.

Thommen, B., Ammann, R. and von Cranach, M. (1988), *Handlungsorganisation durch soziale Repräsentationen*. Bern: Hans Huber.

Thommen, B., von Cranach, M. and Ammann, R. (1992), The organization of individual action through social representations: A comparative study of two therapeutic schools. In: M. von Cranach, W. Doise, G. Mugny (eds.) *Social Representations and the Social Bases of Knowledge*. Lewinston N.Y: Hogrefe & Huber. 194–201.

Valach, L. (1990a), A theory of goal-directed action in career analysis. In: R. A. Young, W. A. Borgen (eds.) *Methodological Approaches to the Study of Career*. New York: Praeger Publishers. 107–126.

Valach, L. (1990b), Kulturpsychologische Tendenzen in der psychosozial-medizinischen Forschung. In: C. G. Allesch, E. Billmann-Mahecha (eds.) *Perspektiven der Kulturpsychologie*. Heidelberg: Asanger Verlag. 85–93.

Valach, L., Augustiny, K., Blaser, A., Dvorak, J., Fuhrimann, P., Tschaggelar, W. and Heim, E. (1988a), Coping von rückenoperierten Patienten-psychosoziale Aspekte. *Psychother. med. Psychol*, **38**, 28–36.

Valach, L., Augustiny, K.-F., Blaser, A., Dvorak, J., Fuhrimann, P., Tschaggelar, W. and Heim, E. (1990), Self-attribution of coping and its social adaptability in patients operated for lumbar disc herniation. In: L. R. Schmidt, P. Schwenkmetzger, J. Weinman, S. Maes (eds.) *Theoretical and Applied Aspects of Health Psychology.* Switzerland: Harwood Academic Publishers.

Valach, L., von Cranach, M. and Kalbermatten, U. (1988b), Social meaning in the observation of goal directed action. *Semiotica,* **71**, 243–259.

Valach, L., Kilchenmann, A. and Heim, E. (1992a), Coping in couples with wife's multiple sclerosis. Unpublished paper, Department of Psychiatry, University of Berne.

Valach, L. and Noack, H. (1985), Gender and a reconstruction of an illness career. Institute of Social and Preventive Medicine, University of Berne.

Valach, L. (1992b), Coping after breast cancer surgery in Berne and in Prague. In: H. Schroeder, K. Reschke, M. Johnston, S. Maes (eds.) Health Psychology-Potential in Diversity. Regensburg: S. Rodeer Verlag. 254–263.

Valach, L., Schaffner, L., Kuehne, D. and Heim, E. (1992c), Coping and its social adaptability in breast cancer operated women during the first year after the operation. In: J. A. M. Winnubst, S. Maes (eds.) *Lifestyles, Stress and Health: New developments in health psychology.* Leiden University: DSWO Press. 227–235.

Vingerhoets, A. J. and Van Heck, G. L. (1990), Gender, coping and psychosomatic symptoms. *Psychological Medicine,* **20**, 125–35.

Vygotsky, L. (1978), *Mind in Society. The Development of Higher Psychological Processes.* Cambridge, Mass: Harvard University Press.

Wertsch, J. (1985), *Vygotsky and the Social Formation of Mind.* Cambridge, Mass: Harvard University Press.

Waddell, G. (1987), A new clinical model for the treatment of low-back pain. *Spine,* **12**, 632–644.

Westbrook, M. T. (1979), A classification of coping behavior based on multidimensional scaling of similarity ratings. *Journal of Clinical Psychology,* **35**, 407–410.

Wortman, C. B. and Dunkel-Schetter, Ch. (1979), Interpersonal relationships and cancer: A theoretical analysis. *Journal of Social Issues,* **35**, 120–155.

Zemore, R. and Shepel, L. F. (1987), Information seeking and adjustment to cancer. *Psychological Reports,* **60**, 874.

APPENDIX I: MODES OF COPING (Heim et al. 1987)

1. ACTIVITY AS DIVERSION: 'I'm throwing myself into my work in order to forget my illness.'
2. THOUGHT AS DIVERSION: 'Something else is more important to me than the illness at the moment.'
3. ACTIVE AVOIDANCE: Necessary medical action is not undertaken or is discontinued; e.g. consulting a doctor, medication, rehabilitation, etc.
4. ACCEPTANCE-STOICISM: 'This is simply the way it is. I'm trying to resign myself to it.'
5. ALTRUISM: 'I want to be here for the benefit of my family as long as I can.'
6. REBELLING: 'Why me?'
7. DISSIMULATION: 'It's really not so bad – actually I'm feeling quite well.'

8. EMOTIONAL RELEASE: 'I feel so miserable, at least crying seems to help a bit.'
9. PRESERVING COMPOSURE: 'I have to pull myself together. No one must notice anything.'
10. ISOLATION-SUPPRESSION: 'I'm not in the least worried by the whole thing.'
11. COMPENSATION: 'When I am not feeling well I buy myself something nice, even if I don't really need it.'
12. CONSTRUCTIVE ACTIVITY: 'I am finally taking some time for myself.'
13. OPTIMISM: 'If I only have faith, then everything will surely be better.'
14. PASSIVE COOPERATION: 'They know what they're doing.'
15. PROBLEM ANALYSIS: 'I'm trying to explain to myself what is actually happening.'
16. RELIGIOUSNESS: 'Everyone's time comes, but God is with me.'
17. RESIGNATION-FATALISM: 'I don't believe there's any point in continuing anymore.'
18. SOCIAL WITHDRAWAL: 'I need peace and quiet. I want to be able to find myself.'
19. RUMINATION: 'Is it really so, or isn't it..? I can't get it off my mind.'
20. GIVING MEANING: Through my illness, I've discovered my true self.'
21. SELF ACCUSATION: 'I don't deserve any better.'
22. SELF-VALIDATION: 'I've succeeded in doing other important things up to now. Actually, I've been quite brave about it all.'
23. RELEASE OF ANGER: 'I am so angry that this illness has happened to me.'
24. TACKLING: 'A lot now depends on what I do and how I take part.'
25. ATTENTION AND CARE: 'Up to now there has always been someone who has listened/understood.'
26. RELATIVIZING: 'I'm in relatively good shape compared with others who have lost a leg.'

Subject Index

ACT–UP... *53*

Adjustment to illness... *177–81, 182*

Adult polycystic disease of the kidney... *100, 117*

Advertising... *9, 15, 58–62, 67, 71–3*

Agency... *164, 191, 196, 198, 201, 211, 249*

AIDS *see* HIV/AIDS

Asylums... *106, 107, 147*
    Victorian... *67–8*

Attitudes
    and behaviour... *31*
    and risk... *123–5*
    to disabled people... *67, 68, 82, 84*
    to HIV/AIDS... *124–5*
    to mental illness... *158*

Attribution
    of responsibility for disease... *112, 163–4*
    theory... *94, 101, 163–4, 175*

Barnado... *71*

Beliefs
    Health Belief Model... *103, 115*
    lay... *147, 158*
    scientific... *149*
    shared... *153–8*
    widespread... *8, 73*

Body
    changes in the representation of... *10–12*
    degeneracy of... *49*

face of AIDS... *49–52*
    illnesses of... *149*

Campaign for Real People... *83*

Cause and effect... *99, 142*
    causes of mental illness... *153*
    lay explanations of causes... *167–77, 178, 181–2*
    perceived vs. actual causes... *100, 147*

Charity(ies)... *15, 28, 37–8, 67, 69–71, 87*
    advertisements... *45, 84*
    campaigns... *67*
    poster campaigns... *82*
    see also Down's Children's Association; Down's Syndrome Association; MENCAP; Royal National Institute for the Blind; Royal National Institute for the Deaf; Spastics Society (SCOPE); Terence Higgins Trust

Common sense... *146*
    folk knowledge... *159*
    in relation to science... *97*
    naive psychology... *101*

Community... *153, 211*
    care in... *107, 153, 158*
    residences... *212*
    residential facilities... *226*

Conventions... *253, 259–60*

Coping... *117, 196*
    and social strata... *251–2*
    as a social process... *251, 255*

as an acting of self active
    systems... *257–8*
as gender specific... *252–3*
as jointly reconstructed...
    258–60
definition of... *249*
nature of... *250, 254*
social consequences of... *251,
    256–7*
social dimensions of... *249*
Culture... *7, 8, 93, 98, 99, 112–14,
    145, 164, 182–3, 254*
    context of... *98*

DCA (Down's Children's
    Association)... *33–7, 45*
Deinstitutionalization... *150*
Diabetes... *97–8, 100–1, 164–81*
Dialogical process... *195–6*
Disability... *45, 100*
    definition... *43*
    images of... *67*
    NUJ guidelines... *83*
    UN guidelines for positive
        portrayal... *82*
    vs. handicap... *43–4*
Discourse... *8, 131, 137*
    institutional... *132*
    lay... *149*
Disease... *164*
Down's Children's Association
    (DCA)... *33–7, 45*
Down's Syndrome... *26–7, 33, 37,
    76–8, 197*
Down's Syndrome Association...
    26–7, 77–8, 84–5

Epidemiology... *13–14*
    of representations... *7–8*
Epistemology
    lay... *105, 146, 147*
    professional... *99–105*
    scientific... *147*

Explanations
    lay... *96–8, 163, 165, 167–77,
        181*
    of causality... *99–101*
    of illness... *148*
    probabilistic... *101, 181*
    professional... *97–8*
    scientific... *95–8*

Feminism... *10*

Genetic disorder... *99, 100, 103,
    104, 197*
Goal directed action... *249, 257*
Green revolution... *11, 12*

Haemophilia... *99–100, 111, 117,
    197, 199*
Handicap
    definition... *43*
    image of... *29*
    mental... *28–9, 37, 68*
    physical... *98*
    specific... *29*
    vs. disability... *43–4*
Health
    lay beliefs of... *148*
    representations of... *5, 93*
Health Belief Model... *103, 115*
Health campaigns... *7, 10, 56–8*
Health education... *8, 10, 13, 47,
    49, 57, 58–62, 65, 103, 182*
Health Education Authority...
    41–3, 58–62
Health foods... *5*
Health problems... *133*
Health warnings... *9, 52, 192*
Heterosexuals... *40*
HIV/AIDS... *7, 9, 10, 12–15,
    38–43, 104, 113–14, 122*
    attitudes to... *124–5*
    face of AIDS... *49–65*
    images of AIDS... *38, 60–1*
    in prisons... *117–25*

Homosexuals... *38–43, 52, 199–200*
Huntington's chorea... *104, 197*

IDM (Intravenous Drug Misuse)... *119–20, 125*
Illness... *114, 164*
    adjustment to... *177–82*
    cause of... *5*
    germ theory of... *100*
    lay explanations of causes... *167–77, 178, 181–2*
    mental... *11, 67–8, 145, 151, 159*
    ravages of... *53*
    representations of... *5*
    sin and punishment... *112*
    social dimension of... *145*
Image (s)
    and text... *9*
    in the media... *51–2, 67*
    of AIDS... *38, 60–1*
    of death... *49–51*
    of health... *9*
    of people with learning disability... *67*
    on posters... *33*
    popular... *49*
    role of in advertising... *71–3*
Individualism... *193–5, 200*
Institutional agents... *157*
Institutional discourse... *132*
Institutional experience... *226, 229*
Institutional life... *208–9*
Institutional settings... *132, 147*
Institutions
    for people with learning disabilities... *206–9*
    mental... *153*
    prisons... *117–25*
    total... *105–6, 117, 124*
Intravenous Drug Misuse (IDM)... *119–20, 125*

Labels... *14, 32, 44, 45, 68, 149, 152*
    impact of... *45, 68*
Learning difficulties... *17, 43, 68*
Learning disabilities... *28, 43, 68–9, 73, 79, 82–4*
Legal reform: unintended consequences of... *107–8*
Life satisfaction... *229–30*
Life style... *13, 41, 52, 101, 137–8, 140, 143*
    gay life style... *52*

Madness... *148*
    fear of... *153*
    history of... *148–9*
Mass media of communication... *4, 6, 7–10, 14, 31, 33, 73, 80–4, 93*
    media studies... *4, 9*
    photographic genres... *51–2*
    radio... *64(n.8)*
Medical consultation... *134–42*
Medical discourse... *133*
Medical model... *149, 152, 208*
MENCAP... *16–7, 28, 33–7, 44, 70–2, 73–81*
Mendelian inheritance... *99, 100*
Moral defectives... *68*
Moral degeneracy... *207*
Moral dimension... *52–3*
Moral imbecile... *207*
Moral judgment... *113*
Moral obligations... *198*
Morality... *104, 126, 195*

Normalisation... *69, 87, 210–12*

Optimistic bias... *116, 126*
Otherness... *98, 159, 164*
    "them" vs. "us"... *153*
Others: perception of risk... *111–26*

People First... *45, 88*
Perceptions
    of others... *40, 120–2*
    of self... *32, 40, 120–2*
    public, of disabled people... *67*
Plague... *6, 7, 14*
Poster campaigns... *15–29, 31–47,*
    73, 79, 82
Pre-natal diagnosing... *198–9*
Professional(s)
    in health care... *8, 97, 147,*
       150
    in mental health... *150–2, 158*
    medical... *145*
    practice... *147*
Protection Motivation Theory... *115*
Psychoanalysis... *4, 11–12*

Quality of Life... *5, 28–9, 32,*
    192–3, 197, 202
    and mental health... *225–45*
    and responsibility... *202–3*
    as a social construction... *202*
    definition... *227*
    determinants of... *228–9*
    impact of community care
       on... *227*
    impact of community
       placement... *238–43*
    longitudinal studies of... *228*
    objective assessment
       measures... *201, 227*
    of people with learning
       difficulties... *200–1*
    perceived, in the hospital
       setting... *231–4*
    perception of... *227*
    scale for assessing... *227*
    subjective assessment
       measures... *201, 227*

Representations
    as historical and cultural
       phenomena... *108*

    collective... *3–10, 163–6*
    content of... *157*
    epidemiology of... *7, 9*
    form and nature... *93–5*
    in people's minds... *8*
    in the media... *8*
    of causes... *100*
    of childhood... *106*
    of handicap... *9, 15, 32–3*
    of health and illness... *4–6, 9*
    of HIV/AIDS... *12*
    of mental handicap... *106*
    of mental illness... *98, 105,*
       147–52
    of the human body... *10–2*
    of the mentally ill... *98*
    public and private... *32*
    social... *4, 7, 8, 9, 10, 15, 28,*
       32, 35, 54–6, 71, 73,
       145–60, 163, 249–50
Responsibility... *202–3*
    collective... *193, 202*
    individual... *192, 199*
    mutual... *192–3*
    perceived distribution of... *196*
    societal... *192, 202*
Right (s)
    dialogical concept of... *193,*
       195–6
    individual... *192–4, 198*
Risk
    and attitudes... *123–5*
    and concern... *122–3*
    and control... *124*
    and danger... *102*
    as a social and cultural
       construct... *105*
    behaviour... *111–17, 118*
    concept of... *103*
    of HIV/AIDS... *104*
    perception of risk... *102–5,*
       111–17
    risk appraisal process... *117,*
       126

self-perceived... *110–22*
the term... *102*
theories of... *102–3*
to other... *120–2*
Royal National Institute for the
     Blind (RNIB)... *18, 19, 33–6*
Royal National Institute for the
     Deaf (RNID)... *20, 21, 33–7*

'Safer sex... *38–43, 86*
Science... *181*
     biomedical model... *138, 143*
     immunology... *13*
     medical... *147*
     popularisation of... *149*
     psychosomatic medicine ... *11*
     virology... *13*
     vs. common sense... *96*
SCOPE *see* Spastics Society
Self... *31, 112, 116–17, 159, 164*
     concept of... *6, 38*
     control... *115–16*
     perceptions of... *32, 40,
          120–2*
Self-advocacy... *45, 87–8, 211*
Social construction... *94, 132, 146*
Social movements
     ACT-UP... *53*
     Campaign for Real People...
          83

feminism... *10*
green revolution... *11, 12*
People First... *45, 88*
self-advocacy... *45, 87–8, 211*
Social reform: unintended
     consequences of... *106–7*
Spastics Society (SCOPE)... *22–5,
     28, 33–7, 45, 86, 99*
Stereotypes... *28, 29, 31, 32, 43,
     60, 68–9, 82–4*
Stigma... *11, 14, 52, 98, 149*

Terence Higgins Trust... *41, 86*

Unintended consequences
     of health campaigns... *56–8*
     of legal reform... *107–8*
     of social reform... *106–7*
Utilitarianism... *191*

Voice of medicine... *97, 133, 137,
     138, 140, 142*
Voice of the life-world... *97, 133,
     137, 140, 142*
Voluntary organisations... *7, 28*

Well-being... *192, 198*
     positive self-concepts... *6*